Communication in Nursing

Communication in Nursing

Julia Balzer Riley, RN, MN

President
Constant Source Seminars

Fourth Edition

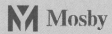 Mosby

St. Louis Baltimore Boston Carlsbad Chicago Minneapolis New York Philadelphia Portland
London Milan Sydney Tokyo Toronto

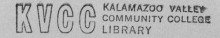

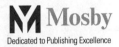
Mosby
Dedicated to Publishing Excellence

Editor-in-Chief–Nursing: Sally Schrefer
Developmental Editor: Jeff Downing
Project Manager: Deborah L. Vogel
Project Specialist: Ann E. Rogers
Book Design Manager: Bill Drone
Cover Art: Laurel Burch

FOURTH EDITION

Mosby, Inc.
A Harcourt Health Sciences Company
11830 Westline Industrial Drive
St. Louis, Missouri 63146

Printed in United States of America

Library of Congress Cataloging in Publication Data
Balzer-Riley, Julia W.
    Communication in nursing.—4th ed./Julia W. Balzer-Riley.
      p.   cm.
    Includes bibliographical references and index.
    ISBN 0-323-00872-0
    1. Nurse and patient.   2. Interpersonal communication. I. Title.
    [DNLM: 1. Nurse-Patient Relations.   2. Communication Nurses'
Instruction.   3. Interprofessional Relations Nurses' Instruction.
WY 87 B198c 2000]
RT86.3.B34 2000
610.73'06'99—dc21
DNLM/DLC
for Library of Congress   99-33660
                                          CIP

99 00 01 02 03 TG/FF 9 8 7 6 5 4 3 2 1

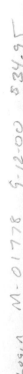

Contributors

Joyce Larson Presswalla, RN, PhD
Culture Counts
Tampa, Florida

James T. Riley
Vice-President, Marketing
Constant Source Seminars
Cumming, Georgia

Reviewers

Mary Alice Dedinsky, MSN, PhD, RN, NCC

Nurse Educator
Milwaukee Area Technical College
Milwaukee, Wisconsin

Kathleen Shannon Dorcy, RN, MN

Lecturer
University of Washington–Tacoma
Researcher
Fred Hutchinson Cancer Research
Tacoma, Washington

Pamela T. Helms, MN, RN

Assistant Professor
University of Mississippi
School of Nursing
Jackson, Mississippi

Alice Kempe, MSN, PhD

Associate Professor
Ursuline College
School of Nursing
Pepper Pike, Ohio

Mary Kunes-Connell, PhD, RN

Associate Professor
Interim Program Chair for Traditional
    Curriculum
Creighton University
School of Nursing
Omaha, Nebraska

Melissa Lickteig, MSN, RN

Faculty
Jefferson School of Nursing
Pine Bluff, Arkansas

Patricia A. Roper, RN, MS

Professor of Nursing
Columbus State Community College
Columbus, Ohio

Introduction

WHY STUDY COMMUNICATION?

Communication is a life-long learning process for the nurse. Nurses make the intimate journey with the client and family from the miracle of birth to the mystery of death. Nurses build assertive communication for this journey. Nurses provide education that helps clients change life-long habits. Nurses communicate with people under stress: clients, family, and colleagues. Nurses deal with anger and depression, with dementia and psychosis, with joy and despair. Nurses serve as client advocates and as members of interdisciplinary teams who may have different ideas about priorities for care. Nurses return to school to specialize, write grants for research proposals, become entrepreneurs. Nurses become administrators, leaders, case managers, infection control specialists, quality experts, and educators. Nurses move into industry in occupational health and into schools and communities to impact the health of large populations and communities. Nurses create new positions where the nurse's voice can affect health care quality. Nurses cross international boundaries to share knowledge to promote worldwide health. Nurses must be assertive to ask the right questions and make their voices heard. Nurses must be assertive to communicate their own needs and be prepared to assert themselves to ensure balance in their own lives. Without such balance, the high-stress environment may diminish the nurse's effectiveness.

Despite the complexity of technology and the multiple demands on a nurse's time, it is the intimate moments of connection that can make all the difference in the quality of care and meaning for the client and the nurse. As nurses refine their communications skills and build their confidence, they can move from novice to expert. Nurses honor the differences in clients with humility and learn and grow in their ability to trust their intuition, to be open to what Martin Buber, a Jewish theologian, calls the I-Thou relationship—the sacred moment of connection when we acknowledge the divine presence in each of us, the essence of each person.

WHAT'S NEW?

This new edition provides information to help the nurse communicate authentically, from information on culture, gender, and age to an introduction to electronic communication. Each chapter includes examples of these "moments of connection." Many of these were contributed by nurses at the annual meeting of The American Society of Pain Management Nurses, 1998, at a workshop conducted by the author, "The Magical Moments of Connection . . . F.O.C.U.S.E.D. on the Healing Presence." In 1998, this text was selected as one of 50 to be included in a study by the City of Hope National Medical Center, through a Robert Wood Johnson Foundation Grant, to "strengthen nursing education for improved end of life care." This led to the decision to include these nurses' "moments of connection." These are the stories through which we can share the meaning of nursing. Through your career, collect your own stories, put them in a journal, share them with colleagues, and submit them for publication. We communicate by the stories we tell. Sharing and celebrating our stories helps us to respirit, reinspire, and revitalize ourselves.

Additional content on assertiveness has been added to this edition to help nurses be more proactive for themselves and for clients and families. Chapters on Spirituality and Humor help add perspective. Active reading skills promote the retention of content. The "Think About It" exercises have been added to each chapter to encourage the reader to reflect on how the content can be applied. Before reading each chapter, note these questions at the end of the chapter, and read the objectives and bold headings. As you read, be thinking about what answers you will write. This will help you keep your attention focused as you read. Pay attention to the "Wit and Wisdom" sections and the proverbs and quotations at the beginning of each chapter that add perspective and involvement with the content. Write your own poems from your clinical experiences. These added features help prevent the "where was I?" thoughts that come when your mind drifts with heavy reading assignments and multiple life commitments.

WHAT'S IMPORTANT?

Honor the sacred nature of your work. Take time each day to connect with your own purpose in your work. A centering exercise* that can help you follows:

1. Before you interact with a client, pause.
2. Let go of any distractions or worries just now.
3. Close your eyes briefly and take a deep breath.
4. Say silently to yourself, "I am here for the greater good of this client and will give my full attention to this moment."
5. Bring to mind someone or something that evokes love and compassion.
6. Hold that feeling of love and compassion, repeating to yourself, "I am present in this moment." (This whole process should take only 5-10 seconds.)

Remember to take time for your own spiritual practice. Remember the body-mind-spirit connection for yourself, too. Remember to take your work seriously but yourself lightly. Remember to laugh and play.

Most of all, remember to listen with the ears, the eyes, your undivided attention, and your heart.

Julia Balzer Riley, RN, MN

---

*Modified from Thornton LM: Self-renewal and nurturing for holistic nurses, *Alternative & Complementary Therapies,* October 1998, pp. 364-366.

Acknowledgments

What a delight it is to recognize the contribution of an artist whose work has been a favorite of mine for many years. Laurel Burch has worked with us to add the magical touch of art to this book. Her whimsical animals and inspiring figures communicate at an intuitive level how we are all connected. Take time to enjoy these creations and let them speak to you. Her own personal commitment to nurses led her to select this project as one she wished to support. I thank her for her talent, her creativity, her time, and her generous, loving spirit. For information, you may contact the Laurel Burch Company at 1-800-280-8156.

Thank you to Guy Zona for opening his work on the collection of multicultural proverbs to me. Look for his books with such titles as *Eyes That See Do Not Grow Old; If You Have Two Loaves Of Bread, Sell One And Buy A Lily;* and *The Soul Would Have No Rainbows If The Eyes Had No Tears.*

Thank you to my editor, Jeff Downing, who was always just a phone call or e-mail away for consultation, direction, advocacy, and good conversation.

Thank you to my husband whose support is never-ending and who made it concrete this time by contributing the chapter on electronic communication! And, as usual, to my cats, who have taken to putting their paws on my lap and their music in my ears to get me to take a break.

Julia Balzer Riley

MOMENTS OF CONNECTION CONTRIBUTORS

Carla Andrews
Alison Baswell
Liz Bilinski
Linda Boernke
Pam Budd
Kathy Cadden
Maryjane Cerrone
Cindy Dixon
Terese M. Donovan
Jeffrey Edwards

Joan Epperson
Lynn M. Friebel
Marcia Guilford
Ann Marie Harootunian
Tamara Herrington
Carol Keck
Gwen Kincaid
Teresa Kirkland
Gwen Kolegne
Carol Lewis

Kathy Mansie
Patricia Meehan
Leah Miller
Lorry Roy
Diana Ruzicka
Ana M. Schreier
Merlynn Henley Smith
Joan Steiner
Carolyn W. Sutherland

CHAPTER   # WILL HELP YOU

Part I: Getting Started

1 Responsible, Assertive, Caring Communication in Nursing

Appreciate the significance of assertiveness and responsibility as fundamental approaches for communicating in a caring way.

2 The Client-Nurse Relationship: A Helping Relationship

Develop a communication approach that has the interests of your clients at heart.

3 Solving Problems Together

Collaborate and validate with your clients at each phase of the nursing process.

4 Understanding Each Other: Communication and Culture

Understand others and recognize the need to incorporate differences in culture, gender, and age in nursing interventions.

5 Electronic Communication

Begin to use electronic communication skills and resources to enrich your work.

Part II: Building Relationships

6 Warmth

Demonstrate to your clients in concrete ways that you are concerned about and interested in them.

7 Respect

Show your clients you consider them to be worthwhile and important.

8 Genuineness

Say what you think and feel so that your clients receive honest communication from you.

9 Empathy

Convince your clients and colleagues that you understand their feelings.

10 Self-Disclosure

Relate your own feelings and experiences in a helpful way.

11 Specificity

Be clear and to the point so that others understand your meaning.

12 Asking Questions

Streamline your interviewing techniques so that your clients understand what information you are seeking and for what purpose.

13 Expressing Opinions

Know when it is appropriate to state your views to your clients.

14 Humor

Use humor to build relationships with clients.

15 Spirituality

Explore the spiritual connection in nursing practice.

Part III: Meeting Challenges

Part IV: Building Confidence

Contents

Communication
in Nursing

Part I

Getting Started:

Basic Communication Competence

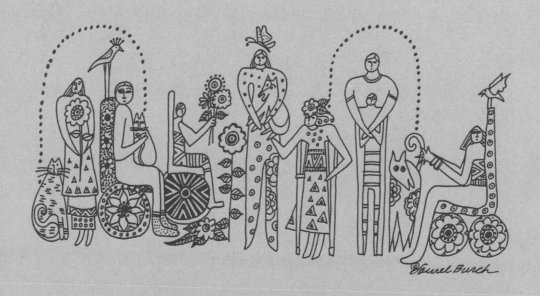

PRACTICE MAKES PERFECT
Getting Started

Welcome to a brand new world. The new millennium sets the stage for a fresh look at communication and its pervasive influence on every part of our lives. Assertive skills are more necessary than ever as we become client advocates and advanced nurse practitioners in an era of managed care. We must learn how to be open to creating moments of connection with clients, family, and colleagues in briefer spaces of time. We celebrate the sacred nature of our work as we commit to understanding diversity in culture, gender, and age of clients so that we can continue to make a difference in lives entrusted to our care. We courageously plunge into the world of electronic communication to keep pace with the information age. Hang on . . . the ride is exciting.

Are you ready to begin? As you read, you will find that you already know some of the basics of communication. Your desire to develop excellence in nursing will motivate you to learn the communication behaviors that are essential to meet that goal. If you haven't already done so, take a moment to read over the table of contents to see what's ahead. Preview each chapter as you prepare to read it, and note the headings and conclusions . . . a secret to increased retention in reading. To make this an active process, ask yourself questions about what you expect to learn from each chapter before you start reading it.

It is important to practice these basic skills as you learn them, and seek to understand their importance, because the skills build on each other. The activities will help you with application and assessment of your level of understanding of each skill. At the end of this book you will find a self-assessment tool. Turn now to the appendix on p. 439 and read the items in the scale. Just as you read course or clinical evaluation objectives at the beginning of a class, knowing what is expected of you sets you up to be successful.

Let's Get Started!

The first step to becoming a better nurse communicator is to build a sound knowledge base about the essential communication behaviors.

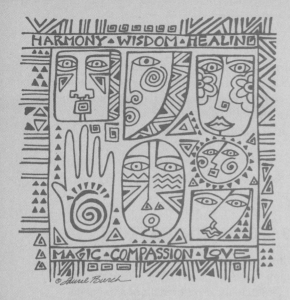

HARMONY · WISDOM · HEALING

MAGIC · COMPASSION · LOVE

Responsible, Assertive, Caring Communication in Nursing

Caring is one of life's essential ingredients; it may be the most essential ingredient.

E.O. Bevis

OBJECTIVES

1. Identify the functions of interpersonal communication in nursing.
2. Distinguish between assertive, nonassertive, and aggressive communication.
3. Identify a three-step process to build assertiveness skills.
4. Identify assertive rights.
5. Identify irrational beliefs that impede assertive communication.
6. Explain the D.E.S.C. script for developing an assertive response.
7. Identify three types of assertions.
8. Identify three essential criteria for presenting an assertive response.
9. Describe the behavior of an assertive nurse.
10. List the advantages of assertive communication.
11. Describe responsible communication in nursing.
12. Discuss the role of caring in nursing.

This book is designed to help you improve your ability to communicate assertively and responsibly with your clients and colleagues. Nursing students can make use of this book as they begin their professional journey. Practicing nurses will also find this work useful as they come to understand that clear communication is an essential ingredient for success in a rapidly changing health care climate. Communication with clients, colleagues, administration officials, and staff members of other community agencies is essential as nurses' roles change and more nurses move into the community to practice.

Before going any farther you need to understand the meaning of four important concepts used in the opening sentence: *communication, assertive, responsible,* and *caring.* These concepts are significant because they form the framework of this textbook.

THE MEANING OF INTERPERSONAL COMMUNICATION

Communication involves the reciprocal process of sending and receiving messages between two or more people. This book will focus on the communication exchange between you, the nurse, and your clients and colleagues. Communication can either facilitate the development of a therapeutic relationship or create barriers (Stuart and Sundeen, 1995).

In general, there are two parts to face-to-face communication: the verbal expression of the sender's thoughts and feelings, and the nonverbal expression. Verbally, cognitive and affective messages are sent through words, voice inflection, and rate of speech; nonverbally, messages are conveyed by eye movements, facial expressions, and body language. Communication by telephone or other electronic media loses the impact of gestures and other nonverbal communication. Powerful nonverbal messages can stand alone: a suspicious glance, for example, or a warm smile or eyes widened with fear.

Senders determine what message they want to transmit to the receiver and encode their thoughts and feelings into words and gestures. Senders' messages are transmitted to the receiver through sound, sight, touch, and occasionally, through smell and taste.

Receivers of the messages have to decode the verbal and nonverbal transmission to make sense of the thoughts and feelings communicated by senders. After decoding the senders' words, speech patterns, and facial and body movements, the receivers encode return messages, either verbally, through words, or nonverbally, through gestures.

In an interaction between two people (e.g., a nurse and a client) each person is both a sender and a receiver and alternates between these two roles. When senders are speaking, they are also receiving messages from the person who is listening. Listeners are not only receiving speakers' messages but are also simultaneously sending messages. Figure 1-1 illustrates this reciprocal nature of the communication process.

At any point in an interpersonal communication we send and receive verbal and nonverbal messages about thoughts and feelings. With little prompting you know that the complex process of interpersonal communication is influenced by many variables that affect how messages are sent and received. Take a few minutes to think of the variety of factors that can affect the exchange of messages between people. Add your own ideas to the following list:

- Environmental factors: formality, warmth, privacy, familiarity, freedom or constraint, physical distance between people, climate, mood, architecture, arrangement of furniture
- Territory and personal space: crowding, seating arrangements, roles, status, position, physical characteristics (size, height)

- Physical appearance and dress: body shape, race, body smell, hair, gender, body movements, body adornments, posture, age
- Nonverbal cues: facial expressions, eye movements, vocal cues
- Intrapersonal factors: developmental stage, language mastery, differences in perception, differences in decision-making processes, differences in values, self-concept
- The use of "I" messages to own your responses, such as, "I don't agree with you" instead of "you" messages, which sound blaming, such as, "You are wrong"

Note that any of the preceding factors has the potential to facilitate communication or to act as a barrier to effective communication, depending on the context of the situation. When these factors are considered, the interpersonal communication process looks something like Figure 1-2.

An important function of communication is to transmit messages from one person to another. The real purpose of communication is to create meaning. Senders of messages wish to convey meaning to receivers, and vice versa. With this intent, senders choose certain words and gestures in a way that they believe is congruent with their intended messages. The sender's objective is to transmit a message that is clear and understandable to receivers.

However, the purpose of communication does not stop there. The real purpose of creating understanding in another person is to influence the other person to effect some change. The sender attempts to persuade the receiver to respond to the sender's requests. Requests from clients and colleagues may be for:

- Understanding
- Action
- Information
- Comfort

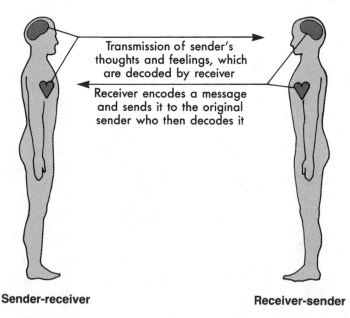

Sender-receiver   **Receiver-sender**

Figure 1-1   Reciprocal nature of interpersonal communication.

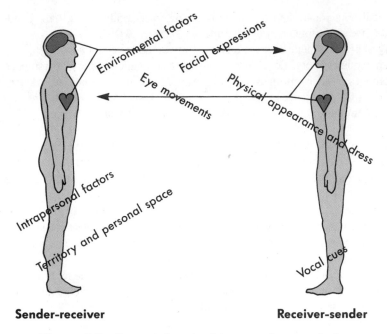

Sender-receiver   **Receiver-sender**

Figure 1-2   Factors influencing interpersonal communication.

Requests may be stated in obvious or indirect ways. The following examples illustrate both direct and indirect requests.

A client has postoperative pain. His physiological need is for pain relief. He asks you: "When is the last time I had my painkiller?" (He winces and holds his wrist.) His direct request is for information about the time of his last analgesic. His indirect request is for information about when he can have more. He is anticipating action (you giving him the medication) so that he will be comforted.

A nursing assistant says at the beginning of the shift: "I have a terrible headache. I was up for 3 hours last night with my sick daughter. Do you have an aspirin?" Her physiological need is for rest and pain relief. Her obvious requests are for understanding (that you will empathize with her pain) and action (that you will give her an aspirin). She is possibly hoping that you will comfort her by making allowances for the fact that she is not at her best.

A nurse, newly hired to a unit, needs to feel that he belongs and fits in with the group. When he asks you to show him around the unit, he is indirectly asking you to understand that he feels alone and unsure. He is directly asking you to take action to orient him and provide him with information about procedures and policy. He is likely hoping that you will make him feel welcome (comforted).

In your interpersonal relationships as a nurse, you will act as both sender and receiver. The purpose of this book is to help you develop your clarity as a sender and your comprehension as a receiver of messages. You will learn how to deliver assertive and responsible messages and to accurately decode messages from your clients and colleagues. You will be able to confidently interpret both direct and indirect requests and make responsible decisions about how to respond assertively (Box 1-1).

Box 1-1	**Important Functions of Interpersonal Communication in Nursing**

- Communication is the vehicle for establishing a therapeutic relationship.
- Communication is the means by which people influence the behavior of others, and thus it is critical to the successful outcome of nursing intervention.
- Communication is the relationship itself, since without it, a therapeutic nurse-client relationship is impossible.

From Stuart GW, Laraia M, 1998.

THE MEANING OF ASSERTIVE COMMUNICATION

Assertiveness is the key to successful relationships for the client, the family, the nurse, and other colleagues. It is the ability to express your thoughts, your ideas, and your feelings, without undue anxiety and not at the expense of others. "If you are clear about your own needs and respectful of others, your style will be naturally assertive" (Communication in Nursing Video Series, 1995).

The assertive nurse appears confident and comfortable. Assertive behavior is contrasted with nonassertive or passive behavior, in which individuals disregard their own needs and rights, and aggressive behavior, in which individuals disregard the needs and rights of others. Assertiveness ". . . involves taking an active role, having a positive, caring, nonjudgmental attitude, maintaining your rights without denying the rights of others and communicating your desires in a clear and direct manner without threatening or attacking" (Scott, 1996) (Table 1-1).

Assertive communication is a lifelong learning skill that requires time and practice. Be willing to accept the fact that you will make mistakes. Be patient. When a person accustomed to behaving passively tries on this new behavior, the results may seem abrupt and abrasive, or shy and tenuous. The goal is not to be continually confrontational. When learning this new skill, you must be assertive all the time or you will be seen as nonassertive. When practicing techniques to learn to become more assertive, it is helpful to begin in a supportive environment with people who are accepting of you. Consider sharing your reading material on assertiveness with a roommate, spouse, or friend with whom you can begin practicing your assertive behavior. Start with small issues such as returning a damaged product to a store or offering a compliment.

Assertiveness is a matter of choice. It is important to feel confident that you can speak up for yourself, yet it is not necessary or even wise to speak your mind in every situation. With each person we encounter in any situation, we have the choice of communicating in an assertive or nonassertive style. The words we choose and the way we express them can be assertive, nonassertive, or aggressive. Realistically, you may not always have the energy or desire to assert your rights or express yourself fully. There are times when people cannot respond rationally, such as when they are experiencing high levels of anxiety, or panic. A person might fear retaliation from a manager or fear the loss of a job. You must choose what issues, when, where, and with whom your assertive behavior is appropriate. Our goal in this text, though, is to help you develop the skills that will enable you to choose to act in the best interests of yourself and your clients.

TABLE 1-1	Assertive and Nonassertive Styles of Communication		
Characteristics	**Assertive**	**Nonassertive**	**Aggressive**
Attitude toward self and others	I'm OK You're OK	I'm not OK You're not OK	I'm not OK You're not OK
Decision making	Makes own decision	Lets others choose for him or her	Chooses for others
Behavior in problem situations	Direct, fair confrontation	Flees, gives in	Outright, assaultive
Verbal behaviors	Clear, direct statement of wants; objective words; honest statement of feelings	Apologetic words; hedging; rambling; failing to say what is meant	Loaded words; accusations; superior, haughty words; labeling of other person
Nonverbal behaviors	Confident, congruent messages	Actions instead of words (not saying what is felt); incongruence between words and behaviors	Air of superiority; flippant, sarcastic style
Voice	Firm, warm, confident	Weak, distant, soft, wavering	Tense, shrill, loud, cold, demanding, authoritarian, coldly silent
Eyes	Warm, in contact, frank	Averted, downcast, teary, pleading	Expressionless, cold, narrowed, staring
Stance	Relaxed	Stooped; excessive leaning for support	Hands on hips; feet apart
Hands	Gestures at appropriate times	Fidgety, clammy	Fists pounding or clenched
Pattern of relating	Puts himself or herself up without putting others down	Puts himself or herself down	Puts himself or herself up by putting others down
Response of others	Mutual respect	Disrespect, guilt, anger, frustration	Hurt, defensiveness, humiliation
Consequences of style	I win, you win; strives for "win-win" or "no lose" solutions	I lose, you lose; only succeeds by luck or charity of others	I win, you lose; beats out others at any cost

Modified from Piaget G: Characterological lifechart of three fellows we all know. In Phelps S, Austin N: *The assertive woman,* San Luis Obispo, Calif, 1975, Impact Publishers, Inc. and Gerrard B, Boniface W, Love B: *Interpersonal skills for health professionals,* Reston, Va, 1980, Reston Publishing Company.

HOW DO YOU GET STARTED?

As you read and think about assertive communication, begin to analyze situations in your life when you think you would like to respond assertively. Think about what is happening, your response to it, what you want to do or have happen, and the consequences of action versus nonaction. Use this three-step process:

Box 1-2	Assertive Rights

1. You have the right to be treated with respect.
2. You have the right to a reasonable workload.
3. You have the right to an equitable wage.
4. You have the right to determine your own priorities.
5. You have the right to ask for what you want.
6. You have the right to refuse without making excuses or feeling guilty.
7. You have the right to make mistakes and be responsible for them.
8. You have the right to give and receive information as a professional.
9. You have the right to act in the best interest of the patient.
10. You have the right to be human.

From Chenevert M, 1993.

Box 1-3	Irrational Beliefs

Irrational beliefs arise when we are anxious about being assertive and focus on possible negative outcomes. The rational counterparts focus on possible positive outcomes.

Irrational Belief	**Rational Counterpart**
If I am assertive, other people will be upset, hurt by it, or angry with me.	The other person may not be hurt or angry. This person might prefer being open and honest, too. This person might feel closer to me and help me solve the problem.
If someone gets angry with me, I will be devastated.	I will not fall apart in the face of anger. The anger is not my responsibility. An angry response is a choice.
Assertive people are seen as cold and self-serving.	Assertive responses are honest and demonstrate respect for the other person's point of view. Assertion builds healthy relationships.
It is wrong for me to turn down legitimate requests.	It is acceptable for me to turn down even reasonable requests. I can consider my own needs first, and it is not possible to please all of the people all of the time!

Modified from Bloom L, Coburn K, Pearlman J, 1975; and Ellis A, Harper RA, 1975.

1. Review the list of assertive rights (Box 1-2) to see which right or rights you are giving up by not asserting yourself.
2. Review the irrational beliefs that interfere with acting in your own best interest (Box 1-3).
3. Review the D.E.S.C. script to formulate an assertive response (Box 1-4).

To build your assertive skills you will need further study and application. Be patient with yourself and remember that becoming assertive is a lifelong journey (Box 1-5).

When you decide to use an assertive response, remember to consider three essential criteria for success:

| **Box 1-4** | **The Anatomy of an Assertive Response** |

A framework for developing assertive responses is known as the D.E.S.C. script. Although not all steps are used in every situation, it is a useful tool.

Describe the situation
Express what you think and feel
Specify your request
Consequences

From Bower SA, Bower GH, 1991.

| **Box 1-5** | **Types of Assertions** |

1. Basic—simple expression of an idea, belief, or opinion; standing up for your rights or the rights of others such as: "I want to . . ." "I don't want you to . . ." "Would you . . .?" "I liked it when you . . ." "I have a different opinion. I think that . . . " "I have mixed reactions. I agree with these aspects for these reasons, but I am disturbed by these aspects for these reasons" (Counseling Center, University of Illinois, 1984).
   • To buy time to consider: "I can give you an answer tomorrow after I have had time to think about it."
   • To deal with an interruption: "Excuse me, I am almost through. I'd like to finish my thought."
   • To return merchandise: "I am not satisfied with this product and I would like a refund."
   • To say no: "I cannot loan you any money."
2. Empathic—conveys sensitivity to the situation while taking an assertive position.
   • "I know the unit is short-staffed, but I have a pressing personal commitment and cannot work a second shift."
   • "I know you cannot tell me the exact time the computer technician will arrive, but I have a full day and would appreciate knowing if it will be in the morning or afternoon."
3. Escalating—when a simple assertion did not accomplish your goals and your rights are still being violated.
   • "I told you that as a nurse I cannot have a social relationship with you. I must insist that you refrain from asking me personal questions."
   • "I asked you not to use my computer without my permission. You have turned it off improperly and some files have been damaged. Please do not use it again."

Modified from Lange AJ, Jakubowski P, 1976.

   • Timing
   • Content
   • Receptivity

Is the person able to hear your concerns at this time, or is this an extremely busy time? Are you phrasing your intervention in a way that demonstrates respect for yourself and for others? Is the person receptive now, or is a cooling off period necessary? Consider this: sometimes the assertive response is to be quiet and listen for more information (Boxes 1-6 through 1-8).

Remember: assertive behavior does not guarantee you get what you want, but it increases the probability. If you want to change shifts with another nurse to be able to go to a family gathering, try asking assertively. Which of the following statements is assertive?

Box 1-6	**What Does It Mean to Communicate Assertively?**

- Being skilled in a variety of communication strategies for expressing your thoughts and feelings in a way that simultaneously protects your rights and those of others
- Having a positive attitude about communicating directly and honestly
- Feeling comfortable and in control of anxiety, tenseness, shyness, or fear
- Feeling confident that you can conduct yourself in a self-respecting way while still respecting others
- Honoring that you and the other person both have rights

Box 1-7	**An Assertive Nurse . . .**

- Appears self-confident and composed
- Maintains eye contact
- Uses clear, concise speech
- Speaks firmly and positively
- Speaks genuinely, without sarcasm
- Is non-apologetic
- Takes initiative to guide situations
- Gives the same message verbally and nonverbally

Box 1-8	**The Advantages of Assertive Behavior**

- It is more likely you will get what you want when you ask for it clearly
- People respect clear, open, honest communication
- You stand up for your own rights and feel self-respect
- You avoid the invitation of aggression when the rights of others are violated
- You are more independent
- You become a decision-maker
- You feel more peaceful and comfortable with yourself

A. "Jim, I was wondering if you would mind . . . it is probably an imposition, but . . . well, uh, if you could switch this Saturday for next so I could go to a family party."

B. "Jim, how many times have I traded with you and you never think of my social life? I insist you trade weekends with me so I can finally have a life, too."

C. "Jim, my family is having a special party this Saturday that I would really like to attend. I would appreciate it if you could trade with me. I would be glad to return the favor."

Did you select C? If so, you understood that this request honored the nurse's right to make a request and the colleague's right to refuse. The language was clear, non-apologetic, and respectful. Refer back to Box 1-4.

Describe: "my family is having a party"
Express: "I would really like to attend"
Specify: "trade with me"
Consequence" "I would return the favor."

Notice that response A is hesitant and apologetic, not straightforward. The wording denies the right of the request. Response B is aggressive and blaming and even a bit whiny.

Nonassertive communication is a failure to stand up for our legitimate rights and possibly for those of others. It means communicating in an uncertain or uncomfortable way. Sometimes being nonassertive gets us off the hook for the moment. We may agree to run an errand for someone because it is uncomfortable to say it isn't convenient. Consider the phrase, "Short-term gain, long-term pain," the next time you consider not speaking up for your own needs. When we are nonassertive, we lose because we fail to show respect for ourselves, which lowers our self-esteem. We begin to feel like a doormat. Our needs are not met, and we invite others to take advantage of us via aggressive behavior.

Aggressiveness is that loud, forceful, often confrontational way of trying to get what we want, even at the expense of others. When we act aggressively, our rights are responded to out of proportion to those of others. Although we may temporarily gloat at our achievement, the experience is short-lived when we realize how we may have embarrassed ourselves or, worse, hurt another person in our determination to get what we wanted. Aggressive behavior frequently results in people becoming angry or resentful and may result in retaliation or passive-aggressive behavior. When an aggressive approach is taken, mutual respect is lacking; others are treated as objects standing in our way. Table 1-1 differentiates among assertive, nonassertive, and aggressive styles of communication.

When you are assertive you feel better about yourself. It may take a while, however, for nurses who have been socialized to put others first to understand that there is a healthy balance between meeting personal needs and responding in a caring way to others. Nurses who have been more aggressive in their style may soon learn that this behavior distances people. It does get easier when you learn you can choose when to speak up and when to remain silent. You can choose lovingly to do something extra for someone, to inconvenience yourself by choice, not because you feel helpless. A good test of whether you have acted assertively is how you feel after the interaction. If you feel good, it's likely you have been assertive. Remember that if you have been passive most of the time, you may still feel guilty for setting your own priorities, but the resentment that builds if you do not will erode the relationship.

Remember: assertive communication skills make interactions more equal. All parties have a right to express their thoughts, feelings, and beliefs. The next time you feel irritated with a "demanding" client, consider that today's clients are not passive recipients of our care but consumers

---

Box 1-9   An Assertive Consumer . . .

- Wants convenience
- Is informed and better educated
- Wants what he wants when he wants it
- Wants to be heard and be involved in the problem-solving process
- Does not want to depend on the "expert"

Modified from Herzlinger R, 1997.

with the expectation of good customer service (Box 1-9). Assertiveness refers to a style of communicating that has positive benefits for you and for others. It builds your self-confidence to know that you can treat others fairly while taking care of your own needs. This experience creates a healthy attitude of mutual respect. Speaking out about your thoughts and feelings provides others with clear, direct messages that are easier to receive than passive-aggressive ones. Assertiveness helps build trust between people.

THE MEANING OF RESPONSIBLE COMMUNICATION

Responsible means, "placed in control of and having to give satisfaction . . . to consider oneself answerable for" (Webster, 1993). As nurses, this accountability may be described as being personally responsible for the outcome of our own professional actions, which are based on knowledge.

Sometimes, responsible communication is a simple statement of caring: "The pain medication will make you feel more comfortable." Other times, responsible communication may be the art of listening; if you don't know what to say, you can just sit quietly with a client.

To communicate responsibly when a problem has to be solved means to communicate in a logical way based on your nursing knowledge and on the facts presented in the situation. Responsible communication demonstrates accurate problem-solving behavior for the particular situation. Nursing process is a systematic means for nurses to demonstrate accountability and responsibility to clients. Discussions of the nursing process offer several different formats, with the steps varying in number. The American Nurses' Association's *Standards of Clinical Nursing Practice* (1991) presents six steps: assessment, diagnosis, outcome identification, planning, implementation, and evaluation. Nurses base their practice on nursing diagnoses, clinical outcomes, and critical pathways. Yet all of the variations are based on a simple model into which all the steps and strategies can fit. The four-step method, easily remembered by "A PIE," can be a useful tool for the nurse to remember when interacting with others.

Assess—collect the essential verbal and nonverbal data about the client's (or colleague's) thoughts and feelings.

Plan—analyze the data to determine the diagnosis and identify outcomes. Include the client and at times the family to create a plan of care that prescribes interventions to attain expected outcomes. Plan your communication strategy . . . what, when, how, and where you will present the plan.

Implement—implement the interventions identified in the plan of care. At this point you respond to your client or colleague. This book encourages you to respond assertively and responsibly.

Evaluate—evaluate the client's progress toward attainment of outcomes. Here is where you check whether your response was assertive and responsible, and whether your objectives (expected outcomes) were achieved.

This problem-solving process becomes a way of examining every client-nurse (or nurse-colleague) interaction. It becomes a natural part of your day. While you are receiving a message, you are trying to determine its meaning. You decide whether you will meet the sender's request, and then you transmit an assertive and responsible message that conveys your decision. As you send your message you observe the effects of your words and gestures on the receiver. During the course of your day, you are sending and receiving messages continuously (Box 1-10).

Wit and Wisdom

Even your silence holds a sort of prayer.

Apache proverb

Box 1-10   A Nurse Who Communicates Responsibly . . .

- Is naturally focused on the nursing process/problem-solving process
- Considers the world of the client and his family (see Chapter 4)
- Includes the role of client advocate
- Appreciates the sacred role of intimate care of the sick
- Maintains a sense of wonder at the human experience and treats each person as an individual
- Is open to learning to trust intuition as another way of knowing about the client

Moments of Connection...
Daring to Care

A nurse worked with a client who was unable to communicate because of a brain tumor. He sat up in bed, rocking back and forth and crying out in pain. His distress was not alleviated by pain medication. The nurse reported that she climbed up into the bed, rocked him, and sang lullabies to him like she sang to her son. He relaxed, became quiet, and "nestled" into the nurse's arms. He was able to go to sleep a bit later and died in his sleep that night. The nurse said never before or since had she been moved to do this and talked about the importance of trusting your intuition. "I guess God must have directed my actions that day. He put me in the right place and time and gave me the courage to step outside the practice . . . to care in a special way" (Riley, 1999).

THE MEANING OF CARING

Caring is the basis of the nursing profession. Your communication may be technically responsible and assertive, but without caring you still may not be able to facilitate a change in behavior. It is important to examine what caring means.

Caring is not an abstract concept; there are explicit ways we as nurses can communicate to show we care. Encompassed in caring is a commitment to the preservation of common humanity and an unrelenting respect for the uniqueness and dignity of each individual we encounter (Delaney, 1990). Caring is an essential ingredient in life and must characterize the nurse-client

Wit and Wisdom

Give me knowledge so I may have kindness for all.

Plains Indian proverb

relationship. Nurses at St. Luke's Medical Center in Milwaukee have created a clinical practice development model that delineates novice, advanced beginner, competent, proficient, and expert behaviors for what they call the domain of caring. Nurses used their own stories to provide a qualitative, narrative approach to defining caring behaviors. The expert level is evidenced by:

- Trusting relationships based on "being with" not "doing to" the client.
- Understanding of the meaning of the experience to client and family.
- Creating an environment of hope and trust (Haag-Heitman and Kramer, 1998).

Caring is the moral ideal that guides nurses through the caregiving process, and knowledgeable caring is the highest form of commitment (Watson, 1995). Nurses can have an extensive command of scientific facts and theories and be technically expert without being caring professionals. In addition, nurses can be technically and scientifically correct but still make moral errors. Although there is satisfaction in being technologically competent, that satisfaction is not as lasting as meaningful moments of connection with clients, family, and colleagues. Caring communication is holistic, taking into account the entire person and demonstrating respect for clients as people, not just as bodies requiring nursing interventions. A study of caring, as lived by critical care nurses, demonstrated that caring involved affective, cognitive, and psychomotor aspects that led to outcomes. The process of caring began in the nurse's feelings and knowledge and moved the nurse to competent actions that contributed to positive outcomes for the client, family, and nurse (Bush and Barr, 1997).

How can you ensure that your communication is caring? If we as nurses consciously desire to generate the feeling of being cared for in our clients and intend our behavior to convey this desire, we must remember that not all intended caring on our part is perceived as caring by our clients. In an extensive review of care research derived from qualitative research methodology, discrepancies were discovered between nurses' and clients' perceptions of the importance of expressive and instrumental behaviors in caring. Nurses identified more expressive behaviors (such as listening, touching, and presence) as indicators of caring. In contrast, clients identified more instrumental behaviors (such as accessibility and monitoring) as indicative of caring. There may be discrepancies in the care nurses consider optimal and that which clients consider important (Tripp-Reimer and Cohen, 1990). Caring is situation-specific. "Caring must encompass knowledge and skills in the ability to identify care needs and nursing actions that will bring about positive change; that is, movement toward the protection, enhancement, and preservation of human dignity" (Delaney, 1990).

The implications are clear. We must find out what is perceived to be important to our clients in their return to health, validate the effect our caring actions are having on them, and adjust our actions in keeping with their needs. Taking these actions is a necessary component of responsible nursing. Eriksson calls nurses to "understand the world of the patient, the suffering human being" (Eriksson, 1997).

Caring communication is equally important with colleagues as with clients. If caring exists between co-workers, that sense of well-being will likely be passed on to clients. Conversely, if there is little caring between colleagues, then nurses will be unlikely to feel complete and satisfied enough to demonstrate a sense of caring with their clients. Caring involves being assertive and responsible. If you let others control you because you are nonassertive, or if you invade others' rights by being aggressive, you cannot act in a caring way. If you care enough for yourself to be assertive, you will know how to care for others.

HOW CAN YOU LEARN TO COMMUNICATE ASSERTIVELY AND RESPONSIBLY?

This book is based on the belief that effective and caring nurse communicators are not born; they are made. You can learn to communicate in competent, caring, and confident ways. You can replace ineffective and non-therapeutic communication habits with helpful interventions. You can continually add to your communications repertoire so that you develop confidence in your ability to communicate effectively in a variety of situations.

Educational psychologists have proposed that learning involves three domains (McCroskey, 1984; Meichenbaum, 1977; Woodruff, 1961). This book attends to the cognitive (understanding and meaning), affective (feelings, values, and attitudes), and psychomotor (physical capability of doing) aspects of your communication learning process.

By following the guidelines in this text, you will learn basic communication skills (cognitive domain); you will build confidence through a belief in the value and impact of positive communication (affective domain); and you will meet the challenge, putting skills into action in the real world (psychomotor domain).

Cognitive Domain: Basic Communication Competencies

Communication competence is your ability to demonstrate knowledge of the appropriate communicative behavior in any situation. Communication competence is demonstrated by identifying behaviors that would be appropriate or inappropriate in an observed interpersonal situation.

Affective Domain: Belief in the Value and Impact of Positive Communication

A belief in the value and impact of positive communication motivates the nurse to seek feedback and practice self-care strategies that build confidence.

Psychomotor Domain: Putting It All Together

Communication skill is your ability to perform appropriate communication behaviors in any given situation. To be considered a skilled nurse communicator, you must be able to successfully implement communication strategies that are assertive and responsible.

Figure 1-3 illustrates how to become a caring nurse communicator by developing skills in all three domains. The negative consequences of incomplete development in all three aspects are also illustrated.

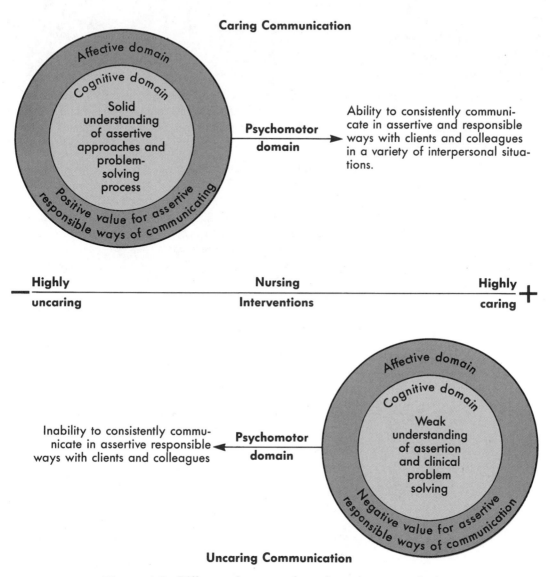

Figure 1-3   Differences between caring and uncaring communication.

Think About It...
What, So What, and Now What?

We know that reading comprehension is improved when the reader is actively asking and answering questions while reading. To build your communication skills, answer the questions in this section in each chapter. Be thinking about how you will write your answers as you read each chapter.

1. **What . . .**   Write one thing you learned from this chapter.

2. **So what . . .**   How will this impact your nursing practice?

3. **Now what . . .**   How will you implement this new knowledge or skill?

THINK ABOUT IT

Wit and Wisdom

Take my heart, friend,
We begin together.
Even stormy times
We can weather.

To be a nurse,
Our heart's desire,
Of practicing skills
We will not tire.

Say what you mean
And ask no less
And you will find
That lives you bless.

Assertive talk
Is a relief you see.
Let's you be you
And me be me.

For as we touch
The lives of others,
We find we all are
Sisters and brothers.

Copyright 1995 Julia W. Balzer Riley.

Practicing Assertive, Responsible, and Caring Communication

Exercise 1

Review Box 1-2. List any rights you have relinquished.
Review Box 1-3. For each right you listed, identify which irrational beliefs you held that interfered with your acting in your own best interest.

Exercise 2

Keep a journal for a week to examine your behavior to build assertive communication skills. Record in the following format:

Event In Which I Was Not Assertive	Was My Behavior Nonassertive or Aggressive?	How Would I Prefer to Have Handled the Situation?

Exercise 3

Observe other students, faculty, staff in your clinical area, colleagues, and family members. Identify one person who could be a role model for assertive communication. Identify one situation in your professional life and one situation in your personal life in which you would have preferred to be assertive. Close your eyes and envision the role model. Ask yourself how this person would have handled the situation and pretend you can see what the person is saying and doing. Write what you imagined and examine the lessons you learn from this to build your own assertive communication skills.

References

Alberti RE, Emmons M: *Your perfect right: a guide to assertive living,* San Luis Obispo, Calif, 1995, Impact Publishers.

American Nurses' Association: *Standards of clinical nursing practice,* Kansas City, Mo, 1991, The American Nurses Association.

Axelrod A, Holtje J, Holtje J: *How to say no gracefully and effectively,* New York, 1997, McGraw-Hill.

Balzer Riley J: *From the heart to the hands . . . keys to successful healthcaring connections,* Ellicott City, Md, 1999, I.M.P.S., Inc.

Bower SA, Bower GH: *Asserting yourself,* Reading, Mass, 1991, Addison-Wesley.

Bloom L, Coburn K, Pearlman J: *The new assertive woman,* New York, 1975, Dell.

Bush HA, Barr WJ: Critical care nurses' lived experiences of caring, *Heart Lung* 26(5):387, 1997.

Chenevert M: *Pro-nurse handbook: designed for the nurse who wants to thrive professionally,* ed 2, St Louis, 1993, Mosby.

Clark S: Rating assertiveness on the road of management, *Philadelphia Business Journal* 15(39):16, Nov 15, 1996.

Communication in Nursing Video Series: *Communicating with clients and colleagues,* St Louis, 1995, Mosby.

Counseling Center, University of Illinois at Urbana-Champaign: *Assertiveness,* 1984.

Delaney C: Computer technology: endangering the essence of nursing? In McCloskey JC, Grace HK, editors: *Current issues in nursing,* ed 3, St Louis, 1990, Mosby.

Ellis A, Harper RA: *A new guide to rational living,* North Hollywood, Calif, 1975, Wilshire Book Company.

Eriksson K: Understanding the world of the patient, the suffering human being: the new clinical paradigm from nursing to caring, *Adv Pract Nurs Q* 3(1):8, 1997.

Guglielmo WJ: Why you should welcome the new assertive patient, *Med Econ* 74(19):96, Sept. 22, 1997.

Herzlinger R: *Market driven health care: who wins, who loses in the transformation of America's largest service industry,* Reading, Mass, 1997, Addison-Wesley Publishing.

Haag-Heitman B, Kramer A: Creating a clinical practice development model, *Am J Nurs* 98(8):39, 1998.

Lange AJ, Jakubowski P: *Responsible assertive behavior,* Champaign, Ill, 1976, Research Press.

McCroskey JC: The communication apprehension perspective. In Daly JA, McCroskey JC, editors: *Avoiding communication: shyness, reticence and communication apprehension,* Beverly Hills, Calif, 1984, Sage Publications.

Meichenbaum D: *Cognitive-behavior modification: an integrative approach,* New York, 1977, Plenum Press.

New Webster's Dictionary and Thesaurus of the English Language, Danbury, Conn, 1993, Lexicon Publications, Inc.

Smith DR, Williamson LK: *Interpersonal communication: roles, rules, strategies and games,* ed 2, Dubuque, Ia, 1981, Wm. C. Brown.

Stuart GW, Laraia M: *Principles and practice of psychiatric nursing,* ed 6, St Louis, 1998, Mosby.

Sundeen SJ et al: *Nurse-client interaction: implementing the nursing process,* St Louis, 1998, Mosby.

Tripp-Reimer T, Cohen MZ: Qualitative approaches to care: a critical review. In Stevenson JS, Tripp-Reimer T, editors: *Knowledge about care and caring: state of the art and future developments,* Kansas City, Mo, 1990, American Academy of Nursing.

Watson J: Postmodernism and knowledge development in nursing, *Nurs Sci Q* 8(2):60, 1995.

Williams SA: The relationship of patients' perceptions of holistic nursing caring to satisfaction with nursing care, *J Nurs Care Qual* 11(5):15, 1997.

Woodruff AD: *Basic concepts of teaching,* Scranton, Pa, 1961, Chandler Publishing Co. An Intext Publisher.

Suggestions for Further Reading

Burley-Allen M: *Managing assertively: how to improve your people skills,* New York, 1995, John Wiley & Sons.

Chenevert M: *Mosby's tour guide to nursing school: a student's road survival kit,* ed 3, St Louis, 1995, Mosby.

This practical guidebook presents a candid, humorous, and helpful description of the experiences all nursing students are likely to encounter. In addition to describing the difficulties and stresses confronting nursing students, the book provides sound advice for coping with these problems.

Chenevert M: *Special techniques in assertiveness training for women in health professions,* St Louis, 1994, Mosby.

Crisp SR, Lloyd M, editors: *Developing positive assertiveness,* New York, 1995, Crisp Publications.

Davidson J: *The complete idiot's guide to assertiveness,* New York, 1997, Macmillan General Reference.

Forsyth D et al: Can caring behavior be taught? *Nurs Outlook* 37(4):164, 1989.

This article concisely summarizes what the authors consider to be the essential behaviors of caring and describes how they can be successfully taught to nurses.

Kilkus SP: Assertiveness among professional nurses, *J Adv Nurs* 18(8):1324, 1993.

Kirkpatrick H, Forchuk C: Assertiveness training: does it make a difference? *J Staff Devel* 8(20):60, 1992.

Michelli D: *Successful assertiveness,* New York, 1997, Barrons Educational Series.

Pegano MP, Ragan SL, Booten S: *Communication skills for professional nurses,* Newburg Park, Calif, 1992, Sage Publications.

Peiffer V: *The duty trap: how to say "no" when you feel you ought to say "yes,"* Rockport, Mass, 1997, Element Books.

Phelps S, Austin N: *The assertive woman,* 1997, Impact Publishers.

Winderquist J, Davidhizar R: The ministry of nursing, *J Adv Nurs* 19:647-652, 1994.

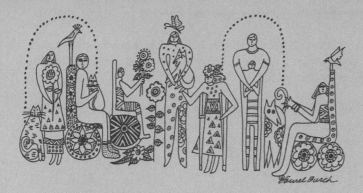

2

The Client-Nurse Relationship: A Helping Relationship

Let people realize clearly that every time they threaten someone or humiliate or unnecessarily hurt or dominate or reject another human being, they become forces for the creation of psychopathology, even if these be small forces. Let them recognize that every person who is kind, helpful, decent, psychologically democratic, affectionate, and warm, is a psychotherapeutic force, even though a small one.

Abraham Maslow

OBJECTIVES

1. Identify the purpose of the client-nurse relationship.
2. Describe the cognitive, affective, and psychomotor abilities that nurses and clients bring to the therapeutic encounter.
3. Discuss clients' rights as consumers of health care service.
4. Identify characteristics of a successful client-nurse relationship.
5. Identify therapeutic communication techniques.
6. Identify nontherapeutic communication techniques.
7. Identify a list of do's and don'ts in the client-nurse relationship.

Encounters we have with our clients can be harmful or helpful. As a compassionate and caring nurse, you will want your interactions with your clients to be helpful and pleasant. This chapter has information that you can integrate and apply to build effective relationships with your clients.

The nature of client-nurse relationships is described so that you can explain the difference from social, collegial, and kinship relationships. The responsibilities of nurses in client-nurse relationships have also been outlined so that you will be able to articulate your roles and interventions at each stage of the helping relationship. You are invited to discover the extent to which you foster a helping relationship in your interactions with clients.

THE NATURE OF THE HELPING RELATIONSHIP

A set of pre-established rules and expectations directs the course of client-nurse interactions. There may be some overlap in these interactions with those involving friends and family, but one factor in particular differentiates helping relationships from social relationships. A helping relationship is established for the benefit of the client, whereas kinship and friendship relationships are designed to meet mutual needs. In particular, the client-nurse relationship is established to help the client achieve and maintain optimal health.

A successful helping relationship between nurse and client represents a different order of interaction than that which occurs in a friendship. This is not because of any superiority in the nurse but because of the mutual trust and the responsibilities for assisting others that characterize true professional relationships.

Nursing actions are planned to promote, maintain, and restore the client's/patient's well-being and health (Congress for Nursing Practice, American Nurses' Association, 1973).

Professional practitioners of nursing bear primary responsibility for the nursing care clients/patients receive (Congress for Nursing Practice, ANA, 1973). Client-nurse relationships are entered for the benefit of the client, but such a relationship is more effective if it is mutually satisfying. Clients are satisfied when their health care needs have been met and they sense that they have been cared for. Nurses feel a sense of accomplishment when their interventions have had a positive influence on their clients' health status and when their conduct has been competent and caring. Client-nurse relationships may be a mutual learning experience, but in general the goals of therapeutic relationships are directed toward the growth of clients (Stuart and Sundeen, 1995).

Never assume that in client-nurse relationships clients play the role of passive receiver awaiting the soothing ministrations of influential nurses. Both clients and nurses bring their respective knowledge, attitudes, feelings, skills, and patterns of behaving to the relationship. Indeed, referring to their interaction as a relationship indicates a sense of affiliation that bonds clients and nurses as well as an interdependency and reciprocity between them.

Clients and nurses alike come to the relationship with unique cognitive, affective, and psychomotor abilities that they use in their joint endeavor of enhancing the clients' well-being. Nurses are responsible for encouraging this interchange of ideas, values, and skills. In an effective helping relationship there is a definite and guaranteed interchange between clients and nurses in all three dimensions.

Standards IV and VI of the American Nurses' Association Standards of Nursing Practice (1991) articulate the importance of clients' participation in their own health care.

Standard IV

The plan is developed with the client, significant others and health care providers, when appropriate. The client/patient and family are continuously involved in planning nursing care.

Standard VI

The client, significant others, and health care providers are involved in the evaluation process, when appropriate. The quality of nursing care depends on comprehensive and intelligent determination of nursing impact upon the health status of the client. The client is an essential part of this determination.

Cognitive, Affective, and Psychomotor Abilities in the Therapeutic Encounter

Following are some of the cognitive, affective, and psychomotor abilities that clients and nurses bring to their therapeutic encounter. Table 2-1 further illustrates that both clients and nurses come with notions and expectations that will influence the course and outcome of their relationship.

Cognitive

Clients and nurses both know something about health and illness in general, and about the individual client's health concerns in particular. Clients have definite notions about what has made them ill and what might improve their health; in turn, nurses have their own views, based on their knowledge and beliefs about what will help their clients. To prevent them from operating in isolation or at cross-purposes, clients and nurses must exchange essential information.

Besides having different ideas, clients and nurses also have preferred ways of observing their worlds and making decisions about what they see. Each of us has a preferred mental process—the one we have developed most highly, the one we use best—that forms the core of our personalities (Lawrence, 1982). Clients and nurses have different ways they prefer to use their minds, specifically, the way they choose to perceive and make judgments (Myers, 1980). Perceiving includes becoming aware of things, people, occurrences, and ideas. Judging includes reaching conclusions about what has been observed.

Some clients and nurses, for example, are primarily practical. They are attuned to immediate experiences, literal facts at hand, and concrete realities. Myers used the word *sensing* to describe this preferred way of collecting data in problem solving. Other clients and nurses prefer to think about what could be, rather than what is. Their intuitive imagination fills their minds with ideas and explanations that do not always depend on the senses for verification. Myers called this preferred way of collecting data *intuitive*.

Consider this situation for understanding the differences in these two ways of perceiving and how they would affect the client-nurse relationship.

> Mr. Zabrick is an 80-year-old resident of a senior citizens' apartment complex where he lives with his retired, widowed sister, age 70. In the past 9 months Mr. Zabrick has had chemotherapy and radiation treatments for lung cancer. His tumor has vanished and his blood levels are stabilized; yet, to his disappointment, he feels lethargic and anorexic.
>
> Eight days ago his sister awoke in the night and found Mr. Zabrick in the bathtub, where he had fallen after mistaking it for the toilet. She noticed that her brother is unsteady on his feet and is losing weight.

TABLE 2-1	Interchange of Knowledge, Attitudes, and Skills Between Client and Nurse in the Helping Relationship

What Clients Bring to the Client-Nurse Relationship	What Nurses Bring to the Client-Nurse Relationship
Cognitive	
Preferred ways of perceiving and judging	Preferred ways of perceiving and judging
Knowledge and beliefs about illness in general and their illness in particular	Knowledge and beliefs about illness in general
Knowledge and beliefs about health promotion and maintenance in general, and information about their own health care activities	Knowledge about their clinical specialty and knowledge and beliefs about health behaviors that prevent illness and promote, regain, and maintain health
Ability to problem solve	Ability to problem solve
Ability to learn	Knowledge about factors that increase client compliance with treatment regimen
Affective	
Cultural values	Cultural values
Feelings about seeking help from a nurse	Feelings about being a nurse-helper
Attitudes toward nurses in general	Attitudes towards clients in general
Attitudes toward treatment regimen	Biases about nursing treatment regimen
Values about preventing illness	Values placed on being healthy
	Value placed on people actively preventing illness or enhancing well-being
Willingness to take positive action about own health status at this time with this particular nurse	Willingness to help clients take positive action to improve their well-being
Psychomotor	
Ability to relate and communicate with others	Ability to relate and communicate with others
Ability to carry out own health care management	Proficiency in administering effective nursing interventions
Ability to learn new methods of self-care	Ability to teach nursing interventions to client

Clients (or family members) and nurses who prefer concrete details, or sensing, would perceive Mr. Zabrick's situation by focusing on the visible evidence that might account for his deterioration. They would notice the lack of saliva under, and the brown furry nature of, the tongue, as well as the unpleasant taste and odor in the mouth. They would see the small, hard stools and the abdominal distention. They would feel the decreased turgor of his skin and the muscle weakness. They would count the amount of fluids and quantity of food consumed by Mr. Zabrick.

Clients or nurses who prefer detailed information would put these pieces together and likely come to the conclusion that Mr. Zabrick is dehydrated. Those who use this way of perceiving prefer information that is measurable, and the thinking process is systematic, taking one step at a time.

Clients (or family members) and nurses who prefer a more intuitive perceiving process might not gather all these data before jumping to a conclusion about what is happening to Mr. Zabrick. They are likely to look for patterns in the data (as opposed to discrete pieces of information); they would start thinking about possible explanations and then work backward to get the facts. They might notice, for example, that Mr. Zabrick has said, "Why bother with trying any more? If I had a chance to do it again, I'm not sure I'd take the treatments," and wonder if his fatigue and grief are consuming him. They might remember that Mr. Zabrick's daughter-in-law died despite rigorous chemotherapy and that his lifelong friend was diagnosed with brain cancer 3 weeks ago, and wonder if Mr. Zabrick's symptoms reflect his doubt about living with such losses. Another theme that intuitive individuals might focus on is the relationship between the assault on Mr. Zabrick's body from treatments, changes in diet, exercise, and sleep deprivation, and the impact of the severe heat and humidity of the past 7 weeks.

These two perceptive processes, sensing and intuitive, are quite different, and it is important for nurses to understand their preferred way of perceiving, and to try to discover which process their clients prefer. Both ways of seeing the world are valuable—one is not better than the other; each simply selects different information on which to focus.

Judging—the way of making decisions about the information collected through perception—is the other mental process in which clients and nurses may differ. Some persons will have logical, orderly, analytical decision-making processes and treat the world objectively (Myers, 1980). Decision makers like these prefer to fit all experience into logical mental systems. Myers called this preference *thinking* and said these people make decisions based on critical analysis of facts, valuing fairness. Other clients and nurses prefer to tune into the subjective world of feelings and values. Myers called this preference *feeling* and said these individuals make decisions by analyzing how they will affect people, valuing harmony.

Each of us prefers one of these decision-making processes to the other (Myers, 1980). Consider this situation to better understand the two judging processes.

> Jossie is a 19-year-old first-year university student who is 8 weeks pregnant and unmarried. She is receiving counseling about her options. She sees three choices and will soon decide whether to have an abortion, continue with the pregnancy and give up her baby for adoption, or carry her baby to term and raise the child herself.

Clients and nurses who prefer a rational, objective way of making decisions would invite Jossie to consider all the facts and then make a logical decision based on them. They would look at the consequences of any decision Jossie might make and judge it using their heads rather than their hearts. They would be able to remain emotionally uninvolved. They have the ability to see the "long view" and would likely encourage Jossie to look pragmatically into her future and act on the most sensible decision (Myers, 1980; Page, 1983).

Clients, family members, and nurses who prefer to consider effects on the people in the situation would likely explore how Jossie feels about each of the choices and how each fits with her values. Such people would likely emphasize the benefits of any plan Jossie considers rather than criticizing it; they would also likely support Jossie's personal convictions (Page, 1983).

This glimpse at two different methods for using our minds alerts us to the misunderstandings that could arise in helping relationships. We cannot assume that clients' minds are guided by the same principles as our own. Clients, their family members, and professional colleagues may reason in the same way that you do, or they may prefer using different ways of perceiving and judging. They may not value the things you value or show interest in the same things you do (Myers, 1980).

We all use different combinations of perceiving and judging, and colleagues and clients with the same preferences are likely to be the easiest to like and understand. They will tend to have similar interests (because they share the same kinds of perceptions) and consider the same matters important (because they share the same kinds of judgment) (Myers, 1980).

On the other hand, it will be harder to understand and predict the behavior of colleagues and clients whose perception and judgment preferences differ from our own. We are likely to take opposite stands on any issue with colleagues and clients who prefer different thinking processes (Myers, 1980). "The therapeutic nurse-patient relationship is a mutual learning experience and a corrective emotional experience for the patient. It is based on the underlying humanity of nurse and patient, with mutual respect and acceptance of ethnocultural differences" (Stuart and Laraia, 1998).

If you would like to learn more about your preferences for perceiving and making decisions, as well as about other personality preferences, arrange with your school's counseling or guidance department to take the Myers-Briggs Type Indicator (MBTI). The aim of the MBTI is to identify, from self-reporting of easily recognized reactions, the basic preferences of people in regard to perception and judgment (Myers and McCaulley, 1985). Learning about your own preferences will make you more aware of how your way of thinking influences your behavior in client-nurse helping relationships.

Affective

All clients and nurses have positive and negative feelings about helping relationships; each also has biases about the other. Both have different priorities for working on particular health concerns. The attitudes of both clients and nurses will greatly affect whether they will work in harmony or discord, whether their respective knowledge will surface or submerge, and whether they will carry out the commitment of improving the health of individual clients.

The major source of our value system is our culture. In America today, the culture is heterogeneous (with a variety of cultural groups), so that nurses and clients are likely to encounter different beliefs and values, particularly as the United States increasingly becomes home to people from all parts of the world. Modern medical and nursing practices become two of the external forces immigrants encounter. This encounter with the American health care system is loaded with choices for immigrants to make in deciding how much of their culture's traditional medical practices they wish to maintain. Cultural patterns are one of the important means by which people adapt to recurrent change in their environments (see Chapter 4).

Psychomotor

Clients need to know what skills nurses have, and nurses need to find out about their clients' ability to participate in their own treatment plan. Both parties must come to an agreement about what their respective tasks will be in their effort to improve the client's health status. Consider a scenario in which a client is more proficient at finding information via the World Wide Web than is the nurse. Can you envision a partnering to share information? The client can find the information and the nurse can help the client understand which sources are most reliable (see Chapter 5).

CLIENT RIGHTS IN THE HELPING RELATIONSHIP

Together nurses and clients share their energy and resources and commit to healing. Together they confront issues of the meaning of illness to the client and family and work toward self-realization and personal growth. As consumers of our health care services, clients have the right to:

- Expect a systematic and accurate investigation of their health concerns by thorough and well-organized nurses.
- Be informed about their health status and have all their questions answered so that they clearly understand what nurses mean.
- Receive health care from nurses who have current knowledge about their diagnosis and are capable of providing safe and efficient care.
- Feel confident they will be treated courteously and that their nurses show genuine interest in them.
- Trust that any issues of personal confidentiality will be respected.
- Be informed about any plans of action to be carried out for their benefit.
- Refuse or consent to nursing treatments without jeopardizing their relationship with their nurses.
- Secure help conveniently, without hassles or roadblocks.
- Receive consistent quality of care from all nurses.

CHARACTERISTICS OF CLIENT-NURSE HELPING RELATIONSHIPS

Client-nurse relationships are special helping relationships that are characterized by the following features:

- A partnership between clients and nurses, both working together to improve the client's health status.
- A philosophy about human nature and what motivates humans in health and illness. As nurses, we should know our beliefs and values and be able to articulate them clearly.
- A purposeful and productive objective. Together, clients and nurses agree about the nature of the health problem in question and they develop and implement a plan designed to reach agreed-upon objectives. Clients and nurses together evaluate the outcomes and decide whether the desired and expected outcomes have been achieved.
- Preservation of the client's present level of health, and protection from future health threats because of the increased knowledge gleaned from the helping relationship.
- Palliation of clients' worries and fears through nurses' reassurances, and easing of pain through soothing comfort measures.
- A psychic or morale booster. Clients perk up from the positive attention and interest they receive from nurses.
- Practicality, offering efficacious, effective, and efficient ways of handling health concerns.
- Portability—taking place wherever and whenever clients and nurses come together.
- A series of phases, with a beginning (initiation), middle (maintenance), and end (termination) to each encounter.
- A personally tailored interaction designed to meet the needs of each particular client.
- Platonic and not passionate expressions of caring. Even though nurses may have strong feelings for their clients, it is expected that they can maintain adequate objectivity and perspective to provide therapeutic assistance.

TABLE 2-2	Summary of Therapeutic Communication Techniques	
Technique	**Definition**	**Therapeutic Value**
Listening	An active process of receiving information and examining one's reaction to the messages received	Nonverbally communicates nurse's interest in client
Silence	Periods of no verbal communication among participants	Nonverbally communicates nurse's acceptance of client
Establishing guidelines	Statements regarding roles, purpose, and limitations for a particular interaction	Helps client to know what is expected of him or her
Open-ended comments	General comments asking the client to determine the direction the interaction should take	Allows client to decide what material is most relevant and encourages client to continue
Reducing distance	Diminishing physical space between the nurse and client	Nonverbally communicates that nurse wants to be involved with client
Acknowledgment	Recognition given to a client for contribution to an interaction	Demonstrates the importance of the client's role within the relationship
Restating	Repeating to the client what the nurse believes is the main thought or idea expressed	Asks for validation of nurse's interpretation of the message
Reflecting	Directing back to the client his ideas, feelings, questions, or content	Attempts to show client the importance of his or her own ideas, feelings, and interpretations
Seeking clarification	Asking for additional input to understand the message received	Demonstrates nurse's desire to understand client's communication
Seeking consensual validation	Attempts to reach a mutual denotative and connotative meaning of specific words	Demonstrates nurse's desire to understand client's communication
Focusing	Questions or statements to help the client develop or expand an idea	Directs conversation toward topics of importance
Summarizing	Statement of main areas discussed during an interaction	Helps client to separate relevant from irrelevant material; serves as a review and closing for the interaction
Planning	Mutual decision making regarding the goals, direction, etc. of future interactions	Reiterates client's role within relationship

From Sundeen SJ et al: *Nurse-client interaction: implementing the nursing process,* St Louis, 1998, Mosby, p. 113.

TABLE 2-3	Summary of Nontherapeutic Communication Techniques	
Technique	**Definition**	**Therapeutic Threat**
Failure to listen	Not receiving client's intended message	Places needs of nurse above those of client
Failure to probe	Inadequate data collection represented by eliciting vague descriptions, getting inadequate answers, following standard forms too closely, and not exploring client's interpretation	Inadequate database on which to make decisions; client care not individualized
Parroting	Continual repetition of client's phrases	The metacommunication is "I am not listening" or "I am not a competent communicator"
Being judgmental	Approving or disapproving statements	Implies that nurse has the right to pass judgment; promotes a dependency relationship
Reassuring	Attempts to do magic with words	Negates fears, feelings, and other communications of client
Rejecting	Refusing to discuss topics with client	Client may feel that not only communication but also the self was rejected
Defending	Attempts to protect someone or something from negative feedback	Negates the client's right to express an opinion
Giving advice	Telling the client what the nurse thinks should be done	Negates the worth of client as a mutual partner in decision making
Stereotyped responses	Use of trite, meaningless verbal expressions	Negates the significance of the client's communication
Changing topics	Nurse directing the interaction into areas of self-interest rather than following the lead of the client	Nonverbally communicates that the nurse is in charge of deciding what will be discussed; possible to miss important topics for individual client
Patronizing	Style of communication that displays a condescending attitude toward the client	Implies that the nurse-client relationship is not based on equality; places the nurse in a "superior" position

From Sundeen SJ et al: *Nurse-client interaction: implementing the nursing process,* St Louis, 1998, Mosby, p. 117.

- A sense of privacy so that clients may disclose intimate details about their lives. Nurses are responsible for protecting their clients' confidentiality.
- Powerful emotions. Clients and nurses can develop attachments for each other, which makes the relationship special for each.

Nurses employ therapeutic communication techniques to implement the nursing process (Table 2-2) as contrasted with nontherapeutic communication techniques (Table 2-3).

POINTERS TO GUIDE YOU IN YOUR CLIENT-NURSE HELPING RELATIONSHIPS

This section offers "do's" and "don'ts" for conducting yourself in client-nurse helping relationships. Here are the "do's."

Do:

- Be prepared mentally, emotionally, and physically to assist your clients in resolving their health care problems.
- Be punctual and polite in your manner of relating to clients.
- Promote clients' well-being, comfort, and increased health status.
- Be philanthropic in your approach to clients by putting their needs and concerns first.
- Be plucky in planning and generating creative solutions to your clients' health concerns.
- Be proficient in the nursing skills required to safely and successfully care for your clients.
- Praise and encourage clients in their efforts to take better care of themselves.
- Be patient and understanding about clients' reactions to their particular health situations.
- Persevere in pursuing your pledge to help clients preserve their health.

Here are the "don'ts."

Don't:

- Patronize clients.
- Preach at or pressure them to change.
- Pigeonhole clients with labels such as "good," "lazy," or "uncooperative," which prevent you from seeing clients as they really are.
- Procrastinate following through on clients' reasonable requests.
- Put down clients by using medical jargon, or in any way making them feel inadequate or estranged.
- Punish clients for acts of omission or commission that have negatively affected their health.
- Reveal prejudices against the race, religion, or creed of clients.
- Be pleasure-seeking or try to meet your own needs through the client-nurse relationship.
- Pretend to have knowledge that you do not in order to avoid looking uninformed. It is the client's health with which you are dealing, and clients have the right to receive honest, forthright communication.

Wit and Wisdom

Good silence is called holiness.

Panamanian Proverb

Being an Effective Nurse-Helper Requires Being Assertive and Responsible

As a nurse, it is your responsibility to ensure that a thorough assessment is made of your clients' health concerns, that suitable nursing actions are chosen and implemented to help your clients, and that an evaluation of the results is carried out. Assuming this leadership does not mean that you take over and do for, or to, your clients. The quality of your nursing care is determined by the completeness of the interchange of knowledge, attitudes, and skills between you and your clients.

To be most helpful to all your clients, make sure that you solicit their knowledge, become aware of their feelings and attitudes, and take into account their strengths and limitations in caring for themselves. You must use this information in order to tailor your nursing care to suit your clients. In addition, you need to be aware of how your knowledge, attitude, and skills affect your ability to be helpful.

Effective nursing requires being assertive and responsible. Your goal is to help your clients achieve their best possible health status and do so in a way that allows expression of your professional competence. It is expected that you attempt to meet both of these desired outcomes.

Wit and Wisdom

*You may light another's candle
at your own without loss.*

Danish proverb

You must act responsibly to achieve your nursing goals. You need to collect pertinent information from your clients and make an accurate assessment on which you will base your nursing care. The interpersonal communication behaviors in this book will help you develop your skills in these areas. The next chapter will show you how to make problem solving a mutual process between you and your clients. Using this approach, you will be an assertive and responsible nurse-helper.

TRUE PRESENCE

And what of technology? What does it mean to be a competent nurse? Remember that the dazzling technology that seems to create miraculous recovery is a means to an end, not an end in itself. Nursing care is person-focused, not technology-focused (Bernardo, 1998). To be truly present is to bear witness to the client's experience, understand the client's perspective, and respect the client's dignity and rights to self-determination.

In a study of the "technologically induced vulnerability and the inherent uncertainty" of clients undergoing bone marrow transplantation, one participant said, "Care was the nurse just being there" (Cooper and Powell, 1998). When clients did not feel like banter or small talk, they could

Moments of Connection...
Some Illnesses Bring Stigma. Beware of Making Assumptions.

A client was admitted because she was dying of liver failure and cirrhosis. She shared her two concerns: embarrassment about her diagnosis because she was afraid people would assume she was an alcoholic, and her fear about dying. "I don't know how to die. I don't know what to do." The nurse reassured her that staff understood there were other reasons for cirrhosis and that they would be there to help her with the dying process every step of the way. The client calmed, and her face relaxed. She died a week later with a nurse at her side.

be "certain of the presence of the nurse" (Cooper and Powell, 1998). The research "depicts a caring presence that appears to transcend the distractions of technology . . . and acknowledged a kinship with patients that derived from an acknowledgment of their shared human experience" (Younger, 1995, in Cooper and Powell, 1998).

The nurse implements the nursing process based on the client's experience and clarifies the client's and nurse's "responsibilities, expectations, opportunities, and accountabilities . . ." (Bernardo, 1998). "True presence is grounded in nursing science, the essence of nursing as a scholarly discipline" (Lynaugh and Fagin, 1988, in Bernardo, 1998). Competency in the technological advances in critical care nursing, however, has been described as a component of caring and is supported by nurse theorists (Orem, 1985, Rogers, 1985, Newman, 1986, and Parse, 1992, in Locsin, 1998). It is suggested that technological competence is another way of knowing more about the client. The helping relationship uses this information to deliver nursing care that focuses on this person in this moment, a person with a desire to live fully as a human being with his own hopes and dreams and vision of himself. The challenge then is to be competent in many ways—to be able to use technology and follow critical pathways to deliver nursing care to a unique person. Building your skills in communication in the helping relationship helps you and the client find meaning in moments of connection.

Think About It...
What, So What, and Now What?

Consider what you read about client's rights and other issues in the client-nurse relationship to answer these questions

What? . . . Write one thing you learned from this chapter.

So what? . . . How will this impact your nursing practice?

Now what? . . . How will you implement this new knowledge or skill?

THINK ABOUT IT

Practicing Helping

Exercise 1

The following questions have been designed to help you think about yourself as a nurse-helper. They are not easy questions, because they focus on your basic beliefs and values about being a helper. To begin, answer the questions on your own. Later, get together with your classmates and discuss your responses. You will learn a lot from each other.

- What does health mean to you?
- What factors positively influence clients to take care of their health?
- Do you think health is a right or a privilege?
- To what extent do you think clients are responsible for the development of their health problems?
- What can you do, as a nurse, to increase the likelihood that your clients will take better care of themselves?

To be an effective helper it is important that you know how your feelings about this role influence how you relate to your clients.

- To what extent do you think clients are responsible for solving their own health care problems?
- What degree of dependence (independence) are you comfortable with in your clients?
- What is it you like most about helping clients?
- What is it you like least?

Nurses are expected to be proficient in carrying out a range of nursing treatments.

- How competent do you feel implementing the most essential nursing interventions in your clinical area?
- How would you rate your ability to teach clients how to take care of their own health?

Exercise 2

You have relationships with colleagues, friends, family members, and clients. How do your relationships with your clients differ from these? How are they the same? To help you answer this question, observe and make notes about the differences and similarities as you actually engage in these relationships. Once you have formulated your ideas, compare and contrast them with the views of your colleagues.

Exercise 3

What knowledge, attitudes, and skills in the nurse create and foster a therapeutic relationship? Think about your response on your own and then pool your ideas with your classmates. Your responses to this question will help point out where your knowledge, attitudes, and skills are conducive to a helping relationship and help you map out areas that need refinement to make you a better helper.

References

American Nurses' Association: *Standards of clinical nursing practice,* Kansas City, Mo, 1991, The American Nurses Association.

Bernardo A: Technology and true presence in nursing, *Holistic Nurs Pract* 12(4):40, 1998.

Congress for Nursing Practice, American Nurses' Association: *Standards of nursing practice,* Kansas City, Mo, 1973, The American Nurses Association.

Cooper MC, Powell E: Technology and care in a bone marrow transplant unit: creating and assuaging vulnerability, *Holistic Nurs Pract* 12(4):57, 1998.

Lawrence G: *People types and tiger stripes: a practical guide to learning styles,* ed 2, Gainesville, Fla, 1982, Center for Application of Psychological Type.

Locsin RC: Technologic competence as caring in critical care nursing, *Holistic Nurs Pract* 12(4):50, 1998.

Myers IB: *Gifts differing,* Palo Alto, Calif, 1980, Consulting Psychologists Press.

Myers IB, McCaully MH: *A guide to the development and use of the Myers-Briggs type indicator,* Palo Alto, Calif, 1985, Consulting Psychologists Press.

Newman M: *Health as expanding consciousness,* St Louis, 1986, Mosby.

Orem D: *Nursing: concepts of practice,* New York, 1985, McGraw-Hill.

Page EC: *Looking at type: a description of the preferences reported by the Myers-Briggs type indicator,* Gainesville, Fla, 1983, Center for Application of Psychological Type.

Rogers M: Science of unitary human beings: a paradigm for nursing. In Wood R, Kekahbah J, editors: *Examining the cultural implications of Martha Rogers science of unitary human beings,* Lecompton, Kan, 1985, Wood-Kekakbah Associates.

Stuart GW, Laraia M: *Principles and practice of psychiatric nursing,* ed 6, St Louis, 1998, Mosby.

Sundeen SJ et al: *Nurse-client interaction: implementing the nursing process,* St Louis, 1998, Mosby.

Younger JB: The alienation of the sufferer, *Adv Nurs Sci* 17:53, 1995.

Suggestions for Further Reading

Balzer Riley J: *Customer service from A to Z . . . making the connection,* Albuquerque, 1999, Hartman Publishing, Inc.

Offers training modules and exercises to build relationships in health care.

Balzer Riley J: *From the heart to the hands . . . keys to healthcaring connections,* Ellicott, Md, 1998, I.M.P.S. Inc.

Features more than 100 stories and tips on nurse-client relationships; order at 1-800-368-7675.

Davidhizar R, Giger JN: When touch is not the best approach, *J Clin Nurs* 6(3):203, 1997.

Hartrick G: Relational capacity: the foundation for interpersonal nursing practice, *J Adv Nurs* 26(3):523, 1997.

Neil RM, Watts R, editors: *Caring and nursing: Explorations in feminist perspectives,* New York, 1991, National League for Nursing.

Pearson A, Borbasi S, Walsh K: Practicing nursing therapeutically through acting as a skilled companion on the illness journey, *Adv Pract Q* 3(1):46, 1997.

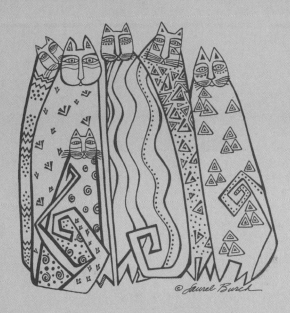

3

Solving Problems Together

Counsel can be given, but not conduct.

Irish proverb

OBJECTIVES

1. Identify the benefits of involving the client in problem solving.
2. Discuss the use of face work and politeness theory in approaching clients.
3. Discuss mutual problem solving to involve the client in the implementation of the nursing process.
4. Complete exercises to practice a mutual problem solving approach to the nursing process.
5. Examine the steps of making contracts with clients.

Moments of Connection...
Setting Goals Together

A nurse was called to a client's room to discuss her therapy options for cancer treatment. As they talked, the client began to clearly understand that this disease was going to be what claimed her life. The client cried the most deep, painful, gut-level crying the nurse had ever experienced with an adult. The nurse held her hand and cried with her. They began to talk when the client relaxed. They set goals of her leaving the hospital and experiencing her next Christmas. The nurse said she felt good that she was able to take the time to let the client cry.

INVOLVING THE CLIENT IN PROBLEM SOLVING

Face Work and Politeness Theory

The outcome of the nurse-client interaction depends on the nurse's ability to engage the client in decision making and share the control and power in the relationship (Roberts et al, 1995, Spiers, 1998). Nurses build their communication skills by studying and practicing techniques, trial-and-error, observing role-models, experience, and gaining comfort with the use of their own intuition. Face work and politeness theory point to the need to consider the client and nurse's "sense of self-esteem, autonomy, and solidarity in conversation" (Spiers, 1998). We speak of "saving face" or helping the other "save face" and mean the preservation of dignity so each party continues to be willing to invest in the interaction without experiencing threat. In the complex nature of problem-solving with the client to promote health, many factors can present barriers, including "perceptions and negotiations about the rules, norms, expectations, and boundaries that can distort both information and interpersonal intent" (Cauce and Srebnik, 1990, and Fox, 1989, in Spiers, 1998). Nurses must "negotiate a mutually acceptable and satisfying level of distance or intimacy, self-disclosure, privacy, and information exchange with a context of power differences, a need for help, and a right to act" (Spiers, 1998). Each party wants to maintain a sense of personal competency and control. An attack on these or on the person's poise or sense of belonging or being liked are called *face threats*.

Consider the actions of the nurse in assessment: questions about the client's behavior, a physical assessment, assessment and intervention in spiritual needs. These are invasive. Polite behavior, more than just our notion of a traditional convention required by mothers, and a part of the consideration of face theory, refers to ways in which nurses ease the interaction to help cover fear, embarrassment, and anger. Polite behaviors lessen the threat of the intimate nature of nursing interventions. Nurses may gently and indirectly encourage the clients' participation in problem solving, whereas a direct order in such a situation would be considered impolite and inappropriate. When discussing a potentially embarrassing situation such as safe sex, the nurse is careful about the language used and asks questions gently to help the client save face. A complicated balance between considerations of face work and politeness and the necessity for client involvement point to the need for further research to supplement successful intuitive strategies that are difficult to teach. Nurses understand the importance of tact in engaging the client's participation. Nursing research validates that treating the client as a unique individual and actively engaging the client in problem solving are associated with increased client satisfaction, an important quality indicator (Roberts et al, 1995).

WHAT IS THE DIFFERENCE BETWEEN PROBLEM SOLVING AND MUTUAL PROBLEM SOLVING IN NURSING?

Problem Solving: The Nursing Process

In Chapter 1 we identified a four-step model of the nursing process, the problem-solving process:

1. Assess
2. Plan
3. Implement
4. Evaluate

We easily remember the steps with a mnemonic, a memory tool, A PIE, a pie.

The Mutual Problem-Solving Process in Nursing

Validation

Validation makes the difference between problem solving *for* clients and mutual problem solving *with* clients. Incorporating validation keeps us focused on the rights and obligations of clients to make their own decisions about their health.

The important activity of validation must be incorporated at each step of the problem-solving process in nursing. Validation means consciously seeking out our clients' opinions and feelings at each phase of the nursing process. Validation means unearthing any questions or concerns our clients have about plans for their health care and securing their understanding and willingness to proceed to the next step. Incorporating validation into our problem solving stops us from forging ahead and doing *to* our clients. It ensures that we obtain complete agreement and commitment from our clients about the nursing care plans being considered for their particular health problems.

A mutual problem-solving process in nursing looks like this:

1. Assess
   A. Collecting data
   B. Analyzing data
   C. Validating interpretation of data with the client
   D. Identifying actual or potential problems with the client
   E. Validating the nursing diagnoses with the client
2. Plan
   A. Setting priorities for resolution of identified problems with the client
   B. Determining expected and desired outcomes of nursing actions in collaboration with the client
   C. Deciding on the nursing strategies to achieve these outcomes in collaboration with the client
3. Implement
   A. Implementing nursing actions with assistance from the client
   B. Encouraging client participation in carrying out nursing actions to meet the outcomes
4. Evaluation
   A. Evaluating the outcomes of nursing care in consultation with the client

Including validation in the nursing process does not necessarily increase the time or energy required to carry out nursing care. Much of the checking can be done quickly and naturally while interacting with clients. Ensuring that clients understand and agree with each step of the nursing process increases the probability that they will do their part to comply with treatment. Clients who have a clear understanding of their health problems, as well as what they and their nurses can do about them, will expend less energy worrying and more energy doing something constructive. Clearly understanding their nursing diagnoses and having a say in how best to handle them gives clients a sense of control.

Validation invites the collaboration that is essential for successful client change. The trust developed from working together is likely to increase the accuracy and validity of the database, enriching the foundation for the rest of the nursing process. The trust growing out of mutuality provides the clients with an "anchor," giving them the support they need to risk changing health behaviors. Collaboration ensures the benefits of two heads working on a health problem; this is essential because nursing cannot exist in a vacuum. We cannot strive for excellence without including the full participation of our clients. Nurse researchers report that "recognition of the client as a unique person and encouragement of active client participation in the nursing encounter are highly associated with client satisfaction, one important indicator of quality care" (Roberts, Krouse, and Michaud, in Spiers, 1998). "Nursing interactions characterized as task oriented and that disregard the client as an equal participant have been related to acts of resistance . . ." by clients (Hallberg et al, in Spiers, 1998).

Many of today's health care customers are speaking up, asking questions, seeking second opinions, demanding alternative health care options, and forming their own self-help groups to take action. Their assertiveness and independence reflect the true meaning of the label "client," designating those who claim the rights and privileges of partnership in health care.

The client contracts for services with a qualified health care provider. This relationship is a negotiated partnership in which the client implicitly agrees to comply with the plan they generate together. The proliferation of Advanced Nurse Practitioners (ANPs) in response to the demands for cost-effective care in a managed care environment demonstrates such a partnership from a holistic perspective. ANPs identify collaboration with clients and other health care professionals as part of their nursing philosophy (Grando, 1998). C. Everett Koop, former U.S. Surgeon General, emphasized that clear communication between clients and physicians could prevent serious medical problems. He reported results from a Louis Harris poll that indicated out of 1000 clients questioned, 25% admitted a hesitancy to talk with their physicians because they seemed rushed or distracted or because the client was embarrassed (Koop, 1998). Nurses can build working relationships between nurses, clients, and physicians by assisting with collaborative communication.

Not all health care customers think of themselves as active, responsible partners in their care. Some do what health care professionals tell them, living out the definition of the label "patient." The passive nature of this role creates an imbalance between the power of the nurse and client. The passivity of this stance creates an inequitable relationship between nurses and others. As nurses, we can help reverse this apathy and listlessness by encouraging our clients to be partners in their own health care (Cooper and Powell, 1998). This means appreciating the worth of our clients and calling on their strengths. We can transform our nursing care into a mutual problem-solving process when we invite, even request, the full participation of our partners, the clients.

Earlier in this century patients were more satisfied with a system of illness care that focused on disease eradication. As the influence of science and technology on health care has increased, discontent has emerged, along with resentment of chauvinistic "all-knowing," health care professionals. Clients began demanding more influence in their health care and requesting more individualized care. Evidence of this movement materialized as early as 1972, with the publication of the Patient's Bill of Rights (presented by the American Hospital Association). This document describes the expectations for respect, knowledge, privacy and confidentiality, and access to any information essential for adequate treatment. Nurses need to focus on the individual's responsibility for health care along with his or her rights. It is important to emphasize what clients can do to take care of themselves, as well as to safeguard their right to quality, informed care. The notion of clients as consumers of health care in the 1970s has moved to the idea of clients and their families as customers. In addition to informed care, nurses must now give attention to customers' expectation of service. Decreased hospital stays, outpatient surgery, and the movement toward home health care make the need for problem solving even more essential, because clients and their families and significant others play a more active role. Since clients are frequently discharged from the hospital before they are able to care for themselves, much client education and care must be done in the home. Clients need to be able to make informed decisions about their choices for insurance. Nurses need to be informed about the differences in choice of providers and services covered by managed care providers to assist clients in selection and in proper procedures for reimbursement.

The following statements from the Standards of Nursing Practice (1991) demonstrate the support of the American Nurses' Association for a mutual problem-solving approach with clients:

Standard IV

The plan is developed with the client, significant others, and health care providers, when appropriate. This standard demands that clients, family, and significant others are kept informed about current health status, changes in health status, total health care plan, nursing care plan, roles of health care personnel, and health care resources. Clients, family, and significant others must be provided with the information needed to make decisions and choices about promoting, maintaining and restoring health; seeking and utilizing appropriate health care personnel; and maintaining and using health care resources.

Standard VI

The client, significant others, and health care providers are involved in the evaluation process, when appropriate. Clients are an essential part of the comprehensive and intelligent determination of nursing's impact upon health status. Clients, family, significant others, and health care providers evaluate nursing actions and goal achievement.

Incorporating Validation Into the Nursing Process

The following example will illustrate suggested methods for ensuring maximal client participation in a mutual problem-solving approach.

Validating Interpretation of Collected Data

From the time clients enter our nursing care, we start asking them questions about their health problems. As we receive information about their situations from the answers they give us, the way they answer our questions, and objective data from laboratory tests and physical assessment, we start to piece together a meaningful picture. That picture is our interpretation of the data; it starts off fuzzy and develops into a clear explanation of our clients' health problem(s).

Nurses are not the only ones who crave a clear picture of what is going on—clients are usually eager to know about their situation as well. Put yourself in the following clinical nursing situation:

Mrs. Cook is 48 years old and has been referred to a home health care agency by her family physician to help establish control of her adult-onset diabetes. She has been on oral hypoglycemic agents for the past 2 years. Her most recent blood sugar was 350 mg/ml.

Mrs. Cook: "Oh, don't worry about me. I'll be fine. You won't need to visit me. I can't be worrying my husband. He wants a healthy wife!"

As you talk, you learn that Mrs. Cook has little knowledge about the special care she must take, how to monitor her nutritional intake, how to pay careful attention to skin care, and how to check her urine daily for sugar. You learn that sickness is "unacceptable" in her family. She has two sisters who are "perfectly healthy" and a husband she calls a "fitness fanatic."

All her life Mrs. Cook has received verbal and nonverbal messages from her parents and husband that she must be a perfect wife and homemaker and that sickness is not tolerated. When the symptoms of hyperglycemia first occurred, Mrs. Cook tried to ignore them and pretend nothing was wrong. Her neighbor insisted that Mrs. Cook see a doctor when her symptoms of increased thirst and appetite were accompanied by diminished strength and weight loss.

You want to share with Mrs. Cook your assessment that she appears to have little knowledge about how to manage her diabetes to prevent complications. You suspect she has never really learned much about diabetes in an attempt to be "healthy" to live up to her parents' and husband's expectations. It was easier to pretend she was healthy than to admit she had a chronic illness. You sense that she may mistakenly assume that she will not be able to live an active and full life as a diabetic. You validate this interpretation of the information with the following statement:

You: "Mrs. Cook, I know you are eager to feel better, and I have some concerns about your ability to continue to feel healthy without learning more about taking care of yourself and managing your diabetes. From what you've told me I know it is important to you and your husband that you are healthy. It is my experience that, with proper self-care, diabetes doesn't have to stop you from doing anything you want, but to accomplish this you must accept the fact that you have diabetes. You can do things to be healthy. Tell me what you think about that."

This validation respectfully lets your client know your assessment of her health situation. Your ending allows Mrs. Cook to argue, disagree, or ask questions about your interpretation of her situation.

Identifying Actual or Potential Problems With the Client

When Mrs. Cook has either agreed with or amended your assessment, you can then formulate and validate the nursing diagnosis.

Mrs. Cook might say: "What else is there to learn? The nurse practitioner in Dr. Wood's office taught me to give myself insulin. I am fine with that."

Her response gives you an opening to teach her about potential problems people with diabetes need to avoid. You could respond:

You: "You have mastered taking your insulin; however, there is more to learn. You need to understand the signs of low blood sugar and have a plan for emergencies. Since diabetes affects the circulation, you would benefit from learning about skin care. Taking care to regulate your calories to adjust to your changing levels of energy is also essential to keep you feeling well. Learning how to manage your daily activities can help you stay healthy and active like your family."

This identification of some of the potential problems of diabetes empowers Mrs. Cook to take charge of her own health. You offer hope that she can live normally.

She might respond: "I thought all I had to do was give myself this insulin every day and I'd be okay. I guess there's more to it. My husband wants me to be healthy, and you have to be to keep up with him. He worries about me but doesn't want me to know. He's due home from work early today. Will you talk with him, too? Will you help him understand that I'm okay?"

Validating the Nursing Diagnoses With the Client

You respond: "I'd be glad to talk with him. You and I have some work to do, too. The three main areas you need to learn about are adjusting your caloric intake to match your activity level, taking special precautions with your skin care—especially your feet—and having a plan to cope with low blood sugar, should that occur. Does that about cover it for you?"

Mrs. Cook: "That sounds like a lot to learn. The thing that surprises me is this talk of skin care. I've always had good skin and I can't imagine having problems with it."

Setting Priorities With the Client for Resolution of Identified Problems

In this case, it is appropriate to start with the problem of interest to the client since there is no current crisis.

You: "OK, let's start with skin care."

This validation gives Mrs. Cook some control of the teaching session.

Determining Expected and Desired Outcomes of Nursing Actions in Collaboration With the Client

You and your client are concerned about outcomes. It is important for each of you to reveal your goals so that you can work together. To begin the negotiation of the plan you can clarify expectations:

You: "We both need to have some idea where we are headed in our work together so we know when we have met our goals. I would expect you to be able to have a plan to prevent skin breakdown and low blood sugar and have a plan if they do occur. As for nutrition, it is my hope you will be able to figure out the number of calories you need to have the energy required for your active lifestyle. This sounds like a lot, but I think it's manageable. I'd like to hear what you think."

These suggestions make it clear what you want to accomplish. Now it is Mrs. Cook's turn to indicate her goals.

Mrs. Cook: It does seem like a lot to learn, but I guess I don't have much choice. I don't want to feel that sick again. I don't think either my husband or I would want to go through that again. What you say makes sense. I'll give it a try."

You: We can start with these goals. I believe you'll feel more in control of your body and that will make it easier for you to accept the differences in your body that diabetes causes. Just knowing there are things you can do can take away much of the fear. It will get easier, and these things will become a part of your routine. If you have questions and can't reach me, there is a 24-hour hotline number for the American Diabetes Association.

With this reply you have given Mrs. Cook another good reason for learning about her condition—to be less fearful.

Deciding on the Nursing Strategies to Achieve These Outcomes in Collaboration With the Client

You and Mrs. Cook agree on your goals, and you have access to the knowledge, people, and material resources to help this client achieve the expected and desired outcomes.

You: "You indicated you would like to start with learning about skin care. I see you have a VCR. We have a video I can bring that has examples of how to ensure that your skin does not break down. We also have booklets on skin care. And I can answer any questions you have. Which would you prefer?"

Mrs. Cook: "Booklets sound too much like school. I'd like to start with the tape and then look at the booklets just to make sure I understand."

You have now made a plan with Mrs. Cook's help to start work on the first goal. When she is ready, you can introduce resources for the other goals and supply her with the 24-hour hotline number for the American Diabetes Association. Later on, you can recommend a support group that might be useful as well.

Implementing Nursing Actions With Assistance From the Client; Encouraging Client Participation in Carrying Out Nursing Actions to Meet the Outcomes

In Mrs. Cook's situation, your main focus is to encourage her participation in the various forms of learning how to manage the diabetes. One way to show your interest and involvement is to ask open-ended questions about her progress. For example:

"What are your thoughts about the tape?"

"What questions do you have about skin care after seeing the tape and reading the booklets?"

The answers reveal areas where additional teaching is needed and offer an opportunity to offer praise and reinforcement.

Evaluating the Outcomes of Nursing Care in Consultation With the Client

After Mrs. Cook uses the resources, you might decide to use a light, humorous approach for evaluation.

You: "Just like being back in school . . . it's time for a quiz! Are you ready to tell me what you have learned and how you are working on meeting our goals?"

Mrs. Cook: "I feel like I've had a home correspondence course like they advertise on television. Ask me anything!"

You: "I know you've been working hard. Tell me what you are doing to prevent skin problems."

Mrs. Cook: "Sure. First, no more tight shoes. They may interfere with the circulation. I threw out my knee-highs. My husband always teases me about those anyway. He says they just aren't sexy. With the rings they leave on my legs, I can see how bad they are for me. The movie showed me how to cut my toenails straight across. I bought toenail clippers. Oh, yes, I remember to pat dry with the towel instead of rubbing hard. Okay, teacher, what grade do I get on skin care 101?"

You: "I'd say an A, and I just happen to be carrying gold stickers. You are a star. You can use them or share them with your children. I want to add that it's important to stay warm enough in this cold weather and to use body lotion to keep your skin from getting dry and irritated. Rubbing the lotion in will improve your circulation."

Mrs. Cook: "I love those stickers and I feel like I've earned an A. My daughter gave me some fancy lotion for my birthday. I'll use that and thank her for making a good choice."

You can continue to review with Mrs. Cook the other expected outcomes you both agreed on and discuss her progress. You can encourage her to share what she has learned with her husband and how good she feels about her ability to manage the diabetes. Mr. Cook may need help adjusting to the idea that his wife has a chronic illness. Think of ways to involve the entire family: perhaps a conference during your next home visit. The family context is where the notion of health and illness is learned and fostered. Any support the family can give will likely enhance Mrs. Cook's health and motivate her to continue with preventive care. Joining a support group might also be useful for Mrs. Cook. Seeing that other people lead productive lives, even if their health is not perfect, may alter the idea that Mrs. Cook's diabetes will set her apart as different and unhealthy.

Benefits of Mutuality That Go Beyond the Client-Nurse Dyad

March (1990) believed that the benefits of the collaborative client-nurse relationship (which she terms *therapeutic reciprocity*) go beyond any isolated meeting and contribute to growth and development for both clients and nurses. The shared meanings about clients' experiences are a natural precursor to the shared control and responsibility for the outcomes of their relationship. Nurses and clients gain trust in each other as human beings, and in their own ability to relate effectively in the helping relationship. This discovery, although of primary value for the health care context, may transfer to other interpersonal relationships as the value of interdependence is demonstrated.

Matheis-Kraft et al (1990) claimed that clients who take more active roles in their treatments recover faster. This benefits hospitals, which are struggling to contain costs of health care. They reported how one American hospital instituted patient-driven health care. The goal of the hospital's patient-centered approach is to create a caring, dignified, and empowering environment in which their clients truly direct the course of their care and call on their inner resources to speed the healing process. The staff encourages client awareness of how their own physical, mental, and spiritual resources can promote healing.

In addition to the endorsement by clients and their families, nurses working in an environment with this philosophy report a number of spin-offs that have boosted their morale:

- Opportunity to bring more nurturing and caring into their profession
- Enjoyment of expanded autonomy and authority, allowing them to make a real difference
- A more equal relationship with physicians, who listen to their recommendations and even seek their counsel
- Satisfaction of being client advocates as they were educated to be (Matheis-Kraft et al, 1990)

Schwertel-Kyle and Pitzer (1990) described their implementation of Orem's self-care model for nursing in a critical nursing care unit as a way of providing optimal care to clients within concise time frames. Originally spurred by the financial restraints of prospective payment systems (decreased length of hospital stay, increased acuity, and decreased care-giving resources resulting from set reimbursement rates), the plan enhanced clients' self-confidence and feelings of accomplishment. The transformation from passive, dependent patient to active partner is one way for America's nursing clients to start taking responsibility for their health care, in addition to securing their health care rights.

Wit and Wisdom

Mutual Problem Solving

I set a goal
You may comply;
You set a goal
At least then, you'll try.

Two heads really are
Thicker than one.
Solve it together
And then it gets done!

Copyright 1995 Julia W. Balzer Riley

How to Make Your Clinical Problem Solving a Mutual Affair

1. Explore what you believe about the issue of clients having an active part in their health care. The extent to which you uphold clients' responsibility for their health will mirror how you involve them in the nursing process.
2. Practice revealing your opinions to clients. Increase your confidence in telling clients about your assessment of their particular situation.
3. Avoid giving nursing care without checking with your clients to see where they would like to start. Do not assume you know best because you are the nurse. Clients usually have personal preferences for where to start working on their health care problems. While you might go from easiest to most difficult, your client may want to work on the most complex problem first.
4. Do not negotiate nursing strategy if there is in fact no choice for your clients. Occasionally the philosophy of the institution in which you work, technical policies, time, and/or staff shortages dictate the prioritization and methodology. Most clients resent being given the false impression that they have some choice.

Moments of Connection...
Partners in Life and Death

A neonatal intensive care unit (NICU) was caring for a premature infant who was near death. The parents were concerned that their baby had never experienced anything but the NICU environment in 7 months of life. The nurse and family decided to take the baby outside to feel the sun on his face, to see the flowers. The nurse bagged the baby while the family introduced him to the family dog. There was a brief rain shower that washed the baby's face. It was a beautiful experience to see their final moments with their baby.

5. Before you do something for your clients, ask yourself: Could my clients be doing this (turning, transferring, making a telephone call, speaking to a relative, making a bed, changing a dressing) for themselves? By doing for our clients we rob them of the opportunity to discover their own power to take care of themselves. Every time we provide clients with the wherewithal (information, equipment, contacts) to do something for themselves, we save ourselves time and energy, two precious commodities in this time of tight restraint on health dollars.

6. Remember to evaluate with your clients. If you have been successful in collaborating through all the steps of the nursing process, then continue your good performance through this last phase. The only way to know if your clients are satisfied with the outcomes of your nursing care is to ask for, and listen to, their opinions.

7. Keep in mind that validating is an assertive act. We are not effective when we hesitate to express our points of view or shy away from seeking those of our clients. Validation does not mean commanding or coercing clients. Mutual problem solving is a two-way street; open communication is exchanged between clients and nurses.

Making a Contract With Your Client

Once you have mastered the skills of validation and mutual problem solving, you will have the basic ingredients for making a contract with your clients. This agreement involves formalizing many of the steps you already carry out in your nursing practice.

A contract is an agreement between you and your client outlining activities and responsibilities for each party (see Box 3-1). The contract is often a motivator for learning for both client and staff (Rankin and Stallings, 1990). Contracts should be realistic, spell out measurable behaviors, have dates of expected completion, be worded positively, and build in rewards for success. In a formal contract both parties would spell out the availability, amount of time, skills, commitment, and area of responsibility they will contribute to the improved health status of the client. This negotiation can usually be covered in a verbal agreement. In some situations you may wish to make a written, signed agreement.

Under the terms of a contract both parties must fulfill their complementary obligations. Nurses have the right to make their clients aware if they have not carried out those tasks to which they

Box 3-1	**Elements of a Client-Nurse Contract**

Here is a list of components of a client-nurse contract for you to adapt to your workplace:

- Names of client and nurse
- Purpose of the client-nurse relationship
- Roles of client and nurse
- Responsibilities of client and nurse
- Expectations of client and nurse
- Specific details such as meeting times and structure for confidentiality
- Conditions for termination

Modified from Stuart GW, Laria M, 1998.

have agreed, and the clients can point out to their nurses if they have reneged on their part of the bargain. Conversely, they are both eligible for praise when they have successfully accomplished their respective tasks.

When nurses and clients have both done their part to fulfill the activities agreed on, they can evaluate the effectiveness of their efforts and determine if their contract is completed. A contract provides standards for evaluation because the expected outcomes are clearly delineated (Rankin and Stallings, 1990). If both parties are satisfied with the results, the contract can be terminated. If clients want more treatment, they must negotiate with their nurses, who may or may not be willing to continue. Conversely, it may be nurses who want their clients to do more for themselves or to reach a higher level of health. If so, they must entice their clients to pursue further treatment and make clear their own part in the extended contract.

Sometimes clients will try to extract a promise from their nurses that certain information is to be held in confidence. This should be a red flag. Nurses can say that they are obligated to share any information that is important to their clients' well-being. Such a request may precede information that clients are planning to harm themselves or others. Such a contract of confidentiality cannot be made before or after such information is disclosed. If you must reveal something your clients have told you in confidence, explain that you cannot withhold potentially harmful information.

Through participation in a contract, clients can take personal control of their health rather than becoming passive recipients of health care directed by the provider. As clients become more assertive about taking an active part in their health care planning, nurses will be forced to respond by renegotiating the terms of their mutual commitment. As nurses become more vocal about our contribution to health care, we become more accountable. Whether for legal, ethical, or philosophical reasons, we are likely to become much more explicit about the terms of contracts with our clients in the years to come.

It is important to remember that life's problems sometimes require the healing power of time for resolution. Nurses, clients, family members, and colleagues all share in common their own humanity . . . this is the beauty and the challenge of the situation!

Think About It...
What, So What, and Now What?

Consider what you read about mutual problem solving in nursing and how you can involve clients in the implementation of the nursing process.

What? . . . Write one thing you learned from this chapter.

So what? . . . How will this impact your nursing practice?

Now what? . . . How will you implement this new knowledge or skill?

— THINK ABOUT IT ———

Wit and Wisdom

If you can't solve the problem, at least have a good laugh together!

Author unknown

Practicing Mutual Problem Solving

Exercise 1

For this exercise, work in threes. One person will play the role of a client, one the nurse, and the third the observer who gives feedback. The purpose of this exercise is to give you an opportunity to practice mutual problem solving and to receive feedback on your performance.

The client will approach the nurse with a specific problem. The nurse will help the client begin solving the problem using the principles of mutuality.

After 10 minutes of discussion, give the nurse feedback on how effective he or she is in making the relationship with the client a mutual problem solving situation. The following questions can be used as guidelines:

As the nurse, did you:

- Allow your client to provide you as much information as possible about his or her health problem(s)?
- Show interest in your client's assessment of the situation?
- Check out your analysis and nursing diagnosis(es) with your client?
- Find out your client's reactions to the health problems?
- Discover what goals your client has for treatment?
- Discuss your hopes and expectations for your client's care?
- Elicit your client's opinions of all possible nursing actions?
- Work out how your client could be more actively involved in implementing treatments?
- Assess together how effective the treatment plans had been?

Review the steps of a mutual problem solving nursing process to see where you were successful and where you could improve. What made it possible for you to validate in some instances but not in others? Compare your experiences with those of your colleagues.

As the client and the observer:

- How well did the nurse follow the steps of mutual problem solving?
- What suggestions would you make for improving the nurse's ability to incorporate validation into the nursing process?

In 10 minutes the nurse and client may not get through all the phases of the nursing process. Review how mutual the problem-solving process was for the stage that was reached.

Switch roles so that you each have a chance to play all the roles.

Exercise 2

For each of the following client situations, describe what you would say to these clients to encourage them to take a more active part in their health care.

1. Mr. Bane is a 33-year-old client newly diagnosed with epilepsy. He has to take medication every 4 hours.

Continued

Practicing Mutual Problem Solving—cont'd

2. Mrs. McNeil is a 63-year-old client with arthritis. She has been urged by her physician to do wrist and finger range-of-motion exercises three times a day.
3. Johnny is a 17-year-old client who has been advised to use specially prepared soap for his facial acne.
4. Beth is a tense young client who has been urged to meditate twice a day to promote relaxation.
5. Mr. Jameson has a high cholesterol level. He has been taught how to reduce the cholesterol in his diet. He selects his own menu daily.

Compare your strategies for approaching each client situation with the suggestions of your colleagues.

Exercise 3

For each of the following case studies write down how you would discuss the fact that your client has broken your mutual agreement about what actions he or she would take to improve his or her health status. Write out specifically what you would say when you approach the topic with your client.

1. Miss Marson is a 19-year-old admitted for investigation of severe, debilitating headaches. She has agreed not to consume any of her own over-the-counter drugs to alleviate her pain while tests are being done to discover the source of her headaches. On your night rounds you find Miss Marson in the washroom swallowing one extra-strength pain reliever tablet and about to take another.
2. Mrs. Dodds is a 22-year-old client admitted for investigation of severe and rapid weight loss. She has agreed to stick to a bland diet while the reasons for her weight loss are being unearthed. On the evening shift you discover her eating spicy chili her visitor brought her from the local deli.
3. Mr. Jones is a 45-year-old who had surgery 5 hours ago. Preoperatively he agreed to do his deep breathing and coughing after surgery, yet now he has been adamant that he has no intention of letting you support his incision so that he can cough. He only wants to sleep peacefully.
4. You are completing a health history on a client who has had chest pain in the past few weeks. She has agreed to bring you the pertinent information about her family's cardiac health history for her appointment today. She comes without the information, telling you that she was too busy with her friends this week to get the information from her aunt.

After you have done this exercise on your own, compare your responses with those of your colleagues in your class. Be aware of the many ways to assertively inform your clients that they are not completing part of the nursing care plan to which they agreed.

Exercise 4

In the following situation you and your client disagree about the priority of the client's health problem. Think about how you would assertively handle such a situation and be prepared to discuss your suggested strategies with your classmates.

Mrs. Boyd is a 30-year-old admitted for a cholecystectomy. She is 2 months postpartum and is eager to continue breast-feeding even though she is about to undergo surgery. You are concerned about her physical health because Mrs. Boyd is lethargic and jaundiced and has dry, itchy skin and severe abdominal pain. She wishes to have her baby brought in to be nursed at his regular feeding periods. You would prefer that she get as much rest as possible and start her baby on formula feedings.

Mrs. Boyd feels strongly that breast-feeding is essential to the health of her baby. She acknowledges that it may be difficult to continue breast-feeding at this time but she fears if she stops she will not be able to restart, and then her baby would suffer. In addition, breast-feeding is a special part of being a nurturing mother for Mrs. Boyd, and she does not want to miss the experience.

Compare your strategy for working out this difference in priorities with Mrs. Boyd to the suggestions of your colleagues.

Exercise 5

The next time you are on the nursing unit where you are doing your clinical course, attempt to practice a mutual problem-solving approach with your assigned clients. Use the following questions to evaluate your ability to validate with your clients:

I. Assess
   A. Assessment
      1. Do you allow clients the opportunity to tell you what they know and believe about their health concerns?
      2. In what ways are your views about health congruent with your clients', and where are they divergent?
      3. What client knowledge gaps surfaced?
      4. What have you learned about your clients' health beliefs, health care habits, and problem-solving abilities?
   B. Validating the Nursing Diagnosis With Your Clients
      1. Do you determine what your clients think their problems are and what they think might be causing them?
      2. Do you inform clients about your assessment of their health problem?
      3. Do you and your clients agree on the assessment?
      4. How do you handle the situation when your views are disparate?
      5. Do you explore how your clients feel about their nursing diagnoses?
      6. How comfortable are you with sharing your views about the nursing diagnoses with your clients?
II. Plan
   A. Determining Desired Outcomes for Your Clients
      1. Are you and your clients in agreement about the desired outcomes?
      2. Are you realistic in your hopes and expectations for your clients' health?
      3. Are you and your clients able to agree on mutually acceptable outcomes?
   B. Choosing Nursing Strategies to Help Your Clients Achieve Their Expected and Desired Outcomes
      1. Do you take into account how your clients feel about the options?
      2. Do you take into account your clients' personal and cultural preferences, schedules, finances, and abilities?

Continued

Practicing Mutual Problem Solving—cont'd

     3. Are you able to inform your clients about the efficacy of the various options?

     4. Are you willing to express your opinions about the various treatment choices?

III. Implement

    A. Implementing a Plan of Action to Help Meet Your Clients' Needs

       1. How much consideration do you give to your clients' ability to carry out the plan themselves?

       2. Do you do for your clients when they could be doing for themselves? Conversely, do you expect too much from your clients without adequately training them?

       3. Do you take the opportunity to find out how your clients feel about carrying out the plan?

       4. Do you make certain your clients are ready and willing to continue with the plan?

       5. Do you make clear what your role, and that of your clients, is?

IV. Evaluation

    A. Evaluating the Outcomes Together

       1. How extensively do you ask your clients their opinions and feelings about the outcomes of treatment to date?

       2. To what extent do you share your views about progress with your clients?

       3. How do you handle situations when you and your clients disagree (they are pleased with the outcomes while you wish to persevere for greater excellence or vice versa)?

       4. How well do you prepare your clients for terminating the client-nurse relationship?

Answering the questions posed previously will crystallize your awareness of how you may already be encouraging mutual problem solving with your clients and can stimulate your anticipation of where you can facilitate even more interchange.

Exercise 6

The next time you are a client (of a lawyer, nurse, pastor, priest, rabbi, physician, or a dentist) make note of how much this professional engages you in mutual problem solving. Notice exactly what the professional does to make you feel included in the planning.

- In what ways does the professional make you feel your opinions are important?
- In what ways could this professional include you more in the problem solving process?
- How do your feelings differ when you are included and when the professional takes over and does not consult you?

Compare your experiences with those of your classmates. What has this exercise taught you about mutual problem solving?

Wit and Wisdom

It is good to be reminded that each of us has a different dream.

Crow Indian proverb

References

American Nurses' Association: *Standards for clinical nursing practice,* Washington, DC, 1991, American Nurses Publishing.

Cauce AM, Srebnik DS: Returning to social support systems: a morphological analysis of social networks, *Am J Commun Psych* 18:609, 1990.

Cooper MC, Powell E: Technology and care in a bone marrow transplant unit: creating and assuaging vulnerability, *Holistic Nurs Pract* 12(4):57, 1998.

Fox RC: *The sociology of medicine: a participant observer's view,* Englewood Cliffs, NJ, 1989, Prentice-Hall.

Grando V: Articulating nursing for advanced nursing practice. In Sullivan T: *Collaboration: a health care imperative,* New York, 1998, McGraw-Hill.

Hallberg IR et al: Cooperation during morning care between nurses and severely demented institutionalized patients, *Clin Nurs Res* 4(1):78, 1995.

Koop CE: Patient-provider communication and managed care, *Med Pract Communicator* 5(4):1, 1998.

March P: Therapeutic reciprocity: a caring phenomenon, *Adv Nurs Sci* 13(1):49, 1990.

Matheis-Kraft C et al: Patient-driven healthcare works! *Nurs Management* 21(9):124, 1990.

Rankin SH, Stallings KD: *Patient education: issues, principles, and practices,* ed 2, Philadelphia, 1990, JB Lippincott.

Roberts SJ, Krouse HJ, Michaud E: Negotiated and nonnegotiated nurse-patient interactions: enhancing perceptions of empowerment, *Clin Nurs Res* 4(1):67, 1995.

Schwertel-Kyle BA, Pitzer SA: A self-care approach to today's challenges, *Nurs Management* 21(3):37, 1990.

Spiers JA: The use of face work and politeness theory, *Qual Health Res* 8(1):25, 1998.

Stuart GW, Laria M: *Principles and practice of psychiatric nursing,* ed 6, St Louis, 1998, Mosby.

 ## Suggestions for Further Reading

Brookfield S: On impostership, cultural suicide, and other dangers: How nurses learn critical thinking, *J Contin Educ Nurs* 24(5):197, 1993.
    The development of critical thinking to assist the problem-solving process.

Christensen PJ, Kenney JW: *Nursing process: application of theories, frameworks, and models,* ed 4, St Louis, 1995, Mosby.

Cookfair JM: *Nursing care in the community,* St Louis, 1996, Mosby.

Edwards BS: When the family can't let go, *Am J Nurs* 1:52, 1994.
    Working with the family of a dying patient.

Henson RH: Analysis of the concept of mutuality, *Image J Nurs Scholar* 29(1):77, 1997.

Knollmueller RN, editor: *Prevention across the lifespan: healthy people for the twenty-first century,* Waldorf, Md, 1994, American Nurses Publishing.

Information for providers of preventive services in partnership with clients. This text is for the student with a knowledge of principles of behavior modification. It is an excellent overview on contracting in general, describing theoretical assumptions, and how to set up a contract.

Kuhar MB: Critical thinking: a framework for problem solving in the occupational setting, *Am Assoc Occup Health Nurs J* 46(2):80, 1998.

Miller MA, Babcock DE: *Critical thinking skills applied to nursing,* St Louis, 1996, Mosby.

Tindall JA: *Peer power workbook: becoming an effective peer helper and conflict mediator,* Muncie, Ind, 1994, Accelerated Development, Inc.

See Module 8 for role-plays and an action plan to build mutual problem-solving skills.

Yura H, Walsh MB: *The nursing process: assessing, planning, implementing, evaluating,* ed 4, Norwalk, Conn, 1983, Appleton-Century-Crofts.

This classic book provides readers with a history of the nursing process. It goes into depth on the components of the nursing process and demonstrates application to individuals, families, and the community.

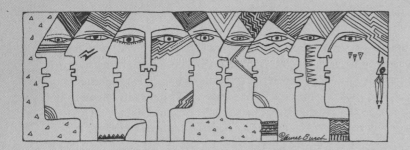

4

Understanding Each Other: Communication and Culture

Joyce Larson Presswalla, RN, PhD

The tongue slow and the eyes quick.

Mexican proverb

OBJECTIVES

1. Define culture, ethnicity, and ethnocentrism.
2. Discuss reasons why nurses need to become informed about the health care beliefs and behaviors of diverse cultures.
3. Discuss two common American values that may interfere with nurses' recognition and appreciation of the health care beliefs and behaviors of diverse cultures.
4. Describe your own cultural background and its influence on your health care beliefs and behaviors.
5. Identify the components of communication suggested for assessment in Purnell's *Model for Cultural Competence.*
6. Discuss techniques that will enhance communicating with clients from diverse cultures.
7. Apply communication techniques to improve the care of clients from diverse cultures.
8. Discuss how the variables of age and gender relate to culture and communication.

Everyone acknowledges the importance of communication because it allows us to interact with our universe. In the American health care setting, nurses understand the importance of communication; however, few recognize the significance of culture. Since nurses spend more time with patients than do other health care professionals, it is particularly important that nurses realize that both communication and culture are inextricably connected to health care. Nurses need to know about culture—their own and their clients'—because it influences both nurses' and clients' health care perceptions and behaviors.

When nursing experts are asked to predict the skills, education, and perspectives that nurses will need to prosper in the coming era, they suggest that nurses will need to demonstrate transcultural competence to employers and consumers (Alexander, Bailey, Curtin, 1998). However, some nurses still ask, "What's culture got to do with it?" After all, according to many Americans, health care is health care; and we've got the best in the world. This ethnocentric attitude interferes with nurses' recognition and appreciation of a broad view of culture and communication. Everyone is familiar with the meaning of communication, but what is culture?

CULTURE, ETHNICITY, AND ETHNOCENTRISM DEFINED

The guru of transcultural nursing, Madeline Leininger, defines culture as the learned and shared beliefs, values, and lifeways of a designated or particular group that are generally transmitted intergenerationally and influence one's thinking and actions. For three decades, Leininger has been an advocate of the need for nurses to become informed about other cultures' health care beliefs and practices.

Ethnicity also needs to be defined because some confuse its meaning with that of culture. According to Leininger (1995), ethnicity refers to the social identity and origins of a social group due largely to language, religion, and national origin; for example, the Amish are an ethnic group. Sociologists and psychologists are more likely to use the term *ethnicity.* The concept of culture is used more by anthropologists and transcultural nurses. Culture is a broader term because it refers to the holistic patterned lifeways of a culture rather than to selected ethnic features or origins (Leininger, 1995).

Ethnocentrism refers to the universal tendency of people to think their ways of thinking, acting, and behaving are the only right and natural ways. Furthermore, ethnocentrism perpetuates an attitude that beliefs that differ greatly from one's own are strange, bizarre, or unenlightened, and therefore wrong (Purnell and Paulanka, 1998).

REASONS WHY NURSES NEED TO BE INFORMED ABOUT CULTURE

There are several compelling reasons why nurses need to be informed about culture (Chrisman, 1993). First of all, care is central to the concept of nursing. If care is to be delivered in a consistent way, it must include assisting the client and family to achieve the goals that they have set up. Goals are strikingly cultural. They vary from culture to culture because of values (for example, maximizing the family versus maximizing the individual). Furthermore, nursing argues that it delivers holistic care. However, all too often, this means using only biophysical and psychosocial data. True holism must include the sociocultural aspect as well. If nurses intend to take care of whole clients, the sociocultural domain is essential. This is particularly true of contemporary nursing in which nurses are on the person's turf—in the household and community. Under these circumstances, to avoid the sociocultural is to truly miss the point of holistic care.

Second, even though the United States has always been a diverse society, this has not always been recognized by health care providers because they have long had the attitude that newcomers should adapt to "us." We as a society are beginning to recognize that this is not desirable; and it will not work. Since our society—and therefore, our client population—is increasingly heterogeneous, it is imperative that nurses be capable of not only understanding, but also of working with that diversity in a productive (health producing) way (Chrisman, 1993). Furthermore, there is serious concern that overall, nursing education does not adequately prepare nurses to work with clients who possess diverse health care beliefs and practices (Lester, 1998b).

Third, health care reform is upon us. Regardless of the final outcome of this process, there are common features. For example, there are managed care conglomerates that compete for patients. Most health care providers believe that the conglomerates that are able to meet people's cultural needs will have a competitive edge. Another aspect of managed care refers to the public health prevention and promotion components of health care. Here again, promoting these parts of nursing requires working in the community and with families. We as nurses are on their turf—at their mercy (Chrisman, 1993).

Finally, the issues of working with elders and with the chronically ill are of immense importance. Chrisman (1993) suggests that there is an increasing number of cases in which health care workers need to work in community settings and with whole families in which the outcomes will not (cannot) be the standard medical outcome of cure. It is clear that nursing outcomes will require working with (versus working *on*) human beings in settings in which the nurse has less control. Consequently, the client and family have more control than does the nurse; and culture has a strong effect on how people act.

In summary, nurses need to know about culture because it influences both nurses' and clients' health care perceptions and behaviors. Also, with health care moving to the community, if nurses expect to be part of this movement, they must know about the culture of diverse clients and communities. To achieve this outcome, nurses must first recognize, and then overcome certain values basic to the American culture.

BARRIERS THAT INTERFERE WITH NURSES' RECOGNITION AND APPRECIATION OF DIVERSE CULTURES

Ethnocentrism interferes with appreciating diverse cultures and their accompanying beliefs and behaviors. Since ethnocentrism is a universal tendency, it is not surprising that it was exhibited at the First International Conference on Holistic Health in Bangalore, India, which I, along with the author of this book, attended in 1989. Many Americans arrived with the perception that the United States had the best health care system in the world. The conference introduced excellent international research that validated many forms of what Americans call "alternative" medicine. The international presenters generally viewed Western health care as delivering topnotch high-tech care; yet lacking because the care was reductionistic rather than holistic. Furthermore, the cost of the care was seen as being exorbitant relative to the outcome. We came home looking forward to investigating the many things we had yet to learn about how culture influences health care practices

Box 4-1	**Identification of Own Health Care Beliefs and Behaviors**

- When you were a child, what were the health care beliefs and behaviors of your family?
- What did your family do to stay healthy?
- What did your family believe caused illness?
- How were specific illnesses treated?
- Who was responsible for deciding the appropriate treatment?
- What health care practitioners outside of the family were used to treat illness?

and perceptions. Recognition of ethnocentrism is necessary to develop an appreciation of diverse cultures. One nurse put it this way: "I always thought of myself as open, flexible, and reasonably unprejudiced; but I am not always! When caring for my friend from Saudi Arabia, I realized that, without knowing, I made value judgments. These judgments reflected in my inability to accept that others handle the same data differently; and their perspectives are equally important as mine."

We recognize that nurses need to know about delivering care to diverse clients, but how do we go about it? First of all, nurses need to become familiar with their own health care beliefs and behaviors because without self-awareness, how can nurses recognize that their beliefs and behaviors are not necessarily common to all? Nurses' lack of knowledge about their own culture can distort their perceptions of the beliefs and behaviors of clients from diverse cultures. It is logical that if a nurse does not understand the reasons for a client's behavior, it is then impossible for the nurse to implement appropriate interventions. Box 4-1 provides guidelines that nurses can use to familiarize themselves with their own cultural health care beliefs and behaviors.

The answers to the questions in Box 4-1 are both interesting and important. For example, consider your answer to the question "What did your family do to stay healthy?" If your family advocated a daily vitamin to stay healthy, how do you view a client who daily drinks a small amount of his own urine to promote health? How do you perceive the Cuban mother who tells you her child is very beautiful and healthy because he is fat?

"What did your family believe caused illness?" If you grew up in the United States, your family probably thought that illness was caused by germs and bacteria. This way of thinking contrasts greatly to that of a client from Thailand who believes her liver cancer is a punishment for a wrongdoing, or a Mexican-American client who believes his illness is a result of witchcraft.

"How were specific illnesses treated?" Americans use medication—over-the-counter or physician prescribed—to treat illnesses. Asian clients often prefer meditation rather than medication to treat illness. They believe that illness is a sign that the body is out of balance, and meditation helps restore the body balance. How do you react when a client refuses morning care or breakfast because it is time to meditate?

"Who was responsible for deciding the appropriate treatment?" Since most Americans place a high value on individualism, the individual adult client usually decides what treatment he or she deems to be most appropriate. How do you perceive a female Hispanic client whose husband decides the preferred treatment for his wife? A nurse notes, "I had always thought the patient was the one making his decision but now I realize that many families, particularly Hispanic and Asian ones, think these are family affairs and not individual choices."

"What health care practitioners outside of the family were used to treat illness?" Most American families eventually consult a medical doctor if illness persists and home remedies do not work. How do you perceive a Mexican-American client who prefers that a *curandero* (folk practitioner), not a physician, treat his liver disease?

It is interesting to compare the health care beliefs and behaviors of your family of origin with those of friends or other health care professionals. It often becomes apparent that your family's ideas and behaviors are not necessarily common to all. This recognition is an important step in not only recognizing, but also in appreciating the health care beliefs and behaviors of diverse cultures.

Because cultures are so diverse, no one can possibly know all the unique aspects of each client's cultural health care beliefs and behaviors. To address this need, nurses and other health care professionals began to develop conceptual and theoretical frameworks for assessing, planning, and implementing culturally appropriate interventions. One of the most popular transcultural theoretical and conceptual frameworks is Leininger's Sunrise Model, which was designed for nursing (Leininger, 1988). Tripp-Reimer and Afifi (1989) suggest two processes that nurses may use to communicate with clients from diverse cultures: cultural assessment and cultural negotiation. *Cultural assessment* refers to the appraisal of a client's health beliefs and behaviors. The information is then used to determine appropriate nursing interventions. *Cultural negotiation* refers to the process of negotiating with the client regarding differences in the lay and professional belief system concerning appropriate care.

On a positive note, there's evidence that culture is "catching on" in nursing. With increasing frequency, a cultural assessment is included as part of the initial client assessment. Consider reviewing the assessment tool that you use when you admit a client. How is the client's culture addressed in the tool? Purnell and Paulanka's (1998) Model for Cultural Competence will give you ideas about other cultural components that may need to be addressed. The twelve domains of culture according to Purnell are communication, family roles and organization, workforce issues, biocultural ecology, high-risk health behaviors, nutrition, pregnancy and childbearing practices, death rituals, spirituality, health-care practices, and health-care practitioners. The domains are interconnected and have implications for health. Box 4-2 details the communication component of the Model for Cultural Competence.

The components of communication listed in Box 4-2 provide the structure for discussion of how culture affects communication in the context of providing health care to diverse clients. When identifying cultural communication similarities and differences, it is important to be cognizant of stereotyping. All cultural groups share some communication practices, but there may well also be broad cultural communication differences. It is dangerous to assume that all members of the same cultural group share the same communication characteristics.

Dominant Language and Dialects

Wouldn't it be great if all of our clients spoke fluent English? It is important to realize that such thinking is grandiose and ethnocentric. Cultural diversity is the current reality. We have an emerging population comprising people from all over the world, whether they be native born or immigrants. As we approach the twenty-first century, nurses are confronted with the challenge of providing health care to these clients. How do you care for clients when communication is significantly impaired because you do not speak the same language? One nurse describes such a situation:

Box 4-2 **Assessment of Parameters of Clients' Communication**

Dominant Language and Dialects

1. Identify the dominant language of this group.
2. Identify dialects that may interfere with communications.
3. Explore contextual speech patterns of this group. What is the usual volume and tone of speech?

Cultural Communication Patterns

4. Explore the willingness of individuals to share thoughts, feelings, and ideas.
5. Explore the practice and meaning of touch in their society; within the family, among friends, with strangers, with members of the same sex, with members of the opposite sex, and with health care providers.
6. Identify personal spatial and distancing characteristics when communicating on a one-to-one basis. Explore how distancing changes with friends versus strangers.
7. Explore the use of eye contact within this group. Does avoidance of eye contact have special meanings? How does eye contact vary among family, friends, and strangers? Does eye contact change among socioeconomic groups?
8. Explore the meaning of various facial expressions. Do specific facial expressions have special meanings? Do people tend to smile a lot? How are emotions displayed or not displayed in facial expressions?
9. Are there acceptable ways of standing and greeting outsiders?

Temporal Relationships

10. Explore temporal relationships in this group. Are individuals primarily oriented to the past, present, or future? How do individuals see the context of past, present, and future?
11. Identify how differences in the interpretation of social time versus clock time are perceived.
12. Explore how time factors are interpreted by this group. Are individuals expected to be punctual in terms of jobs, appointments, and social engagements?

Format for Names

13. Explore the format for a person's names.
14. How does one expect to be greeted by strangers and health care practitioners?

I had a Vietnamese gentleman in for hernia surgery. He had been in this country for two weeks, and his hernia needed to be repaired before he could start work. He spoke no English, nor did his family, and an interpreter was not available. It was with body language and inflection of tone, and hard as that was, we were able to communicate to a small degree. It was very difficult to explain anesthesia. He look scared; he kept his eyes closed most of the time in pre-op. It was like he was pretending he wasn't there. Surgery moves relatively fast, so there wasn't a lot of time prior to induction. I'm sure the recovery process was equally as difficult and frightening for this man.

The nurse in the preceding scenario poignantly identifies the difficulties and anxieties inherent in working with hospitalized clients who are not fluent in English. The clients' anxiety is much greater than the staffs'. Hospitalization is always a crisis. Add to this crisis the anxiety in not being able to communicate your symptoms, perceptions, needs, and questions. The solution is medical interpreters; they are essential to the delivery of culturally competent care. Certification of medical interpreters would help ensure a high quality of care to clients who are not fluent in

---

Box 4-3   Guidelines for Communicating With Non–English-Speaking Clients

1. If there IS an interpreter available
   - Use dialect-specific interpreters, not translators.
   - Give the client and interpreter time alone together.
   - Build in time for translation and interpretation.
   - Avoid using children and relatives as interpreters.
   - Select same-age and same-gender interpreters.
   - Address your questions to the client, not the interpreter.
2. If there IS NOT an interpreter available
   - Use a translator.
   - Determine if there is a third language that is common to you and the client. It is common for clients from diverse cultures to know several languages.
   - Remember that nonverbal communication is more important than verbal.
   - Be attentive to both your own and the client's nonverbal messages.
   - Pantomime simple words and actions.
   - Remember: "a picture is worth a thousand words." Use, and also give to the client, paper and pencil.
   - Talk with administration about the importance of using trained medical interpreters when caring for the non–English-speaking patient.
   - Until medical interpreters are available, use both formal and informal networking to locate a suitable interpreter. If all else fails, owners of ethnic restaurants and grocery stores may be sources for locating interpreters or translators.

English (Lester, 1998a). Until medical interpreters are consistently available, Box 4-3 gives guidelines for communicating with non–English-speaking clients.

Since nurses can expect to care for clients from diverse cultures, it can be expected that the clients' first language will often be something other than English. Professionally trained interpreters are ideal but rare. Clients frequently know at least a little English. Nurses often find themselves in a position to just "go for it" when communicating with a client who knows little English: "I hope I get over it, but I always feel silly when I try to communicate with someone who speaks only a little English. I feel like a little kid—I try to use a lot of gestures. It is really awkward for me; I get so embarrassed. But then I realize how awkward it is for the client to try to speak English. He's got to feel that he's in a place with a lot of foreigners who are responsible for treating him. That's got to be really scary!" Box 4-4 provides guidelines for communicating with patients who speak some English.

There is more to language than understanding the meaning of words. Tone and volume of voice are also important aspects of communication. For example, European-Americans generally talk loudly in relation to people from Thailand. A nurse from Thailand says, "Thai people are very quiet because they believe that talking too much is a sign of stupidity and ignorance. If you talk a lot, you probably don't think a lot." Cuban-Americans are frequently viewed as loud and boisterous because they speak loudly and quickly. A Cuban nurse relates: "Our language (Spanish) is everything to us. We're proud to speak it loudly—we love to socialize anywhere with family and friends." It is important that nurses not misinterpret differences in voice tone and volume; they may be cultural.

Box 4-4	**Guidelines for Communicating With Clients Who Are Partially Fluent in English**

1. Assess the client's nonverbal as well as verbal communication.
2. Keep your eyes at approximately the same level as the client's. This probably means you will sit. Assess if the client is comfortable with eye contact.
3. Speak slowly, and never loudly (unless the client has a hearing impairment).
4. Use pictures when possible (remember: a picture is worth a thousand words).
5. Avoid using technical terms.
6. Ask for feedback. Provide the client with paper and pencil.
7. Remember that clients understand more than they can express—they need time to think in their own language.
8. Remember that stress interferes with the client's ability to think and speak in English.

Cultural Communication Patterns

Communication patterns are an important part of every culture. Box 4-5 offers general guidelines for improving cross-cultural communications.

It is apparent that the nurse must interact with the client to put into practice the guidelines in Box 4-4. This is very important! This is not the time to use the old adage "Don't talk to strangers." All too often, nurses seem to apply this saying to clients from diverse cultures. It is easy to avoid clients whose health care beliefs and behaviors are "different" (Box 4-6).

There are cultural differences in the willingness of individuals to share thoughts and feelings. European-Americans are quite open to discussing feelings on almost any topic. This contrasts with Asian-Americans, who do not value the display of strong feelings and believe that personal thoughts are to be shared only with close friends and family. This fact is respected by the faculty of a college of nursing in California. They no longer require students to keep journals as part of course requirements because it was not a culturally appropriate assignment for their many Asian students.

The acceptability of touch varies considerably among cultures. In Arab and Hispanic cultures, male health care professionals may not touch or examine certain parts of the female body (Andrews and Boyle, 1995). Visitors to France note that both French men and women greet each other with a kiss or kisses on the cheek. Young men in India walk down the street with their arms on each others' shoulders.

Different cultures prefer different degrees of closeness in personal space. People from South America, Africans, Black Americans, Indonesians, and the French prefer a much closer stance than is comfortable for most European-Americans (Sue and Sue, 1990). Americans become uncomfortable when others stand too close. These feelings are associated with a violation of personal space. The United States is a vast country, and historically, Americans are used to a lot of space. In addition, maintaining direct eye contact is an important expectation in American culture. However, this is not a universal standard, as one nurse learned: "Since I am a person who values eye contact, it was interesting to me to find out that this can be cultural. Previously, I assumed a lack of eye contact correlated with a lack of self-esteem."

It is important for nurses to recognize that eye contact is often cultural. For example, the Navajo view direct eye contact as rude and intrusive (Bell, 1994). Muslim-Arab women may not

Box 4-5	Guidelines for Improving Cross-Cultural Communications (L.E.A.R.N.)

Listen with sympathy and understanding to the patient's perception of the problem.
Explain your perceptions of the problem.
Acknowledge and discuss the differences and similarities.
Recommend treatment.
Negotiate agreement.

From Buckwald D, Caralis P, Gany F et al, 1994.

Box 4-6	Avoiding Clients Who Are "Different"

"I've noticed nurses ignore people who are different. I don't think they intentionally do it, but out of frustration over not being able to communicate, they stay out of the room. Recently we treated an older Cuban woman who only spoke Spanish. She wouldn't eat the hospital food and took some strange herbs. Her daughter was the only family member who spoke English. When her daughter was at her side, the interaction was easy—when her daughter wasn't, there was no interaction. She would look at us with big, wide-open, eyes. It was easier to stay out of there than to go in and feel helpless."

have eye contact with males, with the exception of their husband. Hasidic Jewish men have culturally based norms concerning eye contract with women (Andrews and Boyle, 1995).

Facial expressions also vary among cultures. American women smile more often than do American men. However, when the Japanese laugh and smile, it does not necessarily convey happiness; it may mean embarrassment or discomfort. Some Asians believe that smiling suggests weakness (Sue and Sue, 1990).

Variation in greetings is found from one culture to another. Latin Americans shake hands longer, more vigorously, and more frequently (Sue and Sue, 1990). The handshake of an East Indian woman consists of a quick touch of the palms. Most East Indians bow their head, put their palms together and say "namaste" which means "I bow to you—I respect the God in you, I join my hands in prayer for you because I respect you." In American culture, a firm handshake is expected.

Cultural communication patterns take on particular significance for the nurse making home visits (Narayan, 1997). A home visit may be refused if the nurses' communication is viewed as rude or inappropriate. For example, the nurse must keep in mind what social customs are practiced when visiting a person of this culture. It is of the utmost importance that the nurse demonstrate respect for the client. The home is the client's turf—the client has complete control. The following points must be kept in mind: How is respect conveyed in the client's culture? Are shoes removed before entering the home? Do you bow or shake the client's hand? Is a "proper" handshake firm, or just a brief, light touch of the palms? The nurse knows the name of the person he or she is visiting, but how does the client prefer to be addressed?

Temporal Relationships

Americans expect punctuality and generally attach a negative connotation to what is viewed as "lateness." We have an expression "Time is money." The value of punctuality plays out in a strange way with appointments in the health care system. Clients are expected to be on time—often to find that they must wait at least an hour to be seen by the health care professional. Timeliness seems to refer to clients, but not health care providers. This double standard of punctuality needs to change.

The Navajo have a present time orientation. Consequently, they often fail to understand the relationship between one's past activities and present illness (Plawecki, Sanchez, and Plawecki, 1994).

Numerous other cultures are much more flexible regarding time than are Americans: "I've learned from my Filipino friend that I don't have to set a specific time when I need to talk to her. I don't have to announce myself before making a visit. I can drop by her house at any time and it will be accepted in her culture—it's not in mine."

Format for Names

It is important to call a client by the name he or she prefers. Americans are comfortable with calling people by their first name. This is sometimes perceived as not showing respect. It is important to ask a person how they prefer to be addressed because there is considerable cultural variation.

Influence of Age on Communication

The United States is known for valuing youth and beauty; and they are interconnected. Ageism refers to the devaluing of older individuals—and it exists in the American culture.

Aging is generally valued differently in Asian cultures. Increasing age is valued and respected because it brings with it knowledge and experience; the opinions of elders are held in high regard. Evidence of this is seen in India and Thailand, where there are few nursing homes. Elders live with their family and are cared for by them.

Ageism is particularly problematic in American culture because our society is aging. Older adults are avid consumers of health care and average nearly twice as many visits to their physicians as does the general population. Older adults and health care professionals may experience communication problems because of ageism. Examples of ageism include the health care professional using patronizing speech or assuming the older person does not understand. The key to providing effective delivery of health care to the elderly rests on health care professionals' recognition and respect of intergenerational differences (Bethea and Balazs, 1997). Since nurses spend more time with clients than does any other category of health care professional, nurses have the perfect opportunity to practice and then role model care that facilitates communication across generations. Box 4-7 suggests communication strategies that health care professionals can use to improve health care delivery to older adults.

It is commonly accepted that the young do patronize the old in American society. Many nurses have witnessed older clients being addressed in disrespectful terms such as "honey," "sweetheart," "gramps," "granny," and other patronizing forms of speech. The research conducted by Giles and Williams (1994) suggests that patronization is not a one-way street. Older adults also patronize young adults in three distinct speech patterns—nonlistening, disapproving, and parental. This finding suggests the possibility of complex communication problems between health care professionals and clients because of the aging of our society. Not only are clients increasingly older, but health care professionals are also older and are taking care of young adult clients. It becomes clear that it is important for nurses to be aware of the fact that in the American culture, age is often a factor that influences verbal and nonverbal communication patterns with clients. If this is true for you, consider how it influences your delivery of health care.

Box 4-7	**Communication Strategies to Improve Health Care Delivery to Older Adults**

- Develop an increased awareness of ageist stereotyping in the health care professional–older patient interaction.
- View each interaction as a negotiation to reduce miscommunication.
- Develop a unique relationship with each patient (a relational culture unique to each relationship).
- Promote the use of repetition and sensitive interrogation to help older adult patients understand technical jargon, diagnoses, and treatment options.
- Utilize metaphors and examples salient to individual patients' interests to explain medical terms and procedures.
- Enhance the relational interaction on an affective level so patients will be satisfied and remain loyal.
- Develop a holistic understanding of each patient by listening to patient narratives and historical life reviews. Consider the use of a tape recorder to collect patient information and a database management system to refer to patient history before patient visits.
- Understand patients in relation to their cohort membership and its effects on their expectations of the health care professional–patient interaction.

From Bethea L, Balazs A, 1997.

Influence of Gender on Communication

Perhaps the most significant of cultural communication problems are those that exist between men and women because they transcend all cultures. Males and females are socialized differently worldwide, and this is thought to account for differences in behavior.

In the United States the differences in socialization are thought to account for the fact that American women are typically credited with being more expressive and relationship oriented. Women are thought to value intimacy more than do men. Men, on the other hand, are thought to value power and social status, and are more concerned with gathering and processing information. American society provides us with many examples of the frustrations experienced due to the differences in male-female communication values and styles: country western music woefully describes many scenarios where men and women cause each other great grief, television "soap operas" give day-to-day accounts of the triumphs and tragedies (mostly tragedies) that envelop male-female relationships, and a favorite topic of Broadway plays centers around the struggles between men and women. *Defending the Caveman* comically seeks to explain the differences in actions and interactions between the sexes. In the ever-popular *My Fair Lady,* Professor Henry Higgins asks, "Why can't a woman be more like a man?"

Current interest in improving male/female communication is evidenced by the popularity of books that focus on improving male-female relationships. John Gray, in his bestseller *Men Are From Mars, Women Are From Venus: A Practical Guide for Improving Communication and Getting What You Want in a Relationship* (1992), focuses on differences between men and women. He explores how gender differences can create conflicts that prohibit mutually fulfilling loving relationships. This book serves as an excellent guide for developing deeper and more satisfying male-female relationships. The fact that Gray has published a bestseller every year since he wrote *Men are from Mars, Women are from Venus* speaks to the immense interest in the topic of male-female communication.

Another popular author who deals with inter-gender communication is Deborah Tannen. In *You Just Don't Understand: Women and Men in Conversation* (1990), she focuses on patterns of

---

| **Box 4-8** | **Strategies to Improve Nurse-Physician Communication** |

- Level the playing field
- Get to the point
- Use powerful prose
- Exude expertise
- Expect respect

From Woodard E, House B, 1997.

one-to-one conversational style between intimates and friends that are influenced by gender. Her book is based on the assumption that as children growing up we learn styles of communication and that children tend to play in sex-separate groups. The gender differing styles of communication are practiced and reinforced. She focuses on male-female communication as cross-cultural communication. Her later book, *Talking From 9 To 5: How Women's and Men's Conversational Styles Affect Who Gets Heard, Who Gets Credit, and What Gets Done at Work* (1994), focuses on private speaking in a public context—the talk that goes on at work. This book is particularly useful to nurses because it can be used to explore gender differences in communication within the health care environment. Work is a unique place because as we talk to get our job done, we are evaluated in various categories, and the evaluation is often based on how we talk. This presents a special challenge to women because the ways that women are expected to talk at work frequently differs from what is expected in personal relationships. Tannen suggests that no one style of speaking is best and that we need to become aware of and learn from other communication styles and develop flexibility.

Research (Michaud and Warner, 1997) validates Tannen's suggestion that there are consistent gender differences in communication styles used at work—particularly in response to "troubles talk." Men are more likely to tell a joke or change the subject—to be avoidant. Women are more likely to offer sympathy—to be supportive.

Given that the majority of physicians are men and the majority of nurses are women, it is important to be informed about the influence that gender may have on communication. Gender issues may interfere with nurse-physician communication. Learning how to deal with gender issues in the current health care work environment may be one way of improving the delivery of comprehensive nursing care. Box 4-8 provides five strategies to improve communication between nurses and physicians:

Level the playing field: Nurses, who are generally women, need to understand and play by the male rules, rather than spending time complaining about them. *The rules are:*

Get to the point: Simplicity of speech is recommended. "Just the facts" is a valuable communication strategy. Men prefer direct communication with few words. Focus on the goal, not the process. The nurse executive will find that the process skills that are helpful when working with women may be detrimental when working with men.

Use powerful prose: Fear of being viewed as aggressive has stifled many nurses from stating the obvious in client care situations. The use of such phrases as "I'm not sure" and "maybe" are not nearly as interactionally powerful as statements such as "I think so" and "I know." The female nursing executive must behave in competitive, aggressive ways to acquire the resources and influence that the profession of nursing needs. Men expect competition. Women are expected to be "nice." Nurses frequently equate polite behavior with professional respect, an expectation not necessarily shared by males.

Exude expertise: Nurses have information about clients that other members of the health care team need. How this information is imparted is important. A nurse who ends sentences with qualifiers and questions may come across as being unsure of what she is communicating. It is important to speak confidently and present yourself in a manner that makes it clear you do not expect to be refuted.

Women nursing executives may be faced with work environment problems that are part of a male-dominated administration. They can experience short-term success by playing by male rules—be organized, get to the point, seek coaching from the boss, and maintain friendliness. Long-term success requires educating staff about gender differences (Helm, 1995).

Expect Respect: Men interrupt more often than do women. A typical female response to being interrupted is to stop speaking. If nurses believe what they have to say is important, the thing to do is change tactics and keep talking. Nurses must begin all interactions as though they expect respect.

Race may influence respect in the workplace. Prejudicial attitudes about cultural background and or skin color can contribute to a negative workplace atmosphere.

A final way that men and women differ in communication strategies is in that they often bring different rules of behavior to meetings. Men resist being influenced, particularly in public. Men are more likely to have a meeting before the meeting to "get their ducks in a row." Women often prefer to bring their ideas to the meeting for discussion with the group (Helm, 1995).

Given that men and women have been socialized differently, how do we best make use of our gender socialization and differences as we begin the next century in nursing? Nurses' future success will be determined by how we select behaviors, either male or female, that best fit the situation. Male and female health care workers can learn from each other (Cummings, 1995).

Finally, a few words need to be said about how Americans may view the lack of verbal communication, or silence. The meaning of silence in our culture is problematic because we tend to be verbal people. The meaning may be ambiguous; does silence mean client satisfaction or suppressed dissatisfaction? There is also the possibility that silence is cultural. For example, silence is highly valued in the Navajo culture. One who hurries a conversation is thought to be rude. Lengthy periods of silence are used to think so that the spoken word will have significance (Bell, 1994).

A CLOSING THOUGHT

Cultural diversity is the buzzword of the day. This chapter has focused on the importance of nurses recognizing and appreciating health care beliefs and behaviors of diverse cultures. Dealing with differences is important, but there is also something to be said for identifying the commonalties we share as members of the human race. Recognition of commonalties builds bonds (Fogel, 1998). For example, we all value our health and our families, and we all want a better world for our children. Consideration of commonalties emphasizes the sameness of the human species. Recognizing and appreciating commonalties as well as differences offers a holistic or transpersonal way of viewing people. Transpersonal human caring may well be what Florence Nightingale had in mind as reflected in her life's work and writings regarding holistic nursing (Watson, 1998).

Moments of Connection...
Empathy, Respect, and Genuineness

A nurse was assigned to care for an 83-year-old woman from a coastal-mountain fishing village in Thailand. She was diagnosed with liver cancer. Her two daughters served as interpreters. The client's deep religious beliefs in Buddhism were central to her life. Medications and tests were administered at times that were congruent with her schedule for religious practices (e.g., morning prayer, afternoon meditation, and evening devotion). Religious icons were allowed to be placed in close proximity to the patient. It was observed that the patient was drinking only the tea and juice sent on her dietary tray. Negotiations were made, with the advisement of the attending physician, to have the daughters bring traditional foods cooked at home. The nurse was made to feel welcomed when the dietary changes were made. The daughters brought in a huge basket of fruit for the unit staff. While interacting with the family, the nurse mentioned his interest in Oriental cooking and in Buddhism. Soon after, the daughters brought the nurse dumplings and fragrant rice "especially for him." Within a short period of time, the unit was blessed with another huge basket of fruits and what the nurse called, "the most fragrant flowers I have ever beheld." He was called into the room and was given special rare fruits that came from the Far East. The nurse describes his final interaction with the client and her family: "This would be the woman's last night at the unit, and the elderly lady reached out and touched my hand (she had never displayed something like this before). I turned to her family and noticed they were weeping. My throat thickened, and tears filled my own eyes. I bowed to my patient and walked out, knowing what it is like being in the presence of someone so much more aware of life than I will ever be."

Think About It...
What, So What, and Now What?

Consider what you have read about culture and what was new to you.

What . . .   Write one thing you learned from this chapter.

So what . . .   How will this impact your nursing practice?

Now what . . .   How will you implement this new knowledge or skill?

THINK ABOUT IT

Practicing Effective Cross-Cultural Communication

Exercise 1

A. Write what you can remember about at least one client from another culture that you have cared for or observed being cared for where there was a communication problem.

B. Describe the application of a few of the communication techniques suggested in this chapter that may have improved the outcome.

Exercise 2

Write the first words that come to mind when you are assigned to care for an "old" client. Reflect on how your expectations may influence the interaction.

Exercise 3

Identify a workplace interaction problem that may have been caused by gender differences in communication. Review Box 4-8 to identify possible approaches to the workplace problem you identified.

Wit and Wisdom

Differing Gifts

There once was a class, "diversity,"
Taught just to prevent adversity,
But we found there no rifts,
Only differing gifts,
Life being one grand university.

Ask me your questions.
Do not be shy.
I know we're different,
But I know you try.
Ask me your questions,
I don't mind much.
In some ways we're different,
But our lives, they touch.

Copyright 1995 Julia Balzer Riley.

References

Alexander N, Bailey M, Curtin L, et al: What you'll need to succeed, *Nursing 98* 28(5):57, 1998.

Andrews M, Boyle J: *Transcultural concepts in nursing care,* Philadelphia, 1995, Lippincott.

Bell R: Prominence of women in Navajo healing beliefs and values, *Nurs Health Care* 15(5):232, 1994.

Bethea L, Balazs A: Improving intergenerational health care communications, *J Health Commun* 2(2):129, 1997.

Buckwald D, Caralis P, Gany F, et al: Caring for patients in a multicultural society, *Patient Care* p. 105, June 15, 1994.

Chrisman N: Personal communication, December 21, 1993.

Cummings S: Attila the Hun versus Attila the hen: gender socialization of the American nurse, *Nurs Admin Q* 19(2):19, 1995.

Fogel J: Letters, *Am Nurse* May/June 4, 1998.

Giles H, Williams A: Patronizing the young: forms and evaluations, *Int J Aging Hum* Dev 39(1):33, 1994.

Gray J: *Men are from Mars, women are from Venus: a practical guide for improving communication and getting what you want in your relationships,* New York, 1992, Harper Collins.

Helm P: Getting beyond "she said, he said," *Nurs Admin Q* 19(2):6, 1995.

Leininger M: *Transcultural nursing: concepts, theories, research and practices,* Philadelphia, 1995, McGraw-Hill.

Leininger M: Leininger's theory of nursing: culture care diversity and universality, *Nurs Sci Q* 1(4):152, 1988.

Lester N: Cultural competence: a nursing dialogue, 1, *Am J Nurs* 98(8):26, 1998a.

Lester N: Cultural competence: a nursing dialogue, 2, *Am J Nurs* 98(9):36, 1998b.

Michaud S, Warner R: Gender differences in self-reported response in troubles talk, *Sex Roles* 37(7/8):527, 1997.

Narayan M: Cultural assessment in home healthcare, *Home Healthcare Nurse* 15(10 C):663, 1997.

Plawecki H, Sanchez T, Plawecki J: Cultural aspects of caring for Navajo Indians clients, *J Holistic Nurs* 12(3):291, 1994.

Purnell L, Paulanka B: *Transcultural health care: a culturally competent approach,* Philadelphia, 1998, FA Davis.

Sue D, Sue D: *Counseling the culturally different,* New York, 1990. John Wiley.

Tannen D: *Talking from 9 to 5: How women's and men's conversation styles affect who gets heard, who gets credit, and what gets done at work,* New York, 1994, William Morrow.

Tannen D: *You just don't understand: men and women in conversation,* New York, 1990, William Morrow.

Tripp-Reimer T, Afifi LA: Cross-cultural perspectives on patient teaching, *Nurs Clin North Am* 24(3):613, 1989.

Watson J: Florence Nightingale and the enduring legacy of transpersonal human caring, *J Holistic Nurs* 16(2):292, 1998.

Woodard E, House B: Nurse-physician communication: women and men at work, *Orthop Nurs* 16(1):39,1997.

 # Suggestions for Further Reading

Edwards J: Thai cultural assessment for Nursing 4041, "Culture in Nursing Practice," Semester II, 1997, University of South Florida.

Giles H, Coupland N, Coupland J, Williams A, Nussbaum J: Intergenerational talk and communication with older people, *Int J Aging Hum Dev* 34(4):271, 1992.

Haber J, Krainovich-Miller B, McMahon A, Price-Hoskins, P: *Comprehensive psychiatric nursing,* St Louis, 1997, Mosby.

Heineken J: Patient silence is not necessarily client satisfaction, *Home Healthcare Nurse* 16(2):115, 1998.

Hooks B: *Yearning: race, gender and politics,* Boston, 1990, South End Press.

Nance T: Intercultural communication: finding common ground, *J GNN* 24(3):249,1995.

Stevens P, Hall J, Meleis A: Examining vulnerability of women clerical workers from five ethnic/racial groups, *West J Nurs Res* 14(6):754, 1992.

Offers insights into how African-Americans experience problematic interactions with Anglo-Americans.

Spector R: Cultural concepts of women's health and health-promoting behaviors, *J Obstet Gynecol Neonatal Nurs* 24(3):242, 1995.

Tripp-Reimer T, Brink PJ, Saunders JM: Cultural assessment: content and process, *Nurs Outlook* 32(2):78, March-April 1984.

A comparison and description of several cultural assessment guides.

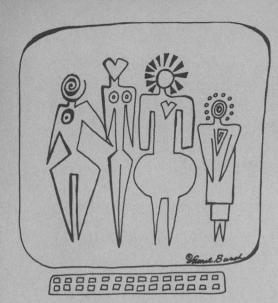

5

Electronic Communication

James T. Riley

OBJECTIVES

1. Identify ways to use electronic mail in health care.
2. Discuss the advantages and disadvantages of electronic mail.
3. Identify the ways in which electronic mail communication varies from face to face or telephone communication.
4. Identify privacy issues in electronic communication.
5. Identify ways to access information via the Internet.
6. Identify clinical applications for electronic communications.
7. Identify applications for electronic communications for the health care consumer.
8. Define and give examples of "Netiquette."

REACHING OUT TO THE WORLD ELECTRONICALLY

Computers are here to stay. The application of electronic communication to health care is changing the practice of the health care provider, but electronic involvement can be fun. Recently a colleague was working on a trivia quiz and needed the birth date of Sherlock Holmes. Finding an answer took less than three minutes on the Internet. (By the way, it's January 9, 1854, in case the question ever arises.) The use of computers at home and in health care is intriguing.

GETTING STARTED

How Do I Get Started?

Most organizations have access to the Internet, and any home computer can have access for a small monthly fee. The new computers almost all have a modem (see vocabulary list) built in to them.

Do I Have to Have State-of-the-Art Equipment?

Electronic equipment changes so rapidly, that it is almost impossible to remain current. You will have to advance your own system at whatever pace makes you the most comfortable. Every change made by the manufacturer does not call for a change from you also. If your word processor is doing the job that you need it to do, then be happy with it; you do not have to upgrade to the next system until you choose.

Is a Separate Telephone Line Necessary for Internet Access?

The use of a modem requires access to a phone line. Although you do not need a separate line, there are some things you must be aware of if you use your regular phone line. Call waiting will have to be disconnected while you are on-line (see vocabulary list); this can be either short term (*70 will discontinue call waiting on most phones and when you sign off it will return to normal operation) or it can be removed from your phone line altogether. You will not be able to make or receive any regular phone calls while you are on-line. You may choose not to have an extra phone line, but as you get more involved you may find that you prefer having separate lines.

What Precautions Should I Take When I Access the World Wide Web?

To protect your computer from unethical people, approach the Internet with care and caution. I believe there are two things you will need to help you get on-line with the least amount of concern: a recent version of **software** (Table 5-1) to scan for **viruses** and clean contaminated files; and a software program that will prevent any other company or individual from collecting information from your computer without your knowledge and permission while you are looking at a **website.** The virus scanner will warn you of any programming that may be hidden within the information you are trying to receive that will harm your computer or your programs. This virus problem is just not on the Internet but also could be in the software programs at your office, or on discs that you receive from others. Using a virus scanner all the time is a good idea, but it is a necessity when you start dealing with the Internet. As you start to use the Internet you will leave an electronic trail back to your computer. Advertisers obtain your electronic address and send you unwanted advertisements. Others can find out your hobbies, physical address, and more information than you would like them to have.

A word of caution: the World Wide Web is a very intriguing place full of wonders and information. It brings far-away places into your home, and puts them at your fingertips. This kind of information is very captivating, and one can be tempted to spend more time and effort than can be spared. Just remember that the 'Net is a tool to be used and not abused.

TABLE 5-1	**Computer Vocabulary**

Term	Definition
Address book	A means to keep a list of the electronic addresses of your friends and colleagues that is provided by most E-mail programs
Attached file	A computer file consisting of text, graphics, or sound sent via the Internet along with an E-mail; the file is then downloaded onto the recipient's computer and opened for access.
Bulletin board	A site where questions can be posed and responses collected
Chat room	A site where on-line conversations can be held by typing text; responses are received in real time
Computer virus	A destructive computer program that can damage or disrupt the normal operation of your computer; anti-virus programs are available at most computer stores
Central processing unit (CPU)	The "brain" of the computer that coordinates its functioning
E-mail	Electronic mail allows rapid transmission of information that is stored until the recipient chooses to read it
Hacker	Person who uses his or her knowledge about computers to access information that was not intended for public access
Hardware	Computer equipment such as the CPU, monitor, and printer (contrast with software)
Internet (the 'Net)	The common name given to the electronic linking of all the computer systems
Keyword	Subjects or categories used in searching the Internet for information
Mailing list	Feature of your E-mail program that allows you to put all the addresses of people who are interested in the same subject together in one place (for sending blanket messages)
Modem	The piece of machinery, "hardware," that is best described as a phone for computers. It sends the information you put into it out to the Internet and brings information back to your computer. Usually installed inside your computer (internal), but can be attached to the outside of your computer (external). Transmission speed is the major concern; the faster data can be transmitted and received, the less time it will take to obtain information
On-line	Connected electronically to the Internet via the World Wide Web
Search engine	A program that allows you to search the Internet by using keywords or topics
Server	Computer or software that delivers a specific kind of service to a client, such as file storage or data transmission
Software	A computer program written to perform a function, such as: word processing software to compose, store, and retrieve documents; or spreadsheet software to collect, tabulate, and retrieve data
Undeliverable	E-mail that the Internet could not find an address to deliver to. These machines will only do what we *tell* them to do, not what we *want* them to do
Website	A collection of pages related by topic or organization maintaining them, perhaps an educational institution, government agency, business, or even an individual
World Wide Web	The universe of hypertext servers (HTTP servers) that allows text, graphics, and sound files to be mixed

Where Can I Learn More?

Many software packages provide a help function or frequently asked questions (FAQ) section. Also consider the purchase of a computer reference book. Something from the "Dummies" series makes a quick, easy-to-use resource.

ELECTRONIC MAIL IN HEALTH CARE

Electronic mail (E-mail) is a form of rapid communication and, at this time, is the number one activity on the Internet. E-mail is used to send, receive, and manage your electronic communication. You can attach files to a message to send information to others, exchange ideas, request information, reply to messages, forward, and even print messages. E-mail can even be fun, playful writing to a friend, advertising to get a good home for kittens, or anything you would like (Box 5-1).

Why have people become so enamored with E-mail? It is immediate. We send it out one day and most times we get some kind of answer that same day. At times you can send out a message and get an answer back within minutes. That makes it valuable in nursing because time is often critical to the well-being of our clients.

Consider that we can say things in a manner that would not be used if we were present. This is also the place that could cause the most problems. We can get into trouble over writing things that are not appropriate. At work, a good rule to follow is that if you cannot say it out loud at a staff meeting, then do not write it. The lack of emotional contact can cause you to be more open, or to be so brief as to appear abrupt and unfeeling (Hallowell, 1999) (Box 5-2).

E-mail erases time and space. You can send a message anytime and it will be received when the recipient chooses. Distance does not make a difference. It is possible to seek help or information from Japan with no difference in effort than if the request was made of a local colleague. You can send a note to a friend, a colleague, or a government official as long as you have their electronic address.

Collaboration with peers makes it easier to solve problems and handle issues. Nurses can get help with pressing problems and give help to those who can use our expertise. Just the ability to get immediate feedback from someone we trust about a problem we are having will make that problem less likely to escalate into something critical.

E-mail is one of the fastest ways to spread knowledge. We have never before had such a sys-

---

Box 5-1 | **Uses for E-Mail**

- Distribute the agenda and minutes of a meeting
- Send and receive newsletters
- Send motivational quotations
- Provide prompt feedback for a job well done
- Share information over long distances, even internationally
- Attach files such as documentation, bibliographies, presentations from programs such as Power Point, or photographs
- Print messages or download attached files

tem. Knowledge discovered in Spokane, Washington, in the morning can be communicated to Portland, Maine, that same morning. Documentation can be attached to any message that will give the receiver access to all the information the sender possesses. Any additional information, improvements, and changes can be returned to the sender within hours.

This is also true of the clients, families, and colleagues with whom we work. Clients and families can have access to the Internet and may become much more aware of their condition and learn new ways to handle their situation. We must attempt to stay current in our work yet understand that with the vast amount of information available, clients and family may have valuable information to contribute. It is important to be open and not defensive or patronizing in our approach. Instead we become partners with clients and families and can help them learn how to discriminate between reliable and unreliable information.

The Advantages and Disadvantages of E-Mail

The main advantage of E-mail is speed. Nurses can connect with someone in the next cubicle or many miles away within seconds. This speed of transfer of information lends itself to spontaneity of thought and brainstorming. We can address our E-mail to as many people as we choose all at one time and get as many answers to our inquires as we need. This then leads to creative thinking. The group will be connected through common needs and interests. The spontaneity and creative thought will provide new ways to solve problems and new approaches to common issues (Box 5-3).

The creation of a peer group, or trusted individuals who can be called on to help solve problems, will provide more universal answers to issues. In all of your training sessions, make it a point to get all the E-mail addresses of the participants and make copies for everyone. This gives you a ready-made mailing list of people who have a common connection. If we just want to

---

Box 5-2 **The Do's and Don'ts of E-Mail**

Do's

- Do make sure you type the address correctly, copying it exactly
- Check to make sure you type the correct case; some programs are case sensitive, and not capitalizing would make mail undeliverable
- Do make a list of addresses frequently used and save them in the address book in the E-mail program
- Save time by compiling mailing lists for different committees, or groups with whom you correspond
- Do save, date, and number all drafts in a project for future reference to avoid confusion and track the progress/development. Some people add the time when a project is passing quickly from person to person

Don'ts

- Don't write anything you would not want your employer to read; E-mail is easily accessible and is not confidential
- Don't use E-mail at work for personal communication
- Don't forward messages indiscriminately
- Don't send a message you would not want forwarded

explore our philosophical thinking about a problem or if we have a real problem that needs to be solved, the more diverse answers we have to compare the more integrated product we will have to work with. The analysis of your situation, whether it is to solve a current problem or collect data to track trends for future planning, will be better enhanced by the inclusion of several other views. Also the E-mail approach will allow you to select the responses to any situation. You have the freedom to use as much or as little of the feedback as you choose.

E-mail allows you to attach documentation to support your answers or suggestions. Attach bibliographies, graphs, PowerPoint presentations, articles, photographs, anything that can be produced on or scanned into your computer. This is a powerful tool to spread knowledge and to get accurate interpretations of the evidence you present. There is no guesswork. The actual documentation is there for all to see and analyze.

The use of E-mail promotes collaboration and enhances problem solving. E-mail can be used for business, but remember that E-mail can be used for fun. Many people have friends that they write to every day, they also can write on-line to anyone they choose. This is a very convenient way to connect to others, but especially your family and your friends.

A major disadvantage is that you must have access to E-mail to participate. This is becoming less of a problem. More and more organizations are providing access for their employees, and the increasing number of personal computers in the home has made E-mail a household word.

Another drawback is the use of incompatible software. No matter how popular a particular software program is, you will have to deal with people who do not use that software. As we hear things about a giant software company that has taken over the computer world, you will still run into people who do not use that brand, and you may have problems sending files or solving prob-

---

Box 5-3 **The Advantages and Disadvantages of E-Mail**

Advantages

- It's fast
- It is cost-effective
- It can be written and sent any time
- A reply can be sent easily and quickly
- Messages can be forwarded easily
- Prompt updates on current problems can be provided
- Brain-storming/creative thinking is encouraged
- For some people it may be easier than verbal communication
- The recipient has time to think through a response

Disadvantages

- Not everyone has access
- Some people are reluctant to use computers
- It is a new skill to learn and can be frustrating
- Some problems exist with software compatibility in receiving E-mail or downloading attached files
- Some E-mail systems can be used only within the organization and do not allow wider access
- Computers do not always function perfectly, causing frustration and what seems like wasted time
- Verbal and nonverbal signals are not available to help clarify the meaning of the message

lems. Even within the same organization, compatibility problems can arise. Departments may be using different versions of the same software program. A more recent version is likely to be able to use data from an older version but the converse is not true. These problems do occur and we must be creative in finding strategies to solve them.

Wit and Wisdom

So . . . computer technology saves you time, right?

A one-liner delivered to wild laughter and applause

Another problem is the frustration that occurs when an instant reply is not received to help you solve your problem immediately. Try to remember not to take the nonresponse as a personal rebuke. There are several reasons for a nonresponse, not the least is that the person that you sent the E-mail to has no answer, and feels challenged that you asked him or her for one. Also, using the computer is not an exact science. The other person may not have received the message. Sometimes messages are delayed for days with no explanation. We joke and say they were "lost in cyberspace." One comedian suggested they resided in the same space as single socks missing from the dryer. The simplest thing to do with no response is to send the message again. Some E-mail systems have the capability to return a receipt to you when the E-mail is received. Try to use that feature when possible. When you do receive an "undeliverable" message, it is usually because an address has been typed incorrectly.

We always have an accelerated sense of time when we are waiting for something. We all know that whomever we send a message to is just waiting to reply to us. We all think that people just wait at their computer knowing that we will send them a message and expect a reply with all the right answers within minutes, but sometimes that does not happen. Sometimes people have other things to do. Sometimes they do not even think that our message is that important. Just try to remember that people will get back to you within their time frame, not yours, and a lot of the anxiety will be gone. If you find yourself getting frustrated, a recent book entitled *Technostress* assures us we are not alone (Weil and Rosen, 1997). Occasionally, just as with any form of communication, the response itself will not be what we expected. You cannot know the current situation of the writer (Box 5-4).

Box 5-4 Reasons Why an E-Mail Message Has Not Been Answered

- You are too eager! Just because you have sent it does not mean it has been read.
- It may be undeliverable because the address was incorrect or is no longer valid; usually you will receive a message if it could not be delivered.
- The receiver may not yet have opened your mail.
- The receiver may be considering the reply or collecting more information before replying.

The last thing to consider is that a response could be delayed when someone chooses not to be the decision maker for the group. There are many reasons for that, ranging from false modesty to just not wanting to take the responsibility for making decisions. A project proceeds more smoothly if roles are assigned early on: someone who can do the review, the person who will collect all the data, and the one to formulate the response. This enables everyone to query the right people and proceed at the best pace possible to get the project done or the problem solved.

ELECTRONIC COMMUNICATION DIFFERS FROM FACE-TO-FACE OR TELEPHONE COMMUNICATION

Nurses value face-to-face communication. The intimate connection with clients and family is at the heart of nursing care. Trusted collegial relationships are based on experience over time, at the bedside, in offices, and in other settings. Yet E-mail is increasingly a part of health care. We must understand the limitations that exist with this form of communication, knowing that all forms of communication have limitations.

E-mail lacks the softening effect of face-to-face contact. The message is received only in print. These messages are interpreted as literal communication, missing many familiar components. This means that receiving the message could be a harsh experience.

We do not have any body "language" to help us interpret the messages we are receiving. How many messages do we receive each day that we interpret through what we see, the nonverbal behavior? Often we listen not so much to what is being said, but how it is being said. We hear and understand the words, but the tone of those words, the inflection on certain syllables, makes it clear to us what the other person is trying to communicate. These cues that we trust are missing in electronic communication. Remember that the person to whom we send our E-mail has the same limitation. We must be very clear in what we write to help offset these limitations.

The KISS principle (Keep it Short and Simple) applies here. Use these guidelines with E-mail or when leaving voice mail messages:

- Start with a brief statement of the purpose of the message. You can use the "Subject" category as an attention-getter in an E-mail. On voice mail identify yourself immediately and use your full name. Do not assume the person will recognize your voice or know you by your first name
- Be sure to include your telephone number (on voice mail, repeat it a second time so the extra time for replay might not be needed)
- Recap important points at the end; try numbering points in an E-mail
- Take time to write brief notes of what you want to include to avoid lengthy, rambling messages that are not respectful of others' time (Weil and Rosen, 1997)

There is an old saying dealing with E-mail: if you can produce it electronically, it can be reproduced electronically. People who have deleted something from their computer screen believe that it is gone forever, but that is not necessarily true. Computer programs have been developed to recover E-mails and other data that have been deleted. E-mail messages have been subpoenaed in court cases. Remember to write only what is necessary to convey the message to the receiver.

Box 5-5	Networking At Its Finest

- Collect business cards at professional meetings
- Add relevant E-mail addresses to your address book in your E-mail program
- Use E-mail to thank someone for an interesting conversation, to pass on a reference of interest, or report a promised referral
- Collaborate with colleagues
- Compliment a speaker at a conference
- Write to an author whose work you admire
- Say Happy Birthday to someone
- Share a compliment about someone's work
- Send information that you may think will be of some value to the individual

E-mail is an effective tool to enhance communication with people you already know. However, seminars, meetings, and other face-to-face networking are still an integral part of professional growth. Even a single personal encounter puts a face to a name, which offers data on which we base judgments about people's reliability. It is possible to develop E-mail relationships, but sometimes it takes a while. Real meaning can be lost or confused unless the communication is very direct. It is wise to consider making a follow-up call if the message is of a very critical nature. Electronic communication can enhance professional relationships through networking (Box 5-5).

In the future we will have visual electronic communication. A camera and a microphone on your computer will send your picture and spoken words to someone else as quickly as E-mail. The development of this technology is being hastened by the present lack of voice and view of the individual from whom we are receiving E-mail messages. The lack of dependable sources of communication verification has produced a demand in the marketplace. It will soon be filled and, as with all technology, at an increasingly affordable price.

PRIVACY ISSUES IN ELECTRONIC COMMUNICATION

We have touched on some of this already. As soon as you send an E-mail, it becomes accessible to everyone with the technical knowledge and the intent to retrieve it. By that, I mean it is no longer your private property. The U.S. Postal Service is working on a method to keep E-mail messages private but has not worked out a safe and secure system yet. There may never be a perfectly safe way to send electronic messages, so it is safest to assume that all messages can be retrieved.

The person or persons to whom you send your message may make copies of the message and distribute it anywhere they choose. A message that was not meant for the world to see could end up on a bulletin board. People write things in jest that could be considered threatening or slanderous.

These messages could be used in litigation. Remember to follow the same rules of confidentiality for this medium as you would for any other. Attached files containing identifying client data could be retrieved.

The first enforcement action on Internet privacy was made against GeoCities because it misled users about how personal information was used. Legislation concerning privacy laws is being considered by Congress (Miller, 1998).

Moments of Connection...
Electronic Communication

Most users of E-mail have access from home. Although not a substitute for a handwritten note, E-mail is more and more being used for personal contact. A CEO of a hospital talked about a director whose wife had just had a baby. The CEO had not had time to congratulate the proud father face-to-face and reluctantly settled for an E-mail. To his surprise, his remarks were more personal and thoughtful in a medium where he could take his time to say what he wanted and feel comfortable. This same phenomenon is sometimes encountered when we talk over the phone to someone and we are able to say things that we would be more reluctant to say face to face.

ACCESSING INFORMATION VIA THE INTERNET

The simplest way to get information from the Internet is to join a provider group. AOL, Compuserve, and Mindspring are all examples of providers for access to the Internet. They also provide access to special Interest groups (nurses, golfers, trekkies) and make it easier for a person to make contact with others who have the same interests.

These companies also allow you access to **search engines,** which make it possible to search by **keywords,** or phrases, that describe what you are looking for. If you would like to find out about "Nurse Speakers," you would type those words into a search engine and all places where those words appear will be listed for you. Yahoo is a search engine that looks for items indexed by topics, and does not actually search the text of each web page so if you searched for "Nurse Speaker" all things connected with "Nurse" would be pulled up, then all things with "Speaker " would be pulled up. Alta Vista is a search engine that uses the words connected by a + sign to search the text of each web page for the connection. So if you were looking for "Nurse Speaker" you would look for it by "Nurse+Speaker." Your search results depend on how general you want to start and how specific you want to get.

There are many private organizations that have databases on line, so you may find the information that you seek. General Motors, Microsoft, and religious organizations are just examples of the myriad groups willing to share information about their products or services. Not only the big companies, but many small entrepreneurial sites are also on-line.

Government agencies and educational institutions were the original users of the Internet. The biggest contributor to the Internet is still the U.S. government. The Library of Congress, the Smithsonian, all elected Representatives, and the White House can be reached by the Internet. The public information sector is also well represented. You can find out about National Parks and even make reservations for your vacation, or visit the Supreme Court or Congress all on-line. You can rent a car, learn how to eat healthfully, grow a garden, and follow a soccer match all on the Internet. The wonder and fun of the 'Net is just being explored and developed. Get involved and you will be surprised at the information that is available to you (Table 5-2).

TABLE 5-2	**Useful Internet Sites**

Getting Started

Fast ways to search	http://www.msn.com/access/allinone.asp
	http://www.askjeeves.com
	http://www.cyber411.com

Nursing Sites

American Journal of Nursing	http://www.ajn.org
American Nurses Association	http://www.nursingworld.org
Healthstream	http://www.healthstream.com

Nursing Management

The Nurse Practitioner, Nursing 98 Drug Handbook	http://www.springnet.com
The University of Tennessee, Knoxville nursing and medical information	http://nightingale.con.utk.edu/

Pain Management Sites

Pain Management On-line	http://www.painmngt.com
World Wide Congress on Pain	http://www.pain.com

H.I.V. Site

Roxane H.I.V. Resource Center	http://hiv.roxane.com/

Government Sites

AHCPR	http://www.ahcpr.gov
Directory and information about U.S. House of Representatives and the U.S. Senate including many E-mail addresses	http://policy.net/capweb/SenateCom/AP.html
National Institutes of Health	http://www.nih.gov
National Library of Medicine; access to MEDLINE and links to many journals	http://www.ncbi.nlm.nih.gov/PubMed/

Research Sites

Resources for qualitative research	http://www.ualberta.ca/~jrnorris/qual.html
	http://www.healthfinder.gov
	http://igm.nlm.nih.gov
	http://www.kidshealth.org/
	http://www.ama-assn.org/
	http://www.hon.ch/

THE INTERNET FOR THE HEALTH CARE PROVIDER AND HEALTH CARE CONSUMER

Consumer Education on the Internet

Clients and families have access to many sources of health education. Just pick up a newspaper and check the technology section. *USA Today* compared three consumer health sites, www.thriveonline.com, www.betterhealth.com, and www.healthfinder.gov for entertainment value, usefulness, and ease of use (July 29, 1998, p. 5D) The nurse or client can type in a keyword, such as *diabetes,* and find a site for the American Diabetes Association with information about educational materials and membership. Chat rooms or bulletin boards help people learn from each other about chronic diseases or other medical problems. A word of caution is in order, though: anyone can create a web site and claim to have medical information. Consumers need to be discerning in their collection of information from the Internet. Just because someone writes credentials after their name does not mean they are genuine.

Clinical Applications of Electronic Communication

A variety of clinical applications of electronic communication offer exciting opportunities for improved nursing care. Caregiver Interventions via Telecommunications (CIT) provides two-way communication for caregivers of elders with dementia. Using telephone or videoconferencing equipment, professionals can provide consultation to supplement home visits. The client's caregiver must have a private telephone line, not a cellular telephone. Contacts are scheduled at mutually convenient times. Video equipment is on a closed system to provide for privacy (Wright, 1998).

Pagers are used by intensive care unit staff to reach family members when necessary. Other departments in outpatient or inpatient settings use pagers to allow the client or family mobility while waiting for diagnostic studies or procedures.

The field of nursing informatics is a "combination of computer, information, and nursing sciences" (Nagelkerk, Ritola, and Vandort, 1998) "Nursing informatics is 'the legitimate access to and use of data, information, and knowledge to: standardize documentation, improve communication, support the decision-making process, develop and disseminate new knowledge, enhance the quality, effectiveness, and efficiency of health care . . .'" (Simpson, 1992a, in Nagelkerk, Ritola, and Vandort, 1998). Computer systems help nurses provide point-of-care documentation via bedside computers. Laboratory data can be available immediately. In addition, analysis of research data is quicker via computer (Nagelkerk, Ritola, and Vandort, 1998).

Software is available to assist in decision making. These programs are based on the processes of experts making decisions about a clinical problem. These processes are analyzed and computerized. The nurse user of this software types in client data and receives a printout of information about further data to be collected (Nagelkerk, Ritola, and Vandort, 1998).

Occupational nurses can use the Internet to access information from the Centers for Disease Control and Prevention or poison control centers and government health requirements from organizations such as the Occupational Safety and Health Administration (OSHA) (Knuth, 1998).

Educational Applications of Electronic Communication

Internet courses create a virtual classroom for students and staff at all levels. The Indiana Higher Education Telecommunications Systems' R.N. to B.S.N. education progressed from distance learning one-way video and two-way video conferences to communication via home computers or loaner laptop computers. By connecting via modem to the Internet students can access courses; connect to a university mainframe; communicate with faculty, other students, or colleagues via E-mail; and transfer files to turn in assignments or exchange information. E-mail access to faculty can increase communication between faculty and off-campus students (Carltol, Ryan, and Sikberg, 1998). Having word processing skills and the ability to share data in spreadsheets make academic work faster and more professional in presentation. Clayton State University students in Georgia are loaned laptop computers as part of their tuition and fees and given a keyword for access to databases via the Internet.

Nurses can use the Internet to locate resources online and find nursing networks to broaden their sources of support and information. Courses can be offered on-line or can be sent via E-mail (Plank, 1998). Nurses can recommend online client support groups (Bachman and Panzarine, 1998).

Nurses can participate with other disciplines in diagnosis and consultation via telemedicine or two-way videoconferencing for access to clients and client information. Continuing education can be offered via videoconferencing such as the program developed by a consortium for education for rural nurses in a demonstration project at Edinborough University (Weber and Lawlor, 1998). Other uses of videoconferencing include courses for academic credit and post-clinical conferences for students whose clinical experience is a long distance from the university.

Computer-assisted instruction (CAI) provides education in hospitals. Staff development departments provide portable computer equipment and programs for convenient use of staff for orientation and mandatory inservices.

WHAT IS NETIQUETTE?

Netiquette—from the words '*Net* and *etiquette*—is the social code of behavior—guidelines for common courtesy and common sense on the Internet. There are several good references to help you understand what is proper behavior on the 'Net, such as Virginia Shea's *Netiquette*. You can also search for "netiquette" on-line (Box 5-6).

Box 5-6   Common Sense on the Internet

- Write in a normal narrative manner; writing IN ALL CAPS gives the impression of shouting.
- *Flaming* refers to sending insulting or controversial messages with the intention of starting or escalating an argument.
- Remember that it is just as easy for you to misunderstand a criticism as for anyone else. Try not to reply when you are angry and always work toward understanding.
- Try to cover only one subject at a time and state it clearly in the subject line of the message. This should help everyone keep track of the messages and in business settings helps with storing and forwarding information.
- If you are at home using your own facilities and equipment, you can do what you like—explore the net or run a business. However, using your organization's facilities and equipment for purposes other than work is unethical.
- Always be careful with what you copy or download from the 'Net. Viruses can be very destructive.

Think About It...
What, So What, and Now What?

Consider what you read about electronic communication and how you might use it in your professional and personal life.

What? . . . Write one thing you learned from this chapter.

So what? . . . How will this impact your nursing practice?

Now what? . . . How will you implement this new knowledge or skill?

━━ THINK ABOUT IT ━━

Practicing Electronic Communication

Exercise 1

Quickly write 5 clinical issues about which you have had questions lately. Write keywords you might use to research these topics. Go on-line and see what you find. Print one resource and share it with a colleague.

Exercise 2

See Table 5-2 (Useful Internet Sites). Search for the names and E-mail addresses of your members of the U.S. House of Representatives and U.S. Senate. File this information so you can communicate your concerns about upcoming health care legislation.

References

A healthy competition on line: *USA Today* p. B1, Wednesday, July 29, 1998.

Bachman JA, Panzarine S: Enabling student nurses to use the information superhighway, *J Nurs Educ* 37(4):155.

Carlton K, Ryan ME, Sikberg L: Designing courses for the Internet, *Nurse Educat* 23(3):45, May/June 1998.

Hallowell E: The human moment at work, *Harvard Bus Rev* p. 57, Jan-Feb 1999.

Incredibly useful sites, *Yahoo Magazine* 4(7):86, 1998.

Knuth G: Web site developer and nurse: an essential business partnership, *Am Assoc Occup Health Nurs J* 46(1):47, 1998.

Miller L: First Internet privacy action raps GeoCities, *USA Today* p. B1, August 14, 1998.

Nagelkerk J, Ritola PM, Vandort PJ: Nursing informatics: the trend of the future, *J Contin Educ Nurs* 29(1):17, 1998.

Overview of netiquette, Ultranet, July 1998. (http://37.com/)

Plank RK: Nursing on-line for continuing education credit, *J Contin Educ Nurs* 29(4):165, July/Aug 1998.

Weber RW, Lawlor AC: Professional nursing series by videoconferencing, *J Contin Educ Nurs* 29(4):161, July/Aug 1998.

Weil MM, Rosen LD: *Coping with technology @work @home @play,* New York, 1997, John Wiley & Sons.

Wright LK, Bennet G, Gramling L: Telecommunication interventions for caregivers of elders with dementia, *Adv Nurs Sci* 20(3):76, 1998.

Suggestions for Further Reading

Andolsek K: Medical information exchange using the Internet, *Am Fam Physician* 55(5):1899, April 1997.

American Society of Pain Management Nurses Website Task Force: Computer technology. Presented at the national ASPMN conference, April 27, 1998, Orlando, Florida.

Bass DM, McClendon MJ, Brennan PF, McCarthy C: The buffering effect of a computer support network on caregiver strain, *J Aging Health* 10(1):20, 1998.

Bowles KH: The barriers and benefits of nursing information systems, *Computers in Nursing* 15(4):191, 1997.

Broffman G: How can pediatric care be provided in underserved areas? a view of rural pediatric care, part 2, *Pediatrics* 96(4):816, Oct 1995.

Brooks S: Net results, *Contemp Longterm Care* 19(1):32, 1996.

Bunting SM, Russell CK: Use of mail (email) for concept synthesis: an international collaborative project, *Qualitat Health* Res 8(1):128, 1998.

Cassell MM: Health communication on the Internet: an effective channel for health behavior change? *J Health Commun* 3(1):71, 1998.

Clark C: Internet opens up secret world of medicine, *Malaria Trop Dis Week* 5, July 9-16, 1997.

Cupito MC: Intranets: communication for the internal universe, *Health Manage Technol* 18(7):20, June 1997.

Evers WD: Enlarging your professional community through electronic communications, *J Nutr Educ* 28(1):47b, 1996.

Fabian N: Internet, cyberspace, information highway, computers, and all that good stuff, *J Environ Health* 57(4):5, Nov 1994.

The flora health club: for the practice nurse and her patients . . . get connected to the Internet, *Pract Nurs* 13(8):484, 1997.

Focus on the Internet: the nursing world at your fingertips, *Nurs Spect* 14(8) July 1998.

Gach G: *The pocket guide to the Internet,* New York, 1996, Pocket Books.

Ground P, Grigaitis M, Thomas, T: A computerized learning tool, *Am J Nurs* 98:11, 1998.

Hales M: Basic Internet facilities, *Lancet* 384(9020):6, July 1996.

Izenberg N, Lieberman DA: The web, communication trends, and children's health, *Clin Pediatr* 37(3): 153, 1998.

Kennedy A: *The Internet: the rough guide* 1999, New York, 1998, Penguin.

Kiley R: *Medical information on the Internet: a guide for the health professionals,* New York, 1998, Harcourt.

King I: Nursing informatics: a universal nursing language, *Fla Nurse* 46(1):1, 1998.

Levine JR, Young ML: *More Internet for dummies,* Foster City, Calif, 1996, IDG Books Worldwide, Inc.

Lore WK, Bennet G, Gramling L: Telecommunication interventions for caregivers of elders with dementia, *Adv Nurs Sci* 20(3):76, 1998.

McAfooes J: Why nurses need to know about information technology, *FITNE/Healthnet* 10(4): 2, 1997.

Nagle LM, Ryan SA: The superhighway to nursing science and practice, *Holistic Nurs Pract* 11(1):25, Oct 1996.

Shea V: *Netiquette,* San Francisco, 1994, Albion Books.

Sparks S, Rizzolo M: World Wide Web search tools, *Image: J Nurs Scholar* 30(2):167, 1998.

Travis R, Brennan PF: Information science for the future: an innovative nursing informatics curriculum, *J Nurs Educ* 37(4):162, 1998.

Tweney D: *Traveler's guide to the information highway,* Emeryville, Calif, 1994, Ziff-Davis Press.

Warburton B: Research technology, electronic mail, *Mod Midwife* 6(11):30, 1996.

Ward R: Network implications of computer networking and the Internet for nurse education, *Nurs Educ Today* 17(3):178, 1997.

Whitehead P, Maran R: *Internet and World Wide Web simplified,* Ontario Canada, 1997, IDG Books Worldwide, Inc.

Part II

Building Relationships

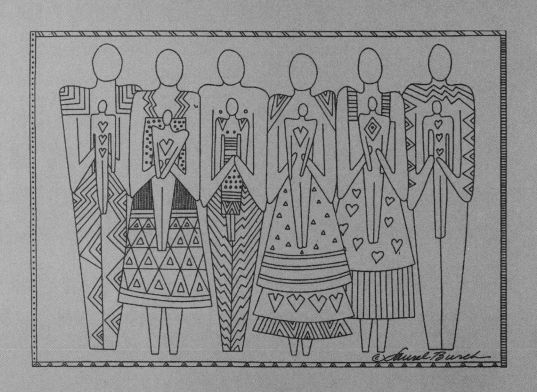

In Part I you learned skills to help you work assertively with clients, to appreciate differences, and to use electronic communication to enrich your work. Here you will look at the essential ingredients of nurse-client and nurse-family relationships. What does it mean to demonstrate warmth, respect, genuineness, and empathy in your communication? How can you appropriately use self-disclosure, spirituality, and humor to enrich professional relationships? Why is it important to pay attention to specificity and how you ask questions and give opinions? Read on.

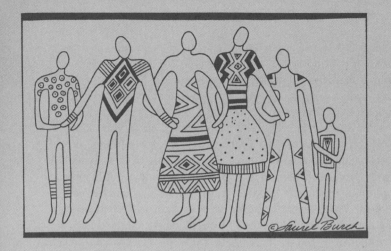

6

Warmth

Unfading are the gardens of kindness.

Grecian proverb

OBJECTIVES

1. Discuss the benefits of warmth in communication with clients and colleagues.
2. Identify behaviors that demonstrate warmth.
3. Review a tool to analyze warmth in interpersonal communications.

After studying this chapter you will be able to describe a variety of ways in which warmth is displayed and articulate the importance of warmth in human interactions. You will be encouraged to become aware of opportunities to embellish your life with warmth in day-to-day encounters with clients and colleagues.

THE BENEFITS OF WARMTH FOR YOUR CLIENTS AND COLLEAGUES

Warmth is the glue in the bonding between people and the magnetism that draws us to a closer intimacy with others. It is a special ingredient, even a catalyst, in our human relationships. Warmth in people makes us feel welcomed, relaxed, and joyful. Although clients may not be able to judge our "intelligence, certifications, or degrees," they can judge our heart by the care we give, the warmth we demonstrate (Carver, 1998).

Warmth has been identified as an essential attribute in psychotherapists. The therapist's warmth, along with empathy and genuineness, contribute to client improvement and lead to more open, full relationships for clients in and out of therapy. Warmth sets the tone for clients, families, and colleagues to share their own stories. Baker and Diekelmann (1994) called these "connecting conversations." Most of you will not be psychotherapists. Your expression of warmth to your clients, however, will make them feel welcomed and not judged. These positive emotions will foster feelings of well-being and likely promote healing. The warmth communicated in family support has a direct effect on the well-being of clients since family members can often offer better support than staff (Cooper and Powell, 1998). Caring acts that show warmth and genuineness have been associated with increasing hope in clients with cancer (Koopmeiners et al, 1997). In a study to develop and validate the dimensions for caregiver reciprocity in intergenerational exchanges, warmth and regard were found to be important factors (Carruth, 1996). Clients who sense your warmth are more likely to engage in dialogue and provide information about their health condition. This communication helps the nurse to make a nursing diagnosis, determine expected outcomes, work out a nursing care plan, and mutually evaluate the progress of nursing care.

Wit and Wisdom

Warmth, kindness, and friendship are the most yearned-for commodities in the world. The person who can provide them will never be lonely.

Ann Landers

Exchanging warmth with colleagues makes the workplace a more pleasant environment. Warmth enhances closeness, which has social and work-related benefits. A study by the American Management Association (Ekeren, 1994) found eight traits that often lead to failure for executives. The first two were "insensitivity to co-workers" and "aloofness and arrogance." Extending our warmth to our colleagues makes us more approachable. Increased communication among colleagues ensures that important messages about clients or unit policies and procedures will be transmitted.

Although we often refer to others as warm, as a human quality it is difficult to pin down. Warmth is one of the most difficult interpersonal communication behaviors to learn. Warmth involves not only attitudinal and psychomotor behavior, but also a total way of offering oneself to another person. Showing warmth to others means conveying that you like to be with them and accept them as they are. In this sense warmth is a way of showing respect to clients and colleagues.

Warmth is not communicated in isolation; it enhances and is enhanced by other facilitative communication behaviors you will learn about in later chapters (such as respect, genuineness, and empathy). By itself warmth is not sufficient for building an effective helping relationship, developing mutual respect, or problem solving, but warmth enhances these processes.

Levine and Adelman (1982) reported that a study conducted in the United States discerned that 93% of a message is transmitted by tone of voice and facial expression, and only 7% by words. It is possible that we tune into the nonverbal expression of emotions and attitudes more than the verbal. Because expression of warmth is predominantly nonverbal, it is wise to heed these findings.

How to Display Warmth to Your Clients and Colleagues

Warmth is displayed primarily in a nonverbal manner. Subtle facial and body signs, as well as gestures (small movements of a hand, brow, or eye), convey our inner relaxation and attentiveness to another person (Table 6-1).

There is a lot that you do with your face to convey warmth. When you are talking to another person, attention is largely focused on the face, so it is important to know how to make facial expressions that maximize your warmth.

Your face can communicate information regarding your personality, interests, and responsiveness during interaction, as well as your emotional state. Your facial expression can open or close a conversation. The context, including the relationship, determines the meaning of our facial expressions. Also, the degree of facial expressiveness varies among individuals and cultures. In relationships with clients and colleagues, it is wise to remember that when people from other cultures do not express emotions (such as warmth) openly, it does not mean that they do not experience these emotions.

Americans express themselves in varying degrees. People from certain ethnic backgrounds in the United States may use their hands, bodies, and faces more than others. There are a variety of ways to express warmth, but it is usually considered suspicious to have a "poker face" or "deadpan" facial expression.

We may interpret insufficient or excessive eye contact as communication barriers. No specific rules govern eye behavior except that it is considered rude to stare, especially at strangers. Eye contact can have different meaning in different cultures.

TABLE 6-1	Facial Signals of Warmth
Facial Feature	**How Warmth is Displayed**
Forehead	Muscles are relaxed and forehead is smooth; there is no furrowing of the brow
Eyes	Comfortable eye contact is maintained; pupils are dilated; gaze is neither fixed nor shifting and darting
Mouth	Lips are loose and relaxed, not tight or pursed; there is an absence of gestures such as biting a lip or forcing a smile; jaw is relaxed and mobile, not clenched; smile is appropriate
Expression	Features of the face move in a relaxed, fluid way; worried, distracted, or fretful looks are absent; face shows interest and attentiveness

Your warmth also emanates from your posture. Movements or ways of holding yourself that encourage communication, interest, and pleasure in being with the other person constitute warmth (Table 6-2).

This list manages to sound like your mother telling you to sit up straight at dinner, yet the details provide solid guidelines for communicating the warmth you feel even if you are anxious.

Warmth indicators include a shift of posture toward the other person, a smile, direct eye contact, and motionless hands. In Knapp's study (1980), gestures such as looking around the room, slumping, drumming fingers, and looking glum detract from warmth. In a dialogue situation, positive warmth cues, coupled with verbal reinforcers such as "mm-hmm," are effective for increasing verbal output for the interviewee (whereas verbal cues alone are insufficient). These findings from an early study have implications for nursing, where so much client information is gathered through interviewing.

Purtilo (1990) pointed out that in addition to whole-body posturing and positioning, gestures involving the extremities—even one finger—can suggest the meaning of a message. Think about how the following gestures would affect your message of warmth: shrugging your shoulders, folding your arms over your chest, rolling your thumb, shuffling your foot, or silently clenching your fist. Even if other parts of your body are focused on conveying warmth, these partial gestures might minimize or erase the message of warmth you are trying to send.

Another point to register about gestures in relation to warmth is that not all gestures embody universal meaning; the interpretation of a wink or a hand gesture may not be received in the same mood of warmth in which it is delivered. For example, our "OK" sign (circle made with thumb and forefinger) is a symbol for money in Japan and is considered obscene in some Latin American countries.

The spatial distance or closeness we create between us and our clients and colleagues can affect the warmth received. For Americans, distance in social conversation is about an arm's length

TABLE 6-2	**Postural Signals of Warmth**
Facial Feature	**How Warmth Is Displayed**
Body position	Client is faced squarely, with shoulders parallel to client's shoulders
Head position	Head is kept at same level as client's; periodic nodding shows interest and attentiveness
Shoulders	Shoulders are kept level and mobile, not hunched and tense
Arms	Arms are kept loose and able to move smoothly, rather than held stiffly
Hands	Gestures are natural, with no clenching or grasping of a clipboard or chart; distracting mannerisms like tapping a pen or playing with an object are avoided
Chest	Breathing is at an even pace; with the chest kept open, neither slouched nor extended too far forward in feigned attentiveness; leaning slightly forward shows interest
Legs	Whether crossed or uncrossed, legs are kept in a comfortable and natural position; when standing, knees should be flexed and not locked
Feet	Fidgeting, tapping, or kicking are avoided

to 4 feet. In our exuberance to display warmth, we may invade this unseen but well-defined circumference. Not all clients or colleagues will feel comforted by this gesture; some may feel intruded upon, and others may feel threatened and act defensively.

Touching is another way to affectionately transmit warmth. From the briefest touch on the shoulder to an embracing hug or extended hand, you can convey warmth to others. The warmth in the touch is augmented when you are truly comfortable with the act of touching. Being overly tentative emphasizes your uncertainty and embarrassment rather than your warmth. Being overly jocular or possessive in your touching may engulf and dissolve your warmth. When touching, it is important to be sincere so the warmth intended reaches the other person. A nurse's hands have been called therapeutic tools that can express warmth, caring, and comfort (Talton, 1995).

Warmth can be conveyed verbally as well as nonverbally. The volume of the voice is related to warmth. Softer, modulated tones convey warmth more than loud, aggressive tones that are harsh to the ears. A pitch that seems comfortable for the speaker transmits warmth more than an unnatural pitch that seems to be out of the speaker's range. The pacing of words is also important. Pressured, stilted, or stoic speech detracts from the warmth that can be conveyed through rhythmic speech, whose pacing is in keeping with the speaker's natural breathing. The actual words also have the power to extend warmth to others. Loving, soft words are warmer than harsh, thoughtless words: "So, you've never exercised before and now you think you'll become a 'super-jock' and take up jogging?" is cold and judgmental compared with "You'd like to improve your fitness level so you're taking a new lease on life and learning to jog."

As you may have noticed, many of the features of warmth are those of a relaxed person. In addition to being relaxed, it is only possible to convey warmth when you have a genuine interest in the other person and a wish to convey that welcome and pleasure to him or her. A desire to be warm is based on the belief that each person you encounter is worthy of receiving the acceptance and comfort that your warmth generates.

When you display high-level warmth, you are completely and intensely attentive to the interaction between yourself and your clients or colleagues, making them feel accepted and important. The opposite—cold behavior—conveys disapproval or disinterest.

Stories of Warmth in the Actions of the Nurse

A collection of "moments of connection" stories demonstrates the tapestry that is woven from lessons learned in our professional and personal journey that provide the warmth that is the caring art of nursing.

Moments of Connection...
For Our Loved Ones and Yours in Their Final Hours

"My father died suddenly in 1992, alone in a hospital far from family. I can only hope and pray that a kind nurse was with him, or hopefully, held his hand or said a prayer with him as he passed away. I tend to want to hold my patient's hands or pray—or be kind—so their family members can rest assured that a kind person was with their loved one."

Moments of Connection...
Pain Management: More Than Analgesia

"I was caring for a pain management patient who was reluctant to take medication. After talking with him, I learned he had lost his only child 3 months before in an automobile accident. He needed to talk. He was frightened and wanted a hand to hold. Despite my busy schedule, I knew this was where I belonged. I left when he was more comfortable. As I walked down the hall, I thanked God for giving me the talent and knowledge to help another person."

Moments of Connection...
A Pillow, a Washcloth, and Myself

"As an operating room nurse I had a patient with muscular dystrophy. Her surgery was delayed, and I spent about 30 minutes with her. She was in her twenties and we laughed and joked. I repositioned her arms and legs for her (she was already quite crippled) and gave her pillows and wet washcloths. Our time meant a lot to her, and she asked me if I would see her after surgery. When I did, she was thrilled and asked me to take my hat off so she could see me better. She visited me each time she came to the hospital. Later I learned she and her mother lived alone. She did not have any friends until we met. These comfort measures were just part of my work, but they meant a lot to her."

Moments of Connection...
Off the Clock

"My story is about my own unplanned C-section. I have been a pain management nurse for 5 years and know many people in the hospital. We all know it can be tough to care for another nurse. A special nurse from PACU inserted my Foley catheter for my male RN friend who was the circulating RN that day. Then she clocked out after seeing my nervousness and anxiety in the holding area. She comforted me and followed me through surgery. She did everything for me to provide warmth and comfort, including holding my hand during the epidural. I could just picture that three and a half inch spinal needle! She took the video for my husband so he could enjoy the first moments of our daughter's life . . . she provided comfort not only physically but emotionally as well. I will never forget her caring."

Moments of Connection...
When the Client Is Scared

"I had just begun to work with cancer patients when I met a young woman dying with sarcoma. She required many boluses of medication to relieve her pain, which was worst at night when she was most fearful. I held her hand and patted her shoulder gently to soothe her until the medication took effect."

Moments of Connection...
Showing Our Sympathy

"Working in the chronic pain setting, we do not have many deaths. When someone does die, as Pain Clinic Coordinator, I call the family to offer condolences. We also send a sympathy card. This time a daughter of a patient was killed in an accident and we chose to send flowers. The patient and family expressed their appreciation for this connection to them at a difficult time."

Extending and Withdrawing Warmth

Any time you wish to get closer to one of your clients or colleagues, or give the message that you really care, an expression of warmth is called for. There are degrees of warmth. An attitude of, "I like that client (colleague); I feel warmly toward him with all his strengths and weaknesses," is warmer than, "I don't feel dislike for my client (colleague)." The warmth you express should reflect your genuine feelings. Your expression of warmth to a colleague whom you would like to date will likely be more open and intense than the warmth you might express to a client in your care.

Factors that make it possible to convey warmth are the physical ability to control the facial, postural, tactile, and verbal features of warmth, and the ability to overcome any of the cognitive or affective influences mediating against warmth. What are some of these factors working against the expression of warmth? Any thoughts or feelings that distract nurses' attention from other people block the expression of warmth. Being rushed, overcome with strong emotions, shocked, or judgmental about others' behaviors are distractions that divert nurses' attention. When they are feeling hurried, nurses' concerns are for themselves, and their expression of enjoyment in other people diminishes or disappears.

Occasions may arise when what we feel conflicts with the expression of warmth. It is only natural to withdraw our warmth when we are angry with another person. When we feel hurt, bitter, irritated, or enraged with a client or colleague, it would be insincere to try to convey warmth. At times we may feel insecure about whether we will be received or rejected by another person. Then, we might hide behind a crisp façade until we feel safe enough to allow our warmth to surface.

On the other hand, there may be occasions when we withhold our feelings for fear of being too warm; perhaps we have romantic thoughts about a client or an unavailable colleague. Sometimes we may have very strong negative feelings toward someone. It is likely that we all have encountered someone who has treated us coldly, with disdain, or even with rudeness or contempt. It would be difficult for most of us to be freely warm with those who have treated us in this way. When we want to protect ourselves from perceived or actual uncaring or disinterest, we may withdraw our warmth or refrain from offering it.

Wit and Wisdom

Professionals are those who do their best even when they do not feel like it.

Author unknown

It is assertive to express your warmth to clients and colleagues when you wish to. It is nonassertive to withhold the warmth you feel. In contrast, it is aggressive to exude a warmth beyond the measure of your feelings. When you sincerely convey the warmth you feel, you bring to life the assertive position: "I like myself; I like you." This warmth is non-possessive and allows others room to be themselves.

Wit and Wisdom

Kind hearts are the garden, kind thoughts are the roots, kind words are the flowers, and kind deeds are the fruits.

Hungarian proverb

Think About It...
What, So What, and Now What?

Consider what you read about how to demonstrate warmth and its importance in making real connections with clients. It is easy to become focused on the technical things you are learning to do for clients. Often the small acts of warmth are what embellish our work with who we are and become our signature.

What? . . . Write one thing you learned from this chapter.

So what? . . . How will this impact your nursing practice?

Now what? . . . How will you implement this new knowledge or skill?

THINK ABOUT IT

The following exercises will make you aware of your warmth and give you pointers on how to convey your warmth when you choose.

 ## Practicing Warmth

Exercise 1

Before you start observing or changing your own behavior, take a few days to observe the warmth displayed by colleagues and friends. Keep notes of what you notice and your reactions. What did you notice about:

- Facial expressions
- Posturing
- Verbal expression
- Touching

What felt good? What warmth behaviors would you like to emulate? Compare your observations with those of your classmates. What did you learn from each other about the communication behavior of warmth?

Exercise 2

For a few days, focus on your delivery of warmth. What is it you do to show your loved ones that you care? How is this expression different from your display of warmth to co-workers and to clients? What is the same? Would you like to display more affection for others than you do? Make note of what you could change to be warmer. Find a partner in the class and exchange notes on the self-observations you have made.

Exercise 3

Find a full-length mirror and take a good look at yourself. Make a statement about the warmth your image projects. Does the set of your face convey warmth? Why? Why not? Note how you are holding your facial muscles. Do your eyes twinkle or are they cold? Are your lips softly mobile or are they tightened? Now, change your expression to make it warmer. Note what you do. How does it feel to soften your facial expression? Recall that feeling; you need that memory to call on when you want to convey warmth to another person (when you don't have your mirror handy).

Next, turn away from the mirror and attempt to recapture that same warm facial expression. Then turn to check in the mirror. Have you got it? Or does your head need tilting, your smile broadening, or your eyes crinkling?

If you want to convey warmth, you need to practice these nonverbal gestures so that you will feel confident you are sending out the warmth you want your clients and colleagues to receive.

Exercise 4

Now stand in front of the full-length mirror and look at how you are holding your body in space. Do your slouched shoulders suggest that you are lackadaisical? Do they show disinterest? What are you doing with your hands? Are they on your hips in defiance? Are you twisting them nervously in front of you, or are they comfortably placed? Look at your lower body. Are your knees stiffly locked or in a relaxed stance? What are you learning about the warmth you convey through your facial expression and posturing?

Exercise 5

In front of the mirror, try out a few gestures that you commonly display in your roles as spouse, student, teammate, nurse, and so on. Examine in the mirror what looks comfortable and natural for you.

Exercise 6

Now try shaking hands with your image. Where do your eyes focus? Do you smile when you look at your image? How does it feel to be receiving a handshake from you? Does it feel warm? What might make it warmer? Try it and see! Does your handshake look assertive?

Exercise 7

Obtain an instant camera with film and a large mirror. Sit in a chair and have another person take a picture of you. While it is developing, sit in front of the mirror and keep your eyes on your image in the mirror. What are your reactions to your posture in the chair? Is your slouch disengaging? Is your posture stiff and cold? Or is your position nicely aligned and at ease? What are your feet doing? Are your toes tucked under the chair ready to pounce, or are they placed in a natural line? Try several different positions and judge which look most relaxed and warm to you. Have your partner take a picture of you in this position. Compare the before and after and keep the snapshots to remind you of the differences. Switch roles and take your partner's picture.

Exercise 8

Talk to yourself out loud. How does your voice sound? Is it soft and warm? Try a different tone. Which one sounds warmer to you? You can also record your voice and listen to it.

Exercise 9

In the classroom find a partner with whom to work. Engage in a conversation with each other. The conversation can be about any topic you wish (such as a summer holiday or a movie). In addition to talking and listening to each other, observe what you like about each other's expressions of warmth.

After an exchange of 4 minutes, give each other feedback regarding how warmth was expressed. If there is just one way in which you think your partner could change in order to be warmer, and if your partner would like to hear your idea, make your suggestion. If a change is suggested to you, think about it and if you judge that it could make you come across as a warmer person, act on it.

Exercise 10

Assessing Your Warmth Skills.* This exercise will help you develop skills in assessing warmth and provide you with feedback on your own warmth skills.

---

*From Gerrard B, Boniface W, Love B: *Interpersonal skills for health professionals,* Reston, Va, 1980, Reston Publishing. *Continued*

Practicing Warmth—cont'd

Name of Person Rated: _____ **Name of Rater:** _____

1-Minute Intervals

Interviewer's behavior	1	2	3	4	5	6	7	8	9	10	Total
1. Maintains eye contact											
2. Faces interviewee "squarely"											
3. Leans forward slightly											
4. Open posture: arms											
5. Open posture: legs											
6. Relaxed posture											
7. Nods heads to show interest											
8. Smiles											
9. Jokes											
10. Warm voice tone											
11. Face shows interest, attentiveness											
12. Speech content shows interest											

WARMTH RATING SCALE

Instructions: Place a check mark (✔) in the box beside the rating that indicates how warm you felt the interviewer's behavior was.

4.0 ☐ Very good response: very warm
3.5 ☐
3.0 ☐ Good response: warm
2.5 ☐
2.0 ☐ Poor response: cool
1.5 ☐
1.0 ☐ Very poor response: cold

Figure 6-1 Warmth Content Analysis Sheet. (The exercise on Assessing Your Warmth Skills and the Warmth Content Analysis Sheet are taken from Gerrard B, Boniface W, Love B: *Interpersonal skills for health professionals,* Reston, Va, 1980, Reston Publishing Company.)

Work in groups of four for this exercise. During the week, all group members should make 10-minute videotapes of themselves individually interviewing clients. (If clients are not available, group members can interview each other about a topic of personal significance to the interviewee.)

Each small group meets by itself to view the videotapes. As the group members show their individual videotape to the group, the other members should use the Warmth Content Analysis Sheet (Figure 6-1) to check off the warmth behaviors they see the interviewer demonstrating.

Instructions for the Warmth Content Analysis Sheet

Each time you observe the interviewer demonstrate one of the warmth behaviors listed during a 1-minute interval, place a check mark in the appropriate column. For example, if during the first minute the interviewer smiles, has a warm voice tone, and leans slightly forward, place a check in the 1-minute column beside the appropriate rows. Even if the interviewer engages in a behavior more than once during a 1-minute interval, you still put only one check mark. During each interval you are only checking off whether a behavior occurs—how often it occurs doesn't matter. When a minute is up, move to the next "minute" column and check off any behaviors that occur during that minute interval. During each 1-minute interval you will be making a separate set of ratings. When the interview is over (or when 10 minutes are up), add up your check marks in each row and write the total in the last column.

At the end of the 10-minute interview, after all group members have totaled their scores for their Warmth Content Analysis Sheet, all members should use the Warmth Rating Scale (see Figure 6-1) to rate overall how warm they felt the interviewer's behavior was.

Note that these two scales measure different aspects of warmth. The content analysis sheet provides information on specific behaviors that occurred during the interview. The rating scale provides an overall assessment of the quality of warmth provided by the interviewer.

When the ratings are complete, group members should give each other feedback on their warmth scores; this feedback includes the overall warmth rating and the specific behaviors used to communicate warmth. As the group members complete their feedback, they should finish by telling the interviewer the one thing the interviewer did best to show warmth.

Repeat these steps with each group member until everyone has had a turn receiving feedback.

Exercise 11

Make your warmth assessment and care plan. At this point you have a lot of information about your warmth ability. List those areas where your warmth is strong and in keeping with how you wish to be. You might write something like this:

"Facial and body expression of warmth to others adequate when feeling inwardly calm, respected by the other person, and caught up in my work."

There may be situations when the expression of your warmth is less than you would like. You might write something like this:

"Diminished expression of facial warmth in situations when I'm expecting criticism. Absence of facial warmth (to the point of coldness) and absence of postural warmth (to the point of rigidity) when encountering an angry client because of fear of disapproval or dislike."

Pinpointing areas of concern helps you realize how specific and isolated the occasions for improvement are and directs you to develop a plan for improving.

Continued

Practicing Warmth—cont'd

Exercise 12

Look for ways to evaluate improvements in your expression of warmth. One of the most important barometers of your warmth gauge is your inner feelings. Are you feeling more relaxed and caring with clients and colleagues? Do you feel like you are expressing more affection and engaging more fully with others? Are your expressions of affection flowing more freely?

For an external evaluation, you can monitor the verbal and nonverbal feedback you get from your clients. Do your clients talk more, look at you more, ask questions of you, shift to a relaxing position in the chair, and indicate that they feel cared for by you?

You might wish to receive even more specifically detailed feedback about your warmth ability. One way to secure these comments is to ask a colleague to watch your interactions with clients and colleagues and to let you know those ways in which your warmth is conveyed and where you might improve.

Wit and Wisdom

Flowers leave fragrance in the hand that bestows them.

Filipino proverb

References

Baker C, Diekelmann N: Connecting conversations of caring: recalling the narrative to clinical practice, *Nurs Outlook* 42(2):65, 1994.

Carruth AK: Development and testing of the Caregiver Reciprocity Scale, *Nurs Res* 45(2):92, 1996.

Carver I: Healthcare with a human touch, *Nurs Spectrum* 8(18):7, 1998.

Cooper MC, Powell E: Technology and care in a bone marrow transplant unit: creating and assuaging vulnerability, *Holistic Nurs Pract* 12(4):57, July 1998.

Ekeren GV: Speaker's sourcebook II: quotes, stories, and anecdotes for every occasion, Englewood Cliffs, NJ, 1994, Prentice Hall.

Koopmeiners L et al: How healthcare professionals contribute to hope in patients with cancer, *Oncol Nurs Forum* 24(9):1507, 1997.

Knapp ML: *Essentials of nonverbal communication,* New York, 1980, Holt, Rinehart & Winston.

Levine DR, Adelman MB: *Beyond language: intercultural communication for English as a second language,* Englewood Cliffs, NJ, 1982, Prentice-Hall Regents.

Purtilo R: *Health professional and patient interaction,* ed 4, Philadelphia, 1990, WB Saunders.

Talton CW: Touch—of all kinds—is therapeutic, *Regist Nurs* 58(2):61, 1995.

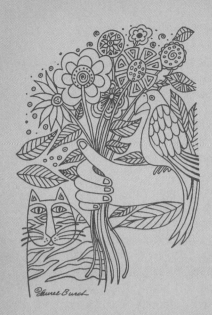

Respect

Unhappy is the man for whom his own mother has not made all other mothers venerable.

Italian proverb

OBJECTIVES

1. Discuss the benefits of respect in the relationships in health care.
2. Identify behaviors that demonstrate respect in relationships.

THE BENEFITS OF RESPECT

Respect is the communication of acceptance of the client's ideas, feelings, and experiences (Haber et al, 1997). When we show respect to our clients and colleagues we are sending them the message, "I value you. You are important to me." Together, warmth and respect form what Carl Rogers (1961) and his successors call unconditional positive regard. When helpers demonstrate they care in a non-possessive way, they transmit unconditional positive regard. This means accepting others for what they are, not on the condition that they behave in a certain way or possess special characteristics.

Receiving respect makes people feel important, cared for, and worthwhile. These examples illustrate such reactions. Your co-worker tells you: "I love going to my new physician. Besides being a good clinician, she makes me feel so important. She's on time for my appointments, her receptionist remembers my name, and she follows up on all my requests." Your neighbor tells you about her recent experience with the nursing staff on the unit where her husband is hospitalized: "The nurses are busy, of course, but they seem to have time to say 'hello' and pause for a few minutes to tell me something new about Jack. They never seem too busy for the little touches that make you feel so special. Not like the unit he was on before where they scowled if you asked for something and gave you the impression that they didn't have time for you."

In contrast, when people do not receive respect, they feel hurt and ignored. For example, a middle-aged woman talks about the health unit coordinator on a busy hospital unit: "She didn't even have the courtesy to raise her head to speak to me when I asked her where Dad's room was. I might as well not have been there." A nurse reports her frustration at the disrespect she encountered: "Boy, I'm glad I don't work there! When I came down to borrow some syringes the two nurses ignored me and kept on talking! It didn't even register that I was in a hurry and needed the stuff quickly." When people feel that they are not being treated with respect they feel angry and rejected.

Experience shows that there is a positive correlation between respect, warmth, empathy, and successful treatment outcomes in psychotherapy clients. Indirect evidence supports the notion that respect, in terms of access to the desired physician, provision of convenient clinics, and reduced waiting times for appointments, has a beneficial influence on client compliance with the therapeutic regimen.

SHOWING RESPECT TO YOUR CLIENTS

Respect is communicated principally by the ways helpers orient themselves toward, and work with, clients. It is respectful to understand and respond to clients' individual responses to grief and catastrophic illness (Bendiksen and Balk, 1998). Although respect starts as an attitude, this mental outlook needs to be translated into behavior in order to demonstrate respect. The behavior that demonstrates respect is acknowledgment.

 Moments of Connection...
Respect for the Sacred Relationships in Marriage

"I was the home health nurse for an elderly woman who was dying. Her husband was her primary caregiver. They had been married for more than 50 years and had always slept together. Now, however, the patient was sleeping in a hospital bed. One day the husband seemed more upset than usual. I asked him what was wrong and whether he needed more help. He began to cry and talked about missing her. I suggested he get into her bed with her and snuggle. He was afraid he would hurt her. I convinced him it would probably mean as much to her as it did to him. At the next visit she was comatose. He confided that he had gotten into bed with her the night before and slept all night with her. She had slept through the night without pain medication. He was so grateful I had made the suggestion."

Acknowledging Clients

It is not enough to feel respect for your clients. They will receive the message that you think they are important and worthwhile only if you deliver the message clearly and directly. The following list provides concrete actions you can take to show respect to your clients.

- Look at your client.
- Offer your undivided attention.
- Maintain eye contact.
- Smile if appropriate.
- Move toward the other person.
- Determine how the other person likes to be addressed.
- Call the client by name and introduce yourself.
- Make contact with a handshake or by gently touching the individual.

Acknowledgment means demonstrating your awareness of your clients as individuals. One nurse wrote about a touching experience with a man sitting in an intensive care waiting room across the hall from where she was struggling with paperwork. Seeing his sadness, she walked over to him, sat down, and asked if she could help. Receiving no response, she simply placed her hand on his and sat in silence with him. After a time of silence, he revealed that both his wife and his son had recently died and now he had been asked to donate his son's organs. The nurse told him she knew this was a difficult time for him and that she was there for him. After more silence, he told her he had made a decision, looked at her sadly, and left.

Simple gestures may communicate when words miss the mark (Taylor, 1994). Copp (1993) identified the waiting room as a place of "lost lessons" and comments that students of nursing could learn about the demonstration of caring by being sensitive to the "weary travelers" who have come long distances, the waiting relatives who feel unsure of how to care for the loved one at home, or the waiting friends or relatives who have put their own lives on hold to be there.

Showing respect involves using verbal and nonverbal skills. Looking at our clients or colleagues as they speak shows attention, but it is the quality of our facial expressions that reveals whether or not we are interested in what our clients or co-workers are saying.

In the United States, introductions are accompanied by a firm, brief handshake. This custom may not be the same in all countries from which clients or colleagues come. In some cultures handshaking is prolonged, and taking our hands away too quickly could be misinterpreted as rejection. Within reason, it is best to allow the patient to end the handshake.

In addition, after opening acknowledgments are made, there usually follows a period of "small talk," during which impersonal and trivial subjects (such as the weather) are discussed to break the ice. Some cultures prolong this period of discussion.

Establishing the Nature of the Contact

After you have acknowledged your client, several actions can convey respect at the outset of a new or ongoing client-nurse encounter.

For a first-time contact:

- Make it clear who you are and what your role is in the agency.
- Wear your name pin or identification badge.
- Ask what the other person needs or wants.
- Be clear about how you can be of help.
- Indicate how you will protect your client's confidentiality.

For an ongoing relationship:

- Ensure that the client recalls who you are and your role in the agency.
- Determine the client's needs at this point.
- Indicate that you recall details about the individual.
- Review the issue of confidentiality.
- Refrain from gossiping about other clients.
- If appropriate, suggest a referral so that the client will receive the required assistance.

As nurses we must remember that the most intensely private and personal moments of clients' lives are revealed in times of crisis and illness, whether in a hospital setting, an outpatient clinic, or the home. At the outset of a client-nurse relationship, we have a duty to tell clients of others with whom we are likely to share the information they give us, so that they understand the parameters of confidentiality in the agency. Some private information may need to be shared with other members of the health care team in developing a treatment plan. We are obliged to diligently protect the confidences of our clients unless required to reveal them by law, or unless our clients give us permission to share these details. Releasing the status of a client's condition to the news media or general public does not create liability exposure, but disclosing more detailed information or a photograph without the client's consent should be avoided. In health care facilities where there is public stigma, such as a psychiatric or drug abuse treatment center, even releasing a client's name would be an automatic invasion of privacy. Clients expect that the information they give will be kept strictly confidential. The need for disclosure should be carefully evaluated before sharing information. Maintaining confidentiality demonstrates respect for the rights of the individual (Erlen, 1998).

Although the following ethical guidelines for confidentiality were written for psychiatric nurse specialists, these principles are applicable guides in any situation where nurses are striving to respect clients by protecting their confidentiality:

- Keep all client records secure.
- Consider carefully the content to be entered into the record.
- Release information only with written consent and full discussion of the information to be shared, except when release is required by law.
- Use professional judgment regarding confidentiality when the client is a danger to self or others. Do not give the client a promise to keep secrets, and acknowledge that you will use your judgment about information shared that might indicate potential harm to the client or someone else.
- Use professional judgment deliberately when deciding how to maintain the confidentiality of a minor. The rights of the parent/guardian must also be considered.

- Disguise clinical material when used professionally for teaching and writing.
- Maintain confidentiality in consultation and peer review situations.
- Maintain anonymity of research subjects.
- Safeguard the confidentiality of the student in teaching/learning situations. (From the Colorado Society of Clinical Specialists in Psychiatric Nursing, 1990.)

Beware of inadvertent breaches of confidentiality. Consider where a report is given and where staff conversations are held or telephone calls are made. Do not use identifying client information in E-mail communication. Be aware of who may be looking at a computer screen with client data.

Establishing a Comfortable Climate

The following list describes the steps necessary to establish a comfortable environment for the patient:

- Indicate at the beginning how much time you have so that your client can gauge the length of the discussion and prepare for your leaving.
- Arrange to meet at another time if the allotted period is too brief for the content to be discussed.
- Ensure privacy before engaging in a discussion of confidential matters.
- Ensure that phones or other people do not interfere with your giving undivided attention to your client.
- Arrange the room so that no barrier, such as a desk, separates you and your client, and avoid standing over a person in a wheelchair.
- Ensure that the environment is comfortable by making space for your client, having a place for a coat and other personal belongings, and adjusting room temperature and lighting.
- Take care to be on time for appointments and try to avoid inconveniencing a client by switching appointments.
- If you are late or have to change an appointment time, explain the reason to your client so that it is clear the delay was unavoidable.

Promptness for appointments is important to Americans, and we consider it irresponsible to miss scheduled appointments. For Americans time is tangible, as is reflected by these phrases: "find time," "spend time," "waste time," "save time," or "kill time." Because clients from other cultures may proceed at a different pace than Americans and have different ways of perceiving, regulating, and dividing time, we may have to be creative about negotiating time customs around appointments. Clients from cultures with different values about time might have to learn about canceling and rescheduling appointments.

An aspect of mutuality is a sense of equality in the partnership. One nonverbal way to achieve an egalitarian relationship with clients is to arrange the seating so you are both at the same height. "Authority can be communicated by the height from which one person interacts with another. If one stands while the other sits, the former has subconsciously placed himself or herself in a position of authority. . . . Height is unwittingly used to project a submissive role onto a patient when he or she is confined to a bed, a treatment table, or a wheelchair" (Purtilo, 1990).

Terminating Contact

How nurses end their discussions with clients is just as important as other phases of the discussion. Following are guidelines for terminating the contact.

- If you have to leave early, prepare your client in advance.
- Summarize what you have discussed.
- Follow through with what you said you would do.
- Make notes of any points you want to remember for future contact.

For ongoing relationships:

- Prepare your client for discharge several visits before termination.
- Allow time and space for the client to talk about the feelings that termination may bring up.
- Express your thoughts and feelings about termination as a way of showing that you care.
- If you are going to be away for a limited period of time, make arrangements for client coverage and be sure to check with your client to make sure that these arrangements are suitable.

To maintain cost-effectiveness in American hospitals, length of stay is decreasing; clients are being discharged earlier. This limits the time for discharge planning, and the transition period from hospital to home is briefer and possibly not as smooth as it once was for clients. Nurses in some hospitals follow a callback system to check on clients at home after discharge for early problem solving. This kind of follow-up demonstrates a respect through a willingness to work with clients by being available and interested in their health care problems. Adopting the mutual problem solving approach is also respectful because it shows good faith in our clients' desire to use their own resources to take care of their health. Learning about issues of diversity to customize care demonstrates respect for the individual.

You can apply many of the above suggestions for showing respect to your colleagues, as well as to your clients. Being courteous, attentive, and mindful of the unique contribution each colleague makes to the total health care team approach are all ways of conveying respect to colleagues.

Attempts to overcome a language barrier with clients and families is another way of demonstrating respect. Check with the hospital's patient advocate or human resources department to identify employees who could serve as interpreters. AT&T Language Line Services can be purchased for over-the-phone interpretation of 140 languages, 24 hours a day, 7 days a week (call 1-800-752-0093 for information).

Being respectful embodies assertiveness. When we show respect we are granting the other person's right to be treated with dignity and consideration, while at the same time not ignoring our own needs to manage our time effectively and carry out the role for which we are qualified. Being respectful means acknowledging others' needs to be attended to, understood, and helped within the limits of nurses' abilities and time.

It is important that we, as nurses, understand the effect we can have on people in every single encounter. Being respectful means showing our finely tuned sensitivity to others with the full realization that we can affect their well-being. As nurses, we need to be aware of the power we have to make our clients and colleagues feel cared for, and, more importantly, to use that power consistently and with good intent. Respect for a client is part of nursing excellence. A study was conducted to examine how the coping behaviors of nurses whose own family of origin was dysfunctional helped build competent caring behaviors. It was concluded that the very behaviors that helped these nurses adapt to their own circumstances were valuable behaviors in fine tuning their sensitivity to clients and their families. One nurse identified her own drive to show clients and families respect because that was what she longed for as a child (Biering, 1998).

One factor that facilitates nurses' showing respect is a strong value that others have the right to be treated with regard for their feelings of worth. Nurses with less well-integrated values of human dignity might be less consistent in demonstrating their respect. If you find you are inconsistent in demonstrating respect, examine which of your values conflicts with being respectful in those situations. What is more powerful in influencing your behavior than your desire to be respectful?

Moments of Connection...
Respect in Quiet Moments

"I work in an out-patient chronic pain center. We needed a piece of equipment that was unavailable, so I went to the ICU to borrow the machine. The nurse told me I could take it from a room where a patient had just died. I went into the room, which was very quiet, with no sounds of talking family or life-sustaining equipment. I stood in the quiet and honored that person who had died, saying a silent prayer. We face sadness, horror, and death, but in this quiet moment I felt peace, respect, and honor for that person—I felt a connection."

Wit and Wisdom

Treasured Moments

I learn your respect
by the way that you
treat me.
I start to sense it
As soon as you
greet me.
Many things I have lost
to the ravages of illness.
Your respect brings comfort
In moments of stillness.

Copyright 1995 Julia W. Balzer Riley.

Think About It...
What, So What, and Now What?

Consider what you read about respect in relationships. How do you demonstrate respect in your relationships with clients, families, and staff?

What? . . . Write one thing you learned from this chapter.

So what? . . . How will this impact your nursing practice?

Now what? . . . How will you implement this new knowledge or skill?

THINK ABOUT IT

Practicing Respect

Exercise 1

Find a partner with whom to work. For the first part of this exercise one of you will talk and the other will listen, and then you will switch roles. When the speaker is talking, the task of the listener is to be blatantly disrespectful. For example, when you first come together, do not acknowledge the other person; give limited attention to the other person's concerns, and demonstrate rude behavior such as reading, looking at your mail, forgetting the other's name, or terminating the conversation abruptly. After 4 minutes, stop talking and discuss the interaction.

As the speaker: How did it feel to receive disrespectful communication?

As the listener: How did it feel to be disrespectful?

Share these feelings with each other as a way of learning about the negative effects of disrespect. Now switch roles so that each of you feels what it is like to be caught in a disrespectful encounter.

Exercise 2

For this exercise work in pairs, one person being the speaker, the other the listener. This time the listener is to show as much respect as possible throughout the interview, by exhibiting the respectful behaviors discussed earlier in the chapter.

After talking for several minutes, pause, and have the speaker give feedback to the listener on how it felt to receive respectful communication. Switch roles and repeat.

In the class as a whole, discuss what doing these exercises has taught you about the importance of respect in interpersonal relationships.

Exercise 3

In your social encounters for the next few days, try to focus on the respect and disrespect you receive from others you meet at work, in the stores, on the street, or in professional relationships. What specific behaviors make you feel worthwhile and which ones humiliate or anger you? In the receiving of respect, does it make any difference whether the relationship is a one-time encounter or an ongoing one? Compare your findings about respect and disrespect with your classmates.

Exercise 4

Consider the factors that prevent you from being as respectful as you would like. For example, you might use your clients' or colleagues' first names without first asking what they would like to be called. List the areas where you would like to improve your ways of conveying respect.

Exercise 5

Review the list of ethical guidelines for confidentiality developed by the Colorado Society of Clinical Specialists in Psychiatric Nursing (see pp. 114-115) and check to what extent your workplace institutes these regulations. What additional guidelines are employed in your unit? To what extent are clients' needs for confidentiality preserved? As a class, share the information from each of your units and learn about the variation in protection of confidentiality in the workplace.

Wit and Wisdom

When people bring us their problems,
they are often asking not for solutions, but for understanding.

Author unknown

References

Bendiksen R, Balk DE: The process of grieving as relearning and resocialization: toward an ethic of respect in caring, *Death Studies* 22(3):296, April-May 1998.

Biering P: "Codependency" a disease or the root of nursing excellence? *J Holistic Nurs* 16(3):320, Sept 1998.

Colorado Society of Clinical Specialists in Psychiatric Nursing: Ethical guidelines for confidentiality, *J Psychosocial Nurs* 28(3):43, 1990.

Copp LA: Teaching site: the waiting room, *J Professional Nurs* 9(1):1, 1993.

Erlen JA: The inadvertent breach of confidentiality, *Orthop Nurs* 17(2):7, 1998.

Haber J, Krainovich-Miller B, McMahon A, Price-Hoskins P: *Comprehensive psychiatric nursing,* St Louis, 1997, Mosby.

Purtilo R: *Health professional and patient interaction,* ed 4, Philadelphia, 1990, WB Saunders.

Rogers CR: *On becoming a person: a therapist's view of psychotherapy,* Boston, 1961, Houghton Mifflin.

Taylor C: Communicating without words: what's left unsaid can make a difference, *Nursing '94* June 30, 1994.

 Suggestion for Further Reading

Olsen DP: When the patient causes the problem: the effect of patient responsibility on the nurse-patient relationship . . . patient's responsibility for the clinical situation, *J Adv Pract* 26(3):515, 1997.

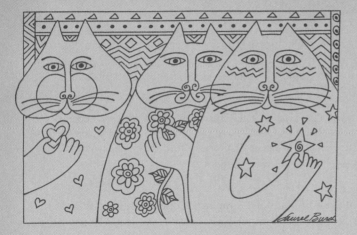

Genuineness

Rather a heart without words than words without heart.

Sudanese proverb

OBJECTIVES

1. Differentiate between genuine and non-genuine behavior.
2. Discuss the importance of being genuine with clients and colleagues.

BENEFITS OF GENUINENESS IN INTERPERSONAL RELATIONSHIPS

Commercial advertising makes millions of dollars claiming that products are "the real thing," "100% all natural," or "the original." If we say a person is genuine, what does it mean? Why is it important to be "your natural self" in human relationships?

Realness and congruence are the two synonyms Carl Rogers (1980), a pioneer in the study of communication, uses for genuineness, which he claims is the basis for the best communication. A fundamental feature of genuineness, in Rogers' view, is the presentation of your true thoughts and feelings, both verbally and nonverbally, to another person. It is not only the words you say or how you say them, but also your facial expression and body posture that make up genuineness. Being genuine means that you send the other person the real picture of you, not one distorted by being different from how you really think or feel. Genuineness is a spontaneous expression conveying an individual's experience (Haber et al, 1997).

In the classic children's story, *The Velveteen Rabbit* (Williams, 1975), toys talk about what it means to be real.

When a child loves you for a long, long time, not just to play with, but REALLY loves you, then you become real . . . by the time you are Real, most of your hair has been loved off, and your eyes drop out and you get loose in the joints and very shabby. But these things don't matter at all, because once you are Real you can't be ugly, except to people who don't understand.

To be real is to be yourself.

In the helping relationship with clients, and in mutually supportive relationships with colleagues in the workplace, being genuine does not mean impulsively dumping your reactions on others; it is aggressive to "hit" clients and colleagues with feelings, then "run." In a therapeutic relationship, genuinely presenting your thoughts and feelings to others can be done assertively and constructively.

As nurses, we make an important judgment call in deciding to genuinely share our inner thoughts and feelings with others. The literature advises nurses to be genuine "when it is appropriate to do so." Appropriateness is linked to whether our revelations will benefit our clients (or colleagues) and/or our relationships. Read carefully the counsel of Peck (1978) on dedication to the truth:

So the expression of opinions, feelings, ideas and even knowledge must be suppressed from time to time in . . . the course of human affairs. What rules, then, can one follow if one is dedicated to the truth? First, never speak a falsehood. Second, bear in mind that the act of withholding the truth is always potentially a lie, and that in each instance in which the truth is withheld a significant moral decision is required. Third, the decision to withhold the truth should never be based on personal needs, such as a need for power, a need to be liked, or a need to protect one's map from challenge. Fourth, and conversely, the decision to withhold the truth must always be based entirely upon the needs of the person or people from whom the truth is being withheld. Fifth, the assessment of another's needs is an act of responsibility which is so complex that it can only be executed wisely when one operates with genuine love for the other. Sixth, the primary factor in the assessment of another's needs is the assessment of that person's capacity to utilize the truth for his or her own spiritual growth. Finally, in assessing the capacity of another to utilize the truth for personal spiritual growth, it should be borne in mind that our tendency is generally to underestimate rather than overestimate this capacity.

We take a risk when we are genuine because sometimes genuineness involves expressing negative thoughts and confronting others with our reactions. When we are genuine, whether expressing negative or positive reactions, the message we give to our clients and colleagues is: "You are strong and worthy of my engaging fully with you." When we are genuine we give careful attention to listening to the other person. We extend ourselves and take the extra step to do the hard work of listening, and oppose the "inertia of laziness or the resistance of fear" (Peck, 1997). We enter into a relationship with a client with a fresh perspective, aware that information we have read or heard about a client could influence our ability to be genuine and see him or her as unique. Focusing on making your own observations of the client's behavior will help you to avoid stereotyping or stigmatizing a client (Sundeen et al, 1998).

Nurses who are genuine seem to their clients to mean exactly what the words they are saying connote, and their accompanying affective behavior matches their words (Arnold and Boggs, 1995). When our verbal message doesn't correspond with our facial expression, posture, tone of

Box 8-1	**Benefits of Nurse Genuineness for Clients and Colleagues**

Nurse Genuineness
- Speaks deep from within without apology
- Expresses thoughts, feelings, and experiences in the here and now
- Shows spontaneity
- Conveys openness

Benefits for Clients and Colleagues
- Feel free to express their true thoughts and emotions
- Develop a feeling of trust for the nurse
- Are provided with information they can use in the relationship here and now
- Can unwind in a relaxed atmosphere
- Enjoy a climate of realness

voice, and body language, clients and colleagues decode the disparity as two distinct and dissimilar messages. It is not hard to imagine that this incongruence of conflicting or mixed messages puts our credibility in question. Furthermore, it is unlikely that a meaningful relationship can ensue when our clients or colleagues doubt our trustworthiness.

As nurses we have expectations about the behaviors that accompany our assumed roles. Some of the behaviors expected of nurse-advocates are providing competent nursing care based on current standards, serving on committees to assure quality care, and coordinating all services used by clients in an attempt to restore, maintain, or promote health. The roles we assume have cultural, gender, and situational performance expectations. These rules are comforting because they provide guidelines for performance. Being genuine means remembering that roles are filled by individuals (Nuwayhid, 1984) with unique personalities, styles, and ideas. Realness means being free from the bonds of the role, and not hiding behind the façade of the role. Being a person and a nurse at the same time involves spontaneity; we cannot weigh every word we say or talk in scripts that seem planned or rigid. Congruence includes an openness to sharing without always waiting to be asked, to express directly what's going on inside us without distorting our messages.

Genuineness is a "what you see is what you get" phenomenon; people receiving your genuineness can trust you because they know you are not sending false signals or hiding something from them. It is this building of trust that is the most important reason for being genuine (Box 8-1). When we believe that we can count on others, we can start to relax in the relationship. We stop worrying about what others might really be thinking and feeling. The energy freed from worrying can be put into the relationship, both deepening and moving it in the direction for which it was established. Being genuine as a nurse is one major step in gaining credibility with clients and colleagues.

INCONGRUENCE

When there is a mismatch between nurses' experiences of their thoughts and feelings and their awareness, this incongruence is called denial of awareness or defensiveness (Rogers, 1961). You may notice, for example, that your colleague looks angry. She is stamping her foot, pointing her finger, becoming red in the face, and raising her voice in an accusatory way. However, when you suggest that she is angry she brushes it off and denies her obvious feelings.

When there is a mismatch between nurses' thoughts and feelings and their communication of this internal experience, it is usually thought of as falseness or deceit (Rogers, 1961). For example, if you disapprove of the new policy to join your unit with another unit in the hospital, but you hide your anger and tell your boss you think the merger is a good idea because you want to make a good impression on her, this is deceit.

If we pretend our thoughts and feelings are different from what they are, then we will say things that we do not believe in. If we act on thoughts and feelings that we do not have, we give people the wrong impression about us, leading them astray. In contrast, expressing our genuine thoughts and feelings about issues makes what we stand for crystal clear to our clients and colleagues. The research findings of Rogers (1957) and Shapiro, Krauss, and Truax (1969) establish that therapist genuineness has positive therapeutic outcomes.

Even if we can control our verbal communication when we are trying to deceive another about our true thoughts and feelings, our nonverbal cues can give us away (Knapp, 1980). Nonverbal behavior can reveal the information we are hiding or indicate that we are attempting to deceive without indicating specific information about the nature of the deception (Knapp, 1980). We are skilled at manipulating our facial expression and our posture to jibe with our verbal message, but the way we move our feet, legs, or hands can betray incongruence with our verbal message—that we are not genuine. Some of the feet and leg movements that might alert others to our incongruence are aggressive foot kicks, flirtatious leg displays, autoerotic or soothing leg squeezing, abortive restless flight movements, tense leg positions, frequent shifts of leg posture, and restless or repetitive leg and foot motions. Revealing hand movements might include digging our hands into our cheeks, tearing at our fingernails, or protectively holding our knees while smiling and looking pleasant. Knapp reports studies revealing that one of the reasons we may not expend much effort inhibiting or dissimulating feet and hand behavior is that, over the years, we have learned to disregard internal feedback, and we don't learn to control areas of our bodies in which we receive little external feedback (Knapp, 1980). Another way we might reveal our incongruence is by neglecting to include the nonverbal action that customarily would accompany the verbal message. Our omission is a signal to clients and colleagues that something is wrong (Box 8-2).

You may ask yourself how anyone could act any way but genuinely. Occasionally it feels risky to reveal what we think and feel to others. What if they do not agree? What if they think we are ignorant? Sometimes we fear that clients or colleagues might reject us if they do not like what we say. We worry that others might laugh at us, argue with us, put us down, or gossip about us. We may be threatened by fears that, if we are honest, a colleague might refuse to work with us or a client may request the services of another nurse.

When feeling vulnerable to rejection, we might modify what we think and feel to make ourselves more acceptable to others. We change in an attempt to give others what we think they wish to hear. In so doing, we begin the entanglement of giving a false impression of ourselves. If others are fooled, they expect the behavior to be repeated, and then we are trapped. We can continue to try to act falsely or we can confess. If our lack of authenticity is spotted, then others will stop trusting us, question our word, or ask for a second opinion. It is ironic that when we behave insincerely to avoid rejection, our worst fears of rejection can occur.

When we are genuine we have no guarantee that our clients or colleagues will accept us or agree with us, but they will usually be touched by our willingness to present ourselves as we are

Box 8-2	**Negative Effects of Nurse Incongruence for Clients and Colleagues**

Nurse Incongruence

- Puts up façade or pretense
- Withholds thoughts or experiences
- Is a mismatch between verbal and nonverbal messages
- Is rigid and contrived and looks as if it is scripted

Negative Effects On Clients and Colleagues

- Distrust for nurse
- Suspicion of nurse
- Strained, tense relationship
- Valuable information missing from the interchange
- Message is decoded as two distinct and dissimilar ones
- Confusion
- They may only believe the nonverbal message
- Credibility of the nurse is questioned
- It is difficult to maintain meaningful dialogue in the presence of mixed messages
- They don't feel they are talking to a real person
- They feel that the nurse is trying to impress rather than reach or connect with them

and our courage to risk rejection. Our honesty is reassuring and refreshing. If others choose to withdraw from a relationship with the genuine us, then they leave us with the satisfaction of knowing we have been honest with ourselves. Being genuine is being assertive; it is an action of standing up for our legitimate rights to express our point of view. When we are authentic our concept of ourselves as assertive nurses is strengthened.

BEING GENUINE WITH CLIENTS AND COLLEAGUES

The following examples illustrate how to be genuine with clients and colleagues.

For several days Joyce, a nurse, has been assigned to care for a client who has been flirtatious. He has asked for her phone number, looked at her seductively, and touched her, as if by accident, as frequently as possible.

Joyce's thoughts: She knows it is her responsibility to behave as a professional. Since the behavior has persisted, she knows she must deal with it. This young man is in a vulnerable position as a patient and needs to have access to a professional who can care for him. A social relationship might alter his ability to make his needs known.

Joyce's feelings: She is attracted to this client but sees his behavior as inappropriate and as a barrier to her giving him the care he needs. She is worried about embarrassing herself and him by behaving inappropriately.

The genuine communication is to explain to the client that her relationship with him is professional, not social.

Genuine response: "Our relationship here is that of client and nurse. I would ask you to think of it that way so I can provide you with the professional care you deserve."

This statement assertively communicates Joyce's thoughts and feelings in a way that is in keeping with her personal and professional values, making her trustworthy. If she had refrained from expressing her point of view, she would have communicated in a nonassertive and nongenuine way.

Nongenuine nonassertive response: "Well, I might go out with you . . . we'll see."

This message does not clarify the professional nature of the relationship. It might invite more of the flirtatious behavior Joyce wants to avoid.

Nongenuine aggressive response: "You guys are all the same. You're a chauvinist . . . you treat nurses like playthings. Cool it, mister! I have a job to do here."

This approach creates bad feelings and may interfere with Joyce's ability to give nursing care.

Consider this situation between colleagues in the workplace:

A fellow nurse tells you that she has told a client her husband could bring in their cat when he comes to visit his wife. She explains to you, "I thought it might cheer up Mrs. Kent; she misses her cat so much. You don't mind, do you?"

The truth is, you *do* mind. The hospital has strict rules about not having pets on the unit and you agree with them. You are in charge on this shift and you do not wish any negative repercussions from breaking the rules.

Your thoughts: It is unfair to show favoritism by breaking the rules for one client. Good reasons exist for excluding animals from the unit.

Your feelings: You are annoyed that your colleague has made this decision without consulting you, since you will bear the brunt of any consequences. You wish to correct your colleague without putting her down.

The genuine way to communicate would be to state your disagreement and disappointment and ask your colleague to reverse her mistake.

Genuine you: "It's unfortunate that you didn't discuss this issue with me first. I feel strongly that we shouldn't show favoritism and I agree with the health unit's rationale for restricting pets from the unit. Will you tell Mrs. Kent that she won't be able to have a visit with her cat while she's in the hospital?"

This assertion makes it clear to your colleague what you think and feel, and does so in a way that respects her feelings.

Nongenuine nonassertive you: "Gee, I don't think we should be allowing a cat on the unit, do you? I guess there's nothing we can do about it now."

By passively allowing the rule to be broken and not expressing your annoyance and opinions in a clear, direct way, you are denying the expression of your genuine reaction.

Nongenuine aggressive you: "You what? Well, forget it. Go and tell Mrs. Kent that you've made a mistake. Don't ever make that kind of decision without consulting me."

This angry outburst is incongruent with your desire to communicate respectfully with your colleagues.

Being genuine is an assertive act. In expressing our thoughts and feelings we need to take care that they are clear, direct, and respectful of the positions of others.

FACTORS INFLUENCING GENUINENESS

Our genuineness springs from three main sources: our self-confidence, our perception of others, and our environmental influences.

When our self-confidence is blossoming, we feel strong enough to risk revealing our true selves. When our self-confidence is withering, it is easier to try to impress others with what we think they want to hear in order to feel accepted and important. Self-confidence is not something we are born with, but we must nourish it. When we risk being authentic, we feel good about being true to our thoughts and feelings. This good feeling is translated into self-confidence.

When we perceive that others have power and influence over us, we might refrain from being authentically ourselves. If we decide that another person is smarter, more deserving, or more worthy, then we are more likely to show off for these people than relate to them in a way congruent with our thoughts and feelings. Learning to take charge and empowering ourselves to trust our own reactions will help us to perceive others as equals with whom we can dare to reveal our true thoughts and feelings.

Environmental variables also influence our ability to be genuine. In front of a large group, many of us might shy away from revealing our true thoughts and feelings. Limited time may prevent us from being genuine. If we know that expression of our thoughts and feelings could cause a reaction in others that would require more than the available time to work out, then we might wait for a better time to express ourselves genuinely.

In one study of patients' perceptions of nurses' knowledge and presence, nurses identify shortened hospital stays, paperwork, and time pressures as barriers to the development of relationships with patients. Both patients and nurses valued the "little things," such as using each other's names or remembering nicknames (Cohen et al, 1994).

To be congruent we need to be aware of our thoughts and feelings (Rogers, 1961). As we get to know ourselves better, expanded self-awareness builds and deepens our self-concept. This greater self-awareness is something we need to relate more genuinely to others (Rogers, 1980).

Wit and Wisdom

> *To be genuine,*
> *To be real,*
> *A thing of beauty*
> *No one can steal.*

Copyright 1995 Julia W. Balzer Riley.

HOW YOU CAN EVALUATE YOUR GENUINENESS

You are the most important judge of your genuineness. If you are behaving in ways that are true to your thoughts and feelings, then you will feel more relaxed and self-assured. The comfort that you feel derives in part from the freedom that comes from living in harmony with yourself. Being genuine protects your right to be integrated. In other words, being genuine is being respectful of yourself.

When you are authentic, it is likely that others will react positively by communicating with you, seeking out your trustworthy companionship, and, in turn, revealing their true feelings and thoughts.

Moments of Connection...
Genuine Grief for Real People

"Some of my sweetest experiences have been going to viewings and funerals of patients who have died. The family members share their grief and hug the nurses who cared for their loved ones. They know we cared with our hearts as well as with our hands and that they don't have to hide their emotions or act 'brave' with us. Although nurses don't go to every funeral of a patient who dies, there are some that give us closure and help us to remember that not all success is measured by patient outcomes. Sometimes success is the ability to connect at a level that is meaningful to the nurse and the patient and family."

Think About It...
What, So What, and Now What?

Consider what you read about what it means to be genuine and relate to the client as a unique individual. It takes courage and focus to be genuine and not to seal oneself off emotionally in the face of the demands of nursing.

What? . . . Write one thing you learned from this chapter.

So what? . . . How will this impact your nursing practice?

Now what? . . . How will you implement this new knowledge or skill?

THINK ABOUT IT

Practicing Genuineness

Exercise 1

For the next several days observe the genuineness in those you encounter daily. When you feel that others are genuine, stop and ask yourself what it is about their communication that makes you arrive at that conclusion. Conversely, when you assess that others' communication is insincere, determine what makes them untrustworthy. Was it what they said or the style in which it was delivered? Making these notations will help you discover more about genuineness and will expand your ability to examine your own authenticity.

After you have each done this exercise on your own, get together as a class and compare your findings about genuineness.

Exercise 2

Assess your reactions to being on the receiving end of genuine and nongenuine behavior. What are the differences in how you feel? Which feels better and why? What do your reactions tell you about how you would like to communicate with others?

In the classroom collate your various observations about your reactions to genuine and nongenuine behavior.

Exercise 3

Find a partner with whom to work. One of you will be the speaker and the other the listener.

As the speaker: Think about an emotionally laden situation that you can discuss. For this part of the exercise the speaker will attempt to be nongenuine: if you feel excited, you will downplay it; if you feel sad, you will minimize it; if you think you should keep the reins on your temper you will lose control. After 5 minutes of being unauthentic, stop your conversation.

As the listener: How did it feel to be on the receiving end of nongenuine behavior? What effects did it have on you? Give this feedback to your speaker.

Reverse roles so that each partner can be a nongenuine speaker. In the class as a whole, compare notes on what doing this exercise has taught you about genuineness.

Exercise 4

Continue working with the same partner, one taking the role of speaker, the other of listener. Reenact the same role play situation as in Exercise 3. This time the speaker will attempt to communicate in a genuine manner. As the listener, note your reactions to receiving genuine communication from your speaker, and offer your feedback. Reverse roles so that each of you has seen the picture from both sides.

In the process of giving and receiving authentic and false communication, you will have learned a lot about the importance of genuineness in interpersonal communication. In the class as a whole, compile what you are learning about genuine communication.

Exercise 5

In your day-to-day activities, notice when you are naturally and easily genuine and when you are untrue to yourself. After several days make note of the factors that make it easier for you to be

Continued

Practicing Genuineness—cont'd

genuine and those that make it more difficult. Assessing your genuineness in this way will make clear where you are congruent and where you need to work harder at being integrated.

Exercise 6

This exercise is the same as Exercise 5 except you observe your behavior at work. Note when you use your courage to be real and avoid hiding behind a professional façade. Observe when it is more difficult for you to be authentic about what you are thinking, feeling, or experiencing. What can you learn about your genuineness in relation to these situations? What information do you get about your genuineness or incongruence from the people in the situation?

After you have completed Exercises 5 and 6, ask yourself if there are any differences in your genuineness when you are on duty and when you are off. What does your answer tell you?

References

Arnold E, Boggs K: *Interpersonal relationships: professional communication skills for nurses,* Philadelphia, 1995, WB Saunders.

Cohen MZ et al: Knowledge and presence: accountability as described by nurses and surgical patients, *J Professional Nurs* 10(3):177, 1994.

Haber J, Krainovich-Miller B, McMahon A., Price-Hoskins P: *Comprehensive psychiatric nursing,* St Louis, 1997, Mosby.

Knapp ML: *Essentials of nonverbal communication,* New York, 1980, Holt, Rinehart & Winston.

Nuwayhid KA: Role function: theory and development. In Roy SC: *Introduction to nursing: an adaptation model,* ed 2, Englewood Cliffs, NJ, 1984, Prentice-Hall.

Peck MS: *The road less traveled and beyond:spiritual growth in an age of anxiety,* New York, 1997, Simon & Schuster.

Peck MS: *The road less traveled: a new psychology of love, traditional values and spiritual growth,* New York, 1978, Simon & Schuster.

Rogers CR: The necessary and sufficient conditions of therapeutic personality change, *J Consult Psychol* 21(2):95, 1957.

Rogers CR: *On becoming a person: a therapist's view of psychotherapy,* Boston, 1961, Houghton Mifflin.

Rogers CR: *A way of being,* Boston, 1980, Houghton Mifflin.

Shapiro JG, Krauss HH, Truax CB: Therapeutic conditions and disclosure beyond the therapeutic encounter, *J Counsel Psychol* 16(4):290, 1969.

Sundeen SJ et al: *Nurse-client interaction: implementing the nursing process,* St Louis, 1998, Mosby.

Williams M: *The velveteen rabbit,* New York, 1975, Avon Books.

Suggestion for Further Reading

Tindall JA: *Peer power workbook: becoming an effective peer helper and conflict mediator,* Muncie, Ind., 1994, Accelerated Development. Exercise on being genuine in Module IX.

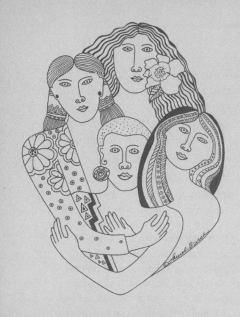

Empathy

Empathy is the single most revolutionary emotion I can think of.

Gloria Steinem

OBJECTIVES

1. Define empathy
2. Identify the preverbal, verbal, and nonverbal aspects of empathy
3. Discuss the benefits of empathy with clients and colleagues
4. Identify six steps to empathic communication

WHAT IS EMPATHY?

Empathy is the act of communicating to our fellow human beings that we understand how they are feeling and what makes them feel that way (Hogan, 1969). Empathy is the ability to "get inside another's skin" and subjectively feel with a client (Haber et al, 1997). Empathy is more complex than the other interpersonal communication behaviors you have mastered so far in this textbook. When we mentally put ourselves in the shoes of others and then verbally convey that we understand what it must be like to wear those shoes, we are being empathic. By the end of this chapter you will understand what empathy is and be able to explain its importance in interpersonal communication. A number of exercises will give you the opportunity to practice demonstrating empathy with supervised feedback. Empathy requires more rehearsal to ensure that it becomes integrated into your communication repertoire. The benefits of empathy for your clients and colleagues outweigh the investment of time that practicing empathy requires.

American psychologist Carl Rogers contributed immensely to the meaning and significance of empathy for helping professionals. He died in 1987 and, in honor of his gifts to us, his direct words are quoted to expand your understanding of the meaning of empathy. This passage is from his book, *A Way of Being* (1980).

An empathic way of being with another person has several facets. It means entering the private perceptual world of the other, and becoming thoroughly at home in it. It involves being sensitive, moment by moment, to the changing felt meanings which flow in this other person, to the fear or rage or tenderness or confusion or whatever he or she is experiencing. It means temporarily living in the other's life, moving about in it delicately without making judgments; it means sensing meanings of which he or she is scarcely aware, but not trying to uncover totally unconscious feelings, since this would be too threatening. It includes communicating your sensing of the person's world as you look with fresh and unfrightened eyes at the elements of which he or she is fearful. It means frequently checking with the person as to the accuracy of your sensing, and being guided by the responses you receive. You are a confident companion to the person in his or her inner world. By pointing to the possible meanings in the flow of another person's experiencing, you help the other to focus on this useful type of referent, to experience the meanings more fully, and to move forward in the experiencing.

A synonym for empathy is communicated understanding. When we are convinced that others fully understand us, without judging us for how we are feeling, questioning why we are reacting that way, or advising us to feel differently, we experience a wonderful sense of acceptance. The process of empathy involves the unconditional acceptance of the individual in need of help; judgments and evaluation of feelings are never offered (Pike, 1990).

This nonjudgmental reception from our fellow human beings is accompanied by feelings of relief and freedom. Once we know we have been understood and accepted, we do not have to struggle to get our point across, nor do we have to justify our reactions to others. When we receive empathic responses we can relax because we no longer fear being misunderstood or rejected. Acknowledgment of our feelings reassures us that we have a right to be who we are. We may wish to change, and we might change our feelings and reactions in the future, but there is nothing so accepting as having others verbally acknowledge that they understand our feelings.

Another skill associated with empathy is active listening. We can listen passively or actively. Listening passively includes attending nonverbally to our clients or colleagues with eye contact, head nodding, and verbally encouraging phrases such as "uh huh," "mm-hmm," "I see," "yeah," or "I hear you." It is easy to delude ourselves that when we listen passively we truly communicate that we understand; passive listening, however, does not include an actual articulation of others' feelings, so it lacks the conviction and reassurance of active listening. The receivers of passive listening have to assume, hope, or pretend that they are being understood. Active listening removes this guesswork; it specifically provides speakers with the knowledge that we know how they are feeling—and understand why. Receivers of active listening feel guaranteed that they have been understood.

Natural empathy is a basic human endowment, an intrinsic ability to understand the feelings of others. Natural empathy contrasts with clinical empathy, a tool or skill that is consciously and deliberately employed to achieve a therapeutic intervention (Pike, 1990). The goal of empathy is to aid in the establishment of a helping relationship. It is not empathy by itself that is beneficial, but the intention of the giver and the perception of the receiver.

If empathy is truly a curative factor, it must somehow be both communicated to, and received by, our clients; it is more than a state of mind or attitude. As a concept, empathy is a "value-neutral tool" that can be used for destructive or manipulative purposes. To be used in a therapeutic or curative way, it must be used to accept, confirm, and validate the total experiencing of others. It must be used with the intention of helping.

As nurses in the changing health care climate come to accept that the business and caring aspects of patient care must be linked, the value of patients' satisfaction with their caregivers becomes essential. Customer service has become another way to look at delivery of excellent patient care. Bell and Zemke (1990) identify empathy as one of five essential ingredients for service recovery when customer service has failed to meet expectations. Patten, in an article about therapeutic hospitality, concludes that "staff interaction skills correlate more highly with patient satisfaction than technical skills" (1994). She discusses the ancient practice of hospitality that has evolved into three levels of depth: public, private, and therapeutic. Therapeutic hospitality involves a high degree of intimacy with a deep personal connection that is therapeutic use of self. Empathy is an important part of this therapeutic use of self.

HOW TO COMMUNICATE EMPATHICALLY

Empathy includes the ability to reflect accurately and specifically in words what our clients or colleagues are experiencing, drawing on the nonverbal behaviors of warmth and genuineness.

Preverbal Aspects of Empathy

In her review of empathy, Pike (1990) summarizes the literature on the mental processes of empathy before the response becomes verbal. Empathy is not total transportation into the world of another, with the self being lost in the process. "While there is momentary abandonment, the empathizer never loses sight of her own separateness; she is always aware that the feelings of the other are not her own." Clinical, therapeutic empathy is not subjective. After experiencing the private world of their clients, nurses achieve objectivity by tuning into their situation. While they understand what the clients' situations feel like, nurses feel tension and discomfort, which prompt them to action. The empathy is transformed into verbal connection with the client for the purpose of being helpful (Pike, 1990). This mental shifting requires flexible ego boundaries. Nurses shift from their world into that of their clients, and then back to a processing part of their mind where they confirm knowledge of their clients' feelings and develop a plan of what to say or do that will be in the clients' best interests.

Verbal Aspects of Empathy

The verbal part of the skill of empathy is reflecting to your clients or colleagues your understanding of their feelings and the reasons for their emotional reaction. The goal is to offer a verbal reflection that is accurate, with no exaggeration or minimizing of what you are being told. Ideally, the feeling words you use match what the speaker intended; the nuance and strength of the feeling need to be expressed. Your reflection of the rationale for the speaker's feelings specifically needs to be what the speaker intended. The two qualities of verbal empathy that have just been described are accuracy and specificity. It is, however, unrealistic to think that after knowing a client a short time that you can always meet these goals. Later you will read about a technique to check out the accuracy of your reflection.

Being empathic does not mean repeating verbatim what others have told you. Parroting only irritates speakers, implying that you have not really processed or understood their situation and subsequent reaction. When you respond empathically you should choose your own words and respond in your own style, yet still be accurate and specific. The following example illustrates how you can accomplish this.

A young patient who has been married for only 6 months has just been told that she has cervical polyps. As she talks, you notice her brow is furrowed, her eyes are glistening, and she hesitantly says, "Can you tell me . . . what I mean is . . . I really love my husband . . . and will these polyps . . . I mean, I hope I can still make love with my husband?"

You pick up several reactions from this young woman. Her stammering and tremulous speech suggest that she is embarrassed about discussing sex. You can most therapeutically deal with her embarrassment by responding in a forthright manner. Her main concern, however, is being able to continue a normal sexual relationship with her husband. You reply empathically with:

"I can see that you are worried that these polyps you have on your cervix will interfere with your sex life with your husband. Let me explain about cervical polyps. I think I can reassure you."

This response meets the criteria for accuracy and specificity. Your use of the word *worry* accurately reflects the verbal and nonverbal clues you picked up. Reflecting the word *fear* would have been too strong, and using the words *wonder about* or *curious about* (the sexual relationship) would have been too neutral for the emotional level she expressed. The feeling words the listener reflects must mirror the nuance the speaker is conveying (Box 9-1). The phrase, "that these polyps you have on your cervix will interfere with your sex life with your husband," specifically captures the reason for her worries.

By using your own words and phrasing things in your own style, you avoid parroting and clearly demonstrate that you have understood her worries. Having felt your understanding before you begin the lesson on polyps will make your client more receptive to the teaching. Hearing understanding from another person gives a sense of relief and leads us to believe that what the listener has to say is trustworthy.

Box 9-1	Choosing the "Right" Empathic Word

Here is a list of adjectives describing feelings of being afraid, tense, or worried (Hills and Coffey, 1982), giving you an idea of the range from which you can select the feeling word or phrase.

Afraid	Disturbed	In a cold sweat	Quivering	Troubled
Agonizing	Dreading	Jittery	Restless	Uncomfortable
Alarmed	Fearful	Jumpy	Scared	Uneasy
Anxious	Fidgety	Nervous	Shaken	Wary
Apprehensive	Frightened	On edge	Tense	Worried
Cautious	Hesitant	Panicky, Petrified	Terrified	
Concerned	Ill-at-ease	Quaking	Trembling	

Nonverbal Aspects of Empathy

The nonverbal features of empathy are equally as important as the verbal aspects. A singer might correctly enunciate each word of a song yet miss expressing the mood of the piece; thus the song lacks vitality. Just as an audience would feel unconnected hearing an emotionless song, so disengagement can occur when empathy is delivered without warmth and genuineness. It is possible to articulate a technically perfect empathic response that meets the criteria for accuracy and specificity but does not positively affect the other person.

It is only when your empathy is accompanied by warmth and genuineness that the true caring and concern for what your clients and colleagues are experiencing comes across. However, it is important not to overplay your warmth to the point that your intended empathy seems gushy or too sympathetic. Being empathic is not equivalent to feeling sorry for another person. Empathy is free of the judgment of condolence; it is a value-free message showing that you understand the other person's point of view. The warmth you express with empathy should convey genuine caring, not honeyed insincerity. An example might clarify the necessity for an appropriate level of warmth:

Your colleague has just told you that she is pregnant and therefore upset because she will not be able to continue her full-time nursing career. If you were to smother her with a hug or become overly solicitous, your attentive warmth would come across as sympathy. Sympathy focuses on your own feelings rather than the other person's. Being too warm in this situation might suggest that you think her predicament is hopeless. Empathy with the appropriate warmth, such as a concerned facial expression and a gentle touch on the shoulder, tells your colleague that you understand; now she can approach her problem unburdened by your overprotectiveness.

It is essential to feel genuine empathy for others. If you decidedly do not care about how your clients or colleagues are feeling, then using an empathic response would be incongruent. Even if the verbal part of your empathy is correct, your nonverbal behavior can give away your lack of caring. Usually our expression of warmth is diminished when we do not genuinely care about the feelings of others. This diminished warmth may speak louder than the words of our empathic response, so that the message received is one of not caring. The mixed message of caring words and uncaring gestures can only be confusing for clients and colleagues.

In summary, empathic communication requires a specific and accurate verbal response accompanied by genuine caring and a receivable level of warmth. These attributes of empathy must be packaged in your own natural style of speaking. In an essay on the lived experience of cancer, a woman writes: "The capacity to recognize and respond to others' distress may be a deep and permeating element of a person's characterological build. For those endowed with the capacity for empathy, its absence is perhaps as unimaginable as color blindness or tone deafness are to those endowed with color perception and perfect pitch" (Charon, 1995).

Wit and Wisdom

Through wisdom a house is built and by understanding it prospers.

Finnish proverb

Moments of Connection...
In the Right Place at the Right Time

"When I was a student nurse, I was in my pediatric rotation and had the opportunity to work with a 17-year-old single mom of a child with a cleft palate and lip. The child was 3 months old and her mom wasn't visiting or holding the child. I asked to speak with her and asked some questions about the baby. I have faint but visible scars from cleft lip surgery, and the mother felt able to talk to me. She told me her parents said the baby was born that way because of the mother's sin of being a single mother. When I asked what she wanted for her child, she replied, to grow up and be able to sing. I was filled with a warm feeling and told her that her little girl could do anything, that I sing . . . and then I sang a little song for her. I told her that God doesn't punish. Sometimes you have to search for the blessing. After our talk, the mother began to visit the baby and take part in feeding and caring for the baby. The baby underwent corrective surgery 3 months later.

WHEN TO COMMUNICATE EMPATHICALLY

Rogers (1980) asserts that there are situations in which empathy has the highest priority of the attitudinal elements, making for growth-promoting human relationships. When clients or colleagues are hurting, confused, troubled, anxious, alienated, terrified, doubtful of self-worth, or uncertain as to identity, then understanding is called for.

Every day nurses encounter clients who are in this kind of pain. Nurses have many opportunities to know their clients' most intimate thoughts and feelings. Dicers (1990) warns that empathy is intrusive and cautions nurses to ask themselves, "How far should I go?" She reminds us that there is a tremendous amount of freedom related to empathy. "Empathy is a concept by intellection, like 'justice' or 'love,' as opposed to a concept by observation like 'chair' or 'bottle.' Such concepts are seductive because there is so much room to play around." It is the clinical and ethical judgment of nurses that guides them when to verbalize empathy. Follow this advice: "Whenever we enter another's mind, we must remember to be respectful and take off our shoes."

Nurses know that we have as much responsibility for clients' need to express their feelings on intimate matters as we do for their privacy. We might ask ourselves: "How much should I encourage my clients to tell me? Am I at risk of crossing the line between facilitating communication (with my empathy) and aggressively pursuing their private reactions?" Being empathic can be helpful or invading, and as nurses we must strive to use our empathic skills with the intent of being helpful.

Dicers (1990) argues: "Empathy is a dangerous notion if it is thought to be mindless, experiential, existential connectedness. Surely every patient encounter requires an openness to the other's experience, for only when one is open to another can one perceive needs. But surely, not every encounter will benefit from empathy; some will require theory, or applied experience, or even translation or consultation."

THE BENEFITS OF EMPATHY FOR CLIENTS AND COLLEAGUES

Clients and colleagues share their thoughts and feelings for the purpose of being understood, but often it is uncomfortable for them to reveal themselves. As listeners, it is not good enough for us to understand how our clients or colleagues feel without verbally sharing that empathic understanding explicitly and accurately. Communicating our understanding has many payoffs for clients and colleagues, and for our relationships with them. In a survey of more than one million clients, "Staff sensitivity to the inconvenience that health problems and hospitalization cause" was found to be the top consideration in a person's decision to recommend a health care facility (*AHA News,* 1997).

Empathy increases the feeling of being connected with another human. This positive feeling of belonging helps reduce negative feelings of loneliness and isolation. Although it has often been said that we are ultimately alone in our journey through life, empathy is a bridge that connects us, giving confidence and hope. A health care administrator compared the changes and stress created by downsizing in health care organizations to climbing a mountain. He commented that he felt the desire to say, "Let's stay close" (Clark, 1996). For colleagues to know they are not alone, to respond to each other with empathy, provides comfort in times of challenging transitions. The knowledge that you understand your clients and colleagues helps them continue on their way, secure that their feelings have been acknowledged as normal human reactions. The companionship you extend through empathy, however brief the engagement, creates a human bond that adds to your clients' or colleagues' personal strength. Rogers (1980) puts it simply: empathy dissolves alienation. Consider, too, the family caregivers with whom you come in contact, those giving full-time care in the home or keeping long vigils at the client's bedside in the hospital. These have been called the hidden patients. Look for signs of exhaustion due to "lack of personal time . . ." problems with "care recipient's behavior," and demands of their own employment (Ostwald, 1997).

Curry (1994) offers these statements of the empathic experience:

When I look at patients, I see friends and loved ones on a battlefield of illness and pain. I see my father in the face of a man who can no longer speak because of a brain tumor, but whose eyes still shine when his grandchildren visit. I feel my mother's hands in those of an elderly woman whose memories have been claimed by Alzheimer's disease. I see my brother in the gaunt young man with AIDS whose family and friends have deserted him.

Empathy can contribute to feelings of increased self-esteem for those to whom you extend it. The fact that you take the time to listen, hear, process, and reflect what your clients or colleagues say makes them feel important. Caring enough to show that you understand makes others feel significant and worthwhile.

It is impossible to accurately sense the perceptual world of another person unless you value that person and his or her world, unless you, in some sense, care. Hence, the message comes through to the recipient that 'this other person trusts me, thinks I'm worthwhile. Perhaps I am worth something. Perhaps I could value myself. Perhaps I could care for myself' (Rogers, 1980).

Your empathy demonstrates that you accept how your clients and colleagues feel and contributes to their trust that you genuinely accept them as they are.

Your withholding of judgment or advice enhances this trust. Empathy is a skill you can use to deepen your relationships with clients and colleagues. When you unconditionally accept others as they present themselves, they can relax and feel free to be who they really are. Your acceptance helps your clients and colleagues to accept themselves.

A consequence of empathic understanding is that others feel valued, cared for, and accepted as the people that they are (Rogers, 1980). " . . . True empathy is always free of any evaluative or diagnostic quality. The recipient perceives this with some surprise: 'If I am not being judged, perhaps I am not so evil or abnormal as I have thought. Perhaps I don't have to judge myself so harshly.' Thus, the possibility of self-acceptance is gradually increased." Finely tuned understanding by others gives us all a sense of personhood and identity. Rogers shows us that empathy gives that needed confirmation.

Your empathy can help your clients and colleagues move on to new feelings and change their behavior.

The acceptance your empathy offers frees your clients and colleagues from having to defend or rationalize their feelings; as a result, they are able to experience alternative reactions, freed of any clinging to defensive feelings. When you do not give empathy, then your clients and colleagues feel they have to justify their feelings.

Receiving empathy helps them to be open and move on to different ways of experiencing. It is perfectly natural for people to change their reactions as new information is processed or if old data are reexamined in a new light. The acceptance you provide through empathy helps your clients and colleagues to remain flexible enough to move to a new awareness. Just as being stuck in one place retards self-growth, so having the option to move on or change fosters self-growth.

In our personal and professional lives we are often in relationships with individuals who must make difficult decisions about their lives. More often than not, that person does not need more information, certainly does not need a judgmental presence, probably does not want the answer or the decision taken from them. What they require from us is real presence that will support them, empower them, and give them the courage to decide (Marsden, 1990).

In some instances your empathic reflection will help your clients or colleagues to comprehend more fully how they are reacting.

Hearing your reflection of their feelings may increase their self-awareness. Not only is this enlightenment satisfying, but it can widen their perspective of their whole situation. Consider this example:

You have just empathically reflected to Douglas, one of your clients in the diabetic clinic, that it just doesn't seem fair that he has diabetes while his roommate's good health allows him the freedom to eat and drink what he wants and to party until all hours of the night.

Douglas: "Yes, you're right! That's exactly how I'm feeling. I hadn't realized how it gripes me that he isn't restricted like I am. I guess I think about the medical expenses that I have, not to mention the time-consuming treatments I have to put up with. No wonder I'm so short with him when I see him having a good time. In fact, sometimes I'm quite miserable to him . . . I'd better not let this situation get out of hand."

Your empathic response increased Douglas' understanding of his behavior and himself. The literature on empathy reports that psychotherapists high in empathy, genuineness, and warmth elicit greater self-exploration in their clients (Shapiro, Krauss, and Truax, 1969).

The insight and expanded self-awareness sometimes triggered by your empathic responses can help your clients and colleagues decide how to handle a situation.

Knowing how one feels about a situation and how those feelings are affecting one's way of coping with a situation are important factors in deciding on a course of action. Good problem solvers take their own feelings into account when confronted with any situation, problem, or issue. Having knowledge of our feelings helps us determine whether the situation should be changed in order for us to feel better, or whether it is more appropriate to change our feelings and outlook on the situation so as to feel better adjusted.

In the previous situation, now that Douglas is aware of his feelings about his roommate's health and freedom, he can use this self-awareness to help him handle his situation. Douglas could consider all kinds of possibilities. In terms of changing his situation, he could get a roommate with a chronic illness so that he would not have to deal with these feelings, or he could brainstorm ways to minimize the restrictions in his diabetic regimen so that he could live his life more naturally. In terms of changing his feelings, he could stop comparing himself to others and augment his gratefulness for the lifestyle he can lead, or he could be hostile toward his roommate until the roommate can no longer tolerate it and decides either to leave or to fight back.

The knowledge of their feelings and awareness of the impact these emotions have on their situation as provided by your empathic response can give clients and colleagues more information with which to generate effective solutions. Your empathy can inspire clients to listen to themselves more empathically.

The non-evaluative and acceptant quality of the empathic climate enables clients to take a prizing, caring attitude toward themselves (Rogers, 1980). Being understood makes it possible for clients to listen with greater empathy for their own reaction to what they are experiencing. This greater understanding and prizing of themselves can open new facets of experience, which bring into their awareness a more accurate picture of themselves and a clearer self-concept.

Research has demonstrated that empathy accounts for improvement in psychotherapy clients (Cartwright-Dymond and Lerner, 1963; Truax et al, 1966; Shapiro, Krauss, and Truax, 1969). Rogers (1980) cites research from the late 1960s and the early 1970s that, in the study of therapist/client relationships, clients who eventually show more therapeutic change (in comparison with those who show less) receive more of the therapist's qualities of empathic understanding, acceptance, and genuineness. Therapist empathy was the most significant of factors distinguished between more and less effective therapists (Lafferty, Beutler, and Crago, 1989). Lafferty's research findings support the significance of the therapist's empathy in effective psychotherapy. Patients of more effective therapists felt more understood than patients of less effective therapists.

It can be argued that empathic responses from nurses can enhance healing and well-being in all clients. Illness and hospitalization cause fear, dependency, and upheaval in clients' daily lifestyle and relationships, whether the health problem is surgical, medical, obstetrical, or psychiatric. Empathic nurses can tune into their clients' feelings in a helpful way. Empathy in health professionals can improve the success of the complete clinical problem-solving process and enhance client compliance because of increased client involvement.

Practicing nurses confirm the benefits of empathy in the workplace. A survey of 67 nurses at an ambulatory surgery conference reports that empathic communication can add joy to the workplace and keep workers enthusiastic about their jobs (Box 9-2).

Box 9-2	**Empathy Is Not Just for Students**

The following are responses from nurses at an ambulatory surgical nursing conference to these two questions:
  1. What would you be willing to do to add joy to the workplace?
  2. What behavior would you like from colleagues to help you look forward to coming to work?

Of the workshop participants, 98% chose to respond in writing to these questions. Answers have been combined since the lists were similar.

- Smile
- Acknowledge each other
- Focus on the positive
- Say thanks for a job well done
- Pitch in and help
- Avoid listening to gossip
- Avoid gossiping
- Tell people how negative comments affect me
- Listen more
- Beware of interrupting colleagues when unnecessary
- Be pleasant even if I'm not a morning person
- Be more positive with new colleagues
- Not complain about changes in the schedule
- End morning report on a humorous or positive note
- Appreciate and accept differences in colleagues
- Send notes to say thank you

Copyright 1995 Julia W. Balzer Riley.

BENEFITS OF BEING EMPATHIC FOR THE NURSE

The preceding points clarify how your use of empathy can benefit your clients and colleagues. Empathy also benefits you, the nurse. The most obvious payoff is the warm feeling of compassion you get when you help others feel understood and accepted. Knowing that you have taken the opportunity to make your clients or colleagues feel better provides immense satisfaction and can augment your feelings of competence.

Nurses want to collect enough information from their clients to accurately assess their concerns and develop the best nursing care plan for treating their health problems. When clients feel accepted, their trust will allow them to open up and provide the information necessary to accurately assess their situation. Having sufficient data to make a correct nursing diagnosis is the first and most important step in the systematic problem-solving approach to nursing care. Whether clients' problems are physical, emotional, or a combination, empathy can be used to acquire sufficient and comprehensive data.

Empathy can be shown at all stages of the problem-solving process. When developing a plan of care, it is essential to determine how your clients feel about the proposed treatment schedule and to empathically reflect your understanding. Acknowledging clients' reactions to treatment regimes, and where possible, adjusting plans accordingly, are likely to increase compliance behavior.

As a nurse you will want to know if your nursing care has been effective. There are many objective measures of success, but one important yardstick is how your clients feel about their treatment outcome. Clients may be sufficiently satisfied and wish to terminate treatment, or they may

Moments of Connection...
When the Tears Come

"I'm a pediatric nurse, a sensitive one. I have always worried about crying too much. I was with a small child who was dying. I was able to do all the nursing care for her, but all the while, tears ran down my face. After she died, the family came to me and told me how much it meant to them that I cried because they did not have a sense of caring from other staff. I no longer worry about my sensitivity to my work!"

want to try an alternative plan to achieve their desired outcome. Clients' input has implications for how to proceed in the client-nurse relationship. Showing empathy lets your clients know that you understand and acknowledge their evaluation of progress.

In your working relationships, being empathic with colleagues augments cohesiveness. Showing that you understand your colleagues not only makes working together more enjoyable, but it helps you prevent and work out difficulties in your relationships.

Ebersole, writing as editor of *Geriatric Nursing* (1993), and having just returned from a 4-month world tour, observes that the world at home got along fine without her. She concludes that "we will all disappear from the lives of those that love us, and they will grieve but will go on. . . . We should define our responsibilities and our pleasures . . . how little it takes to make some people laugh and sing and how much others of us are able to grumble about." When she returned home she found a new awareness of the gift of existence and concluded that some people choose to be impatient while others choose to be patient with others.

OVERCOMING BLOCKS TO EMPATHY

Clearly, empathy has many positive benefits for our clients and colleagues and also has a payoff for us. If we are not conveying empathy at appropriate opportunities in our relationships with clients and colleagues, then it is likely we are relating in ways that are not helpful. What are we doing if we are not communicating empathically when it is warranted, and how can we switch to communication that is more caring?

Several activities might result in our failing to express empathy. Be careful not to judge clients or colleagues. If we question the appropriateness of their thoughts and feelings, then we effectively shut off the unbiased and accepting part of our communication. Being truly empathic means being able to put aside our opinions and tune into how the other person is feeling.

It would be absurd to suggest that we should cancel all judgmental thoughts. It is only human to have preferences and opinions. We are taught throughout life to be selective in our tastes for food, art, clothing, and people. This discriminating behavior is second nature to most of us. We use it every moment of our lives in deciding what to wear in the morning, selecting a strategy to solve a work problem, or choosing what to eat for dinner. It is highly likely that most of us cannot turn off this judgmental thinking in our interpersonal relationships.

Most times our judgments serve a useful purpose in our lives. However, when we verbalize our judgments about other people's thoughts and feelings, we only make them feel criticized and labeled. Clients and colleagues can feel shut out when they have been judged; they may think that acceptance is impossible. Being judged engenders feelings of rejection and defensiveness. Clients and colleagues tend either to withdraw from us to protect themselves from further pronouncements or to aggressively challenge us in an attempt to defend their thoughts and feelings. Whichever response occurs, the verbalized judgment has served to arrest any therapeutic communication.

The following example illustrates the benefits of empathic communication and the detrimental effects of being judgmental.

Your client has come to the physician's office for a colposcopy examination and says to you:

"I'm scared to death of this copos . . . how do you say it? . . . exam . . . the whole idea spooks me. . . ."

You could respond with:

Non-empathic you: "Oh! It's nothing to worry about. You'll be just fine. Lots of our patients have one. By the way, it's pronounced colposcopy."

This response negates your client's fear and belittles her anxieties about this unknown procedure. It is unlikely that this response would make your client feel that you took her feelings seriously. Instead of feeling acknowledged, she likely feels misunderstood and put down by your judgmental reply.

You might have responded with:

Empathic you: "The thought of having a colposcopy exam is really frightening for you. What can I do to relieve some of your fears about it?"

This empathic opening acknowledges her fears about the test, and the accompanying offer demonstrates your desire to help alleviate her fears. It is likely that she will be relieved by this nonjudgmental acceptance of her feelings. Your empathy makes it safe for her to trust you further by asking questions or revealing more of her feelings. Whereas a judgmental response closes lines of communication, an empathic reply opens them.

An example involving a colleague may illustrate further.

You have just started the evening shift on your unit after several days off and the nurse manager on the day shift remarks:

"Boy! Count yourself lucky to have been off for the past 3 days. It's been like a zoo here! We've had two deaths and five admissions, and we've been short-staffed the whole time. I'm wiped out!"

You could respond with:

Non-empathic you: "Well, the time passes quickly when you're busy, and after all, you've been trained to handle hectic situations . . . that's what they pay us for."

This reply undermines your colleague's feelings. Your judgment that she should be coping dismisses her feelings as inconsequential and even inappropriate. A noncaring response like this would only serve to make your colleague hostile and defensive, and would certainly lead to a strained working relationship.

A more understanding response would be:

Empathic you: "No wonder you're tired. It sounds like you've had to handle three times the usual workload with the admissions and deaths . . . and all without enough help. When's your well-deserved time off coming?"

This empathic reply makes your colleague feel she has been heard. There is no doubt that you understand what she has been coping with while you were away. All she desired was for you to register how it has been for her. This response fits that bill.

When we judge others we effectively ignore their point of view. Instead we shift the focus to what we feel or think and emphasize our perspective. As helping professionals we feel sad when we hurt clients or colleagues by ignoring or upstaging them. The desire to communicate in a caring way is motivation to use empathy. Being non-judgmentally empathic requires the desire to show acceptance and the will to focus and concentrate on the concerns of others.

Remember this idea so that as a helping professional you can take care of yourself. It takes courage to be empathic (Pike, 1990). "Entering into a patient's world as if it were his own exposes the nurse to the possibility of pain, despair, anger, fear and hopelessness. Courage is especially called for in situations where the nurse is powerless to cure the patient's distress, pain, or suffering."

The greater the maturity and experience of nurses, the greater is their usable vault of knowledge, attitudes, and learning for enhancing their empathy. But all nurses need one important key to open the vault: access to feelings (Pike, 1990).

Empathy is assertive because it takes into account others' thoughts and feelings and protects your rights to communicate in a caring way. It is responsible to be empathic because it ensures that your clients feel acknowledged enough to engage in all aspects of the nursing process.

SIX STEPS TO COMMUNICATING MORE EMPATHICALLY

How can we nurture our ability to reliably convey empathy on a consistent basis? The following guidelines are based on a systematic problem-solving approach. If you truly want to be empathic, then these six steps will be helpful.

1. *Clear your head of distracting agendas.* In your busy life you will have many thoughts going through your head, such as personal worries, pressure from expanding work, or perhaps feelings of discomfort related to talking with a client or colleague. To the extent that you can put these aside, do so. If you are able to focus on the person you are with, you will streamline communication. Paying attention to other speakers increases the chances that you will deal with their situation more thoroughly and more effectively. Listening empathically means not having to return time and time again to get complete information, and that means one less item on your long list of things to do. Teach yourself to concentrate (Raudsepp, 1990).
2. *Remind yourself to focus on your speaker.* Remember that your priority is to listen and hear your clients or colleagues so that you can verbally convey your understanding. Remind yourself that your purpose is to tune in to what a speaker is saying. Some people find that a physical gesture, such as removing their glasses or adopting a definite listening stance, reminds them to focus. "Don't interrupt," reminds Raudsepp (1990).
3. *Attend to your clients' and colleagues' verbal and nonverbal messages.* Hear the words that speakers are using to describe how they are feeling, and the reasons for their reaction. Look for what your speakers are also saying nonverbally. Take in the whole message that your clients and colleagues are sending you.
4. *Ask yourself "What does this person want me to hear?"* Attempt to pick out the most important message being delivered. What is the predominant theme? Is anguish the strongest feeling?

Is joy the prevailing emotion? Your answer should be what the speaker wants you to hear, and that very seed is the embryo for your empathic response.

5. *Convey an empathic response.* Verbally reflect the speaker's feelings and the reason for them, ensuring that your response meets the criteria for accuracy and specificity. Pay attention to your nonverbal communication. Convey the amount of warmth you deem appropriate and ensure that the expression is congruent with your intentions to be understanding and accepting.

6. *Check to see if your empathic response was effective.* The purpose of being empathic is to make others feel relieved (that we understand them) and cared for (by our genuine interest in their situation). Check it out. Do the speakers nod their head? Do they smile or tell you in other ways that they are delighted you have understood them? Do they visibly relax by letting go of tension or by engaging you in further conversation? These clues will inform you that you have been successful.

If your attempt to be empathic has missed the mark, a speaker will let you know in several ways. More assertive clients or colleagues will tell you outright: "No, that's not quite how I'm feeling. . . . It's more like this . . ." Others may just slowly withdraw from opening up any more with you. It is acceptable most times to explicitly ask your speaker if your empathy is on target. Questions like, "Is that how you are feeling?" or, "Have I understood how it is for you?" are effective.

WHEN TO CONVEY EMPATHY

It is helpful to be empathic any time people share their thoughts and feelings with you. An empathic reply can be used on its own or with another message or communication strategy. For example, empathy can be used with:

Statements: "You feel frustrated because the clinic is not open in the evenings when it would be more convenient for you to come and have your blood pressure checked. There have been several other requests for extended hours, so I will raise this issue with our office manager." In addition to knowing your plan to follow up on such a complaint, it is reassuring for a client to have you acknowledge the situation and the feelings related to it.

Questions: "Yes, I can see that you are pretty excited about being discharged from the hospital earlier than you had expected. Have you had time to arrange for your babysitter to start earlier and give you a hand with your toddler and your new baby?" Your empathic beginning potentiates the effect of your concern for your client's discharge plans.

Alternate Points of View: "You feel pretty adamant that your pack-a-day smoking habit won't harm your health, since your grandfather smoked and lived to be 95. I have a different way of looking at smoking, since I've recently known several clients who have died of lung cancer. The statistics do indicate a high positive correlation between smoking and lung cancer." Most clients and colleagues hear our side of an argument if we give equal recognition to their point of view.

Explanations: "Being moved to a semiprivate room has really upset you and you feel that your privacy has been invaded. Switching rooms truly was our last alternative. We need a single room to carry out isolation techniques for an infectious client in order to protect everyone on the unit." By first acknowledging your clients' feelings, you can help pave the way for acceptance of your decision.

Invitations for more information:

With a client: "You're worried about the sharp pains in your kidney area. Have you had any other unusual signs and symptoms lately?"

With a colleague: "From your point of view our new charting system is cumbersome and pretty frustrating. Do you have any suggestions for streamlining the recording of our nurses' notes?" Most people engage more fully in our request for additional information when they hear that we understand what they have already told us.

Missing opportunities to convey empathy can create a gulf in which speakers feel ignored by listeners. When we do not hear others, a new struggle is created for them. They are disappointed at not being understood and in turn either withdraw with wounded feelings or fight to convince us of their feelings. When empathy is not offered, our clients and colleagues feel cheated, frustrated, and ignored. Including empathy with other communication strategies lets our clients and colleagues know beyond a doubt that they have been heard and understood.

In any therapeutic relationship it is important that our partners feel cared for. Client-nurse relationships are ones in which we have established ourselves as helpers. That label means that we acknowledge and make public our desire to support others. Empathy is one concrete way to show our caring.

Sometimes when stress levels are high we get lost in our own concerns and forget that our colleagues have concerns of their own. Simple acts help get us back on track.

Wit and Wisdom

As One Chronologically Gifted Nurse Said to the Other

After you've been at this a while,
It's hard to stay classy and have some style.
We see life's road bumpy,
Talk tacky and grumpy,
Fix me please, with thanks and a smile.

Sometimes we are lacking in energy
And with each other, we get finicky.
We remember and smile,
Thank each other, that's style.
Our spirits are raised, that's synergy.

Copyright 1995 Julia W. Balzer Riley.

Think About It...
What, So What, and Now What?

Consider what you read about empathy in relationships. How do you demonstrate empathy in your relationships with clients, families, and staff? Does it seem to come naturally to you or will you need to give special attention to slowing down and considering the other person's life view?

What? . . . Write one thing you learned from this chapter.

So what? . . . How will this impact your nursing practice?

Now what? . . . How will you implement this new knowledge or skill?

THINK ABOUT IT

Practicing Being Empathic

Exercise 1

This exercise provides you with several hypothetical situations in which clients or colleagues express thoughts and feelings to you. On your own, write down an empathic response to each of the examples. Remember to meet the criteria of being accurate and specific.

After you have written your initial empathic response, critique it and suggest alternative ways of phrasing your first try to make it more empathic. In your improved response, try to convey complete understanding and phrase it in your natural way of speaking.

Example 1

A nurse colleague says: "I'm not going to be able to get through that job interview with Mrs. Jones for the position of assistant head nurse. I just know I'll be so uptight that I'll blow it like I did the last time."

First attempt at empathy: "You're feeling pretty nervous about that interview."

Critique: This reply lacks specificity. Including a reference to the fact that it is a job interview would have acknowledged the importance of the event for your colleague. Referring to the reason for her worry about the interview would have made a more complete and accurate empathy response.

Suggested alternative: "You're feeling pretty nervous about your job interview for the assistant head position and worried that you might botch it like you feel you have before."

Example 2

A client says: "My first child is retarded. I'd like to have another child . . . but . . . what if that child turns out to be retarded as well?"

First attempt at empathy: "Yeah, it is a big chance to take, isn't it—getting pregnant, I mean."

Critique: This is more of an opinion than an empathic response, and it might feed into her worry. Being more accurate by including a reference to her feelings would make this reply more empathic. Verbalizing her reasons would meet the criteria for specificity.

Suggested alternative: "You have mixed feelings about having another child. On the one hand you'd like another baby, but you're frightened that you may have another mentally impaired child."

Example 3

A client tells you: "I didn't have to take any pain medication last night for my injured back . . . and I slept right through the night. It was the first good sleep I've had in four nights."

First attempt at empathy: "That's great! I'm glad you're sleeping better!"

Critique: This statement is more a judgment than a reflection of the client's feelings. The implied feelings are relief (at not having to take the medication) and joy (at sleeping well). These feelings, and the reasons for them, need to be included to make the response empathic.

Suggested alternative: "Boy! What a relief for you to have been comfortable enough to do without your pain medication, and you look overjoyed that you slept so well."

Now it is your turn! For each of the following situations attempt a written empathic response. Then critique your attempt and suggest how it could be improved.

Continued

Practicing Being Empathic—cont'd

Example 4

A client on unit 2 says to you: "I don't know what to do. My wife is a patient on unit 3 . . . she's just had another small stroke and I don't know how to help her."

Your first attempt at empathy:

Your critique:

Your suggestions for improvement:

Example 5

A client says to you: "My husband died a year ago. It's been the longest and saddest year of my life."

Your first attempt at empathy:

Your critique:

Your suggestions for improvement:

Example 6

A client says to you: "I had a real scare today. My chest x-ray has a spot on it and my doctor has called in a specialist to see what it is. I'm so worried because she told me that cancer can't be ruled out until I've had further tests."

Your first attempt at empathy:

Your critique:

Your suggestions for improvement:

Example 7

A newly hired nurse colleague says to you: "Things are just beginning to fall in place for me since I moved here. I now have a nice place to live in . . . and a reasonable rent. I'm starting to make some friends and beginning to feel comfortable here working on the unit."

Your first attempt at empathy:

Your critique:

Your suggestions for improvement:

Example 8

An 18-year-old client says to you: "I never thought I could be HIV-positive. I'm not gay. I don't use drugs. I've only had sex with one person. My life is over."

Your first attempt at empathy:

Your critique:

Your suggested alternative:

Example 9

A colleague says: "I'm really fed up with having to run all the way down the hall to answer the telephone on evenings when there's no health unit coordinator. Last night it rang five times when I was trying to give out medications at the other end of the unit. Each time I had to lock up my med cart and hurry back to the nurses' station. It's a waste of time and I can't put up with this inconvenience any more."

Your first attempt at empathy:

Continued

Practicing Being Empathic—cont'd

Your critique:

Your suggested alternative:

Example 10

A client is looking forlorn and says: "Oh! I'm just so blue today. I miss my little boy so much . . . he's only 4 . . . I just talked to him on the phone. He wants to know when I'm coming home. I told him I don't know. I will sure be glad when I can go home and be with him again."

Your first attempt at empathy:

Your critique:

Your suggested alternative:

After you have completed the preceding examples on your own, get together with the rest of your class and compare different responses. It will be interesting to see how many different ways an empathic response can be phrased and still meet the criteria of accuracy, specificity, naturalness, warmth, and genuineness.

Exercise 2

This exercise gives you the chance to experience the differences between passive and active listening. Find a partner with whom to work. One of you will be the speaker and the other the listener. The speaker will talk on any subject about which she has strong feelings.

In the first part of the exercise the listener will listen passively, and in the second part she will listen actively. For the first part of this exercise the listener will display attentive nonverbal listening and will offer encouraging responses such as "uh huh," "yes," "I see," and the like. Continue with Part One of this exercise for 4 minutes and then proceed to Part Two.

In the second part the speaker will proceed as she did in Part One. This time the listener will listen actively by responding with empathic statements at every appropriate opportunity. Proceed with this second part of the exercise for 4 minutes.

After completing Parts One and Two, answer the following questions.

As speaker: What differences did you notice between passive receiving and active listening?

As listener: What differences did you notice between listening passively and listening actively?

Switch roles so that each partner will have the chance to both give and receive passively and actively. Then, together as a class, pool all the ideas you have gleaned about empathy from doing this exercise.

Exercise 3

In the next few days observe how others listen to you. Note how you feel when you receive passive listening in contrast to active listening during your conversations with people in your day-to-day activities. What have you learned about empathy from your observations?

Exercise 4

Over the next week, attempt to make an empathic reflection each time others express their thoughts and feelings to you. Try these empathic responses with your grocer, your landlady, the person beside you on the bus, your children, your neighbors—everyone you encounter. This exercise is hard work, but it will provide you with extensive practice in being empathic.

Highly empathic people are socially perceptive to a wide range of personal cues and appear to have an awareness of the impression they make on others. What do you notice about your effect on others when you are empathic? How do others behave when you are empathic with them?

After you have completed this exercise, ask yourself what it has taught you about empathy. Compare your findings with those of your colleagues in your class.

Exercise 5

Take some of the most commonly felt emotions (such as sadness, fear, anxiety, joy, or anger) and for each emotion make a list of the range of words that have similar meanings. Divide the class into small groups and ask each group to take one of the concepts. Have a contest to discover which group will come up with the most synonyms for its feeling concept. Afterwards, compile the lists from all the groups and make copies for all the students. These references will be handy in the future when you are searching for just the right word.

Exercise 6

This exercise gives you a chance to receive supervised feedback on your ability to be empathic. Work in groups of four. One will take the role of speaker, one the role of listener, and the other two will be observers. The speaker will choose a topic about which she has strong feelings. The listener's task is to demonstrate empathic listening to what the speaker has to say during a conversation lasting 4 minutes. The observers will use the Empathy Rating Scale (Box 9-3) to evaluate the speaker's ability to be empathic. Tape recorders or video monitors, if available, provide a valuable asset for self-observation.

Roles should be rotated so that each person in the group has the chance to be speaker, listener, and observer.

The information on the Empathy Rating Scale you will receive as listener will outline your strengths and areas where you need to improve in your ability to communicate empathically. For example, the Empathy Rating Scale may draw your attention to the fact that you neglect to include the rationale for the speaker's feelings, even though you meet the criteria for accuracy, warmth, naturalness, and genuineness. This exercise can be repeated at intervals after practicing empathy so that over time you can see the pattern of improvement.

Box 9-3	Empathy Rating Scale

Response #	Accuracy: matched intensity?	Specificity: rationale included?	Naturalness: own words?	Warmth: verbal? nonverbal?	Genuineness: interest & caring conveyed?
1					
2					
3					
4					
5					
6					
7					

Criteria for Empathy Rating Scale

1. *Accuracy:* Does the intensity of the listener's words match the speaker's intended message?
2. *Specificity:* Does the listener include the rationale for the speaker's feelings?
3. *Naturalness:* Does the listener avoid parroting? Does the listener reflect the speaker's message in a naturally worded style?
4. *Warmth:* Does the listener convey verbal and nonverbal warmth with an empathic response?
5. *Genuineness:* Does the listener convey interest and caring about what the speaker is saying?

Wit and Wisdom

The pen of the tongue should be dipped in the ink of the heart.

Native American proverb

References

Bell CR, Zemke R: *Service breakdown—the road to recovery, in service wisdom,* Minneapolis, 1990, Lakewood Books.

Cartwright-Dymond R, Lerner B: Empathy, need to change and improvement with psychotherapy, *J Consult Psychol* 27(2):138, 1963.

Charon R: Connections that heal, *Sec Opin* 2(1):38, July 1995.

Clark WL: Being there, *Hosp Health Netw* 70(22):28, November 1996.

Curry MC: Nurse Week tribute: what it takes to be a nurse, *Nursing '94* 24(5):33, 1994.

Dicers D: Response to: on the nature and place of empathy in clinical nursing practice, *J Professional Nurs* 6(4):240, 1990.

Ebersole P: Gifts of the moment, *Geriatr Nurse* 14(6):285, 1993.

Haber J, Krainovich-Miller B, McMahon A, Price-Hoskins, P: *Comprehensive psychiatric nursing,* St Louis, 1997, Mosby.

Hills M, Coffey M: On delivering care: an interpersonal skills training manual for nurses, Unpublished manual, 1982.

Hogan R: Development of an empathy scale, *J Consult Clin Psychol* 33(3):307, 1969.

Lafferty P, Beutler LE, Crago M: Differences between more and less effective psychotherapists: a study of select therapist variables, *J Consult Clin Psychol* 57(1):76, 1989.

Marsden C: Real presence, *Heart Lung* 19(5):540, 1990.

Ostwald SK: Caregiver exhaustion: caring for the hidden patients, *Adv Pract Nurs Q* 3(2):29, 1997.

Patten CS: Understanding hospitality, *Nurs Manag* 25(3):80A, 1994.

Pike AW: On the nature and place of empathy in clinical nursing practice, *J Profess Nurs* 6(4):135, 1990.

Raudsepp E: Seven ways to cure communication breakdowns, *Nursing '90* 20(4):132, 1990.

Rogers CR: *A way of being,* Boston, 1980, Houghton Mifflin.

Shapiro JG, Krauss HH, Truax CB: Therapeutic conditions and disclosure beyond the therapeutic encounter, *J Counsel Psychol* 16(4):290, 1969.

Survey: Empathy key to patient satisfaction, *Am Hosp Assoc News* 33(3):5, January 27, 1997.

Truax CB et al: Therapist empathy, genuineness, and warmth and patient therapeutic outcome, *J Consult Psychol* 30(5):395, 1966.

 ## Suggestions for Further Reading

Bennett JA: Caring in the time of AIDS: the importance of empathy, *Nurs Admin Q* 17(2):46, 1993.

Byrne G, Heyman R: Understanding nurses' communication with patients in accident and emergency departments using a symbolic interactionist perspective, *J Adv Nurs* 26(1):93, 1997.

Gibbons MA: Listening to the lived experience of loss, *Pediatr Nurs* 19(6)597, 1993.
Examines the need to be "heard" and how active listening can move us toward understanding.

Morse JM, Proctor A: Maintaining patient endurance: the comfort work of trauma nurses, *Clin Nurs Res* 7(3):250, August 1998.
Offers specific descriptions of the patterns of speech, touch, and postures of nurses in emergency situations.

Proffitt C, Byrne M: Predicting loneliness in the hospitalized elderly: what are the risk factors? *Geriatr Nurs* 14(6):311, 1993.
This article includes a definition of loneliness and strategies to prevent loneliness.

Raudonis BM: The meaning and impact of empathic relationships in hospice nursing, *Cancer Nurs* 16(4):304, 1993.
A naturalistic field study focused on the meaning and impact of empathic relationships with hospice clients.

Roberts KT: Helping older adults find serenity, *Geriatr Nurs* 14(6):317, 1993.
This article includes characteristics of the serene person and potential nursing interventions to promote serenity.

Rolls J: Employee communications has a change of heart, *Human Resources* 38(10):132, 1993.
Strategies for empathic communication in restructuring the organization.

Shearer R, Davidhizar R: Loneliness and the spouse of the geriatric patient, *Geriatr Nurs* 14(6):307, 1993.
Guidelines are given to assess and intervene in loneliness in the spouse.

Stotland E et al: *Empathy, fantasy and helping,* Beverly Hills, Calif, 1978, Sage Publications.
For nurses who have become interested in empathy, this book will broaden their knowledge of the subject. This text is a summary of experimental studies of empathy; it is not a "how to" book. It is clearly written and expands the reader's awareness of issues in measuring empathy.

Summers C: *Inspirations for caregivers,* Mount Shasta, Calif, 1993, Commune-A-Key Publishing.
This is a book of quotes by well-known caregivers on the subject of service.

Tindall JA: *Peer power: strategies for the professional leader, becoming an effective peer helper and conflict mediator,* Muncie, Ind., 1994, Accelerated Development.
Includes exercises on empathy.

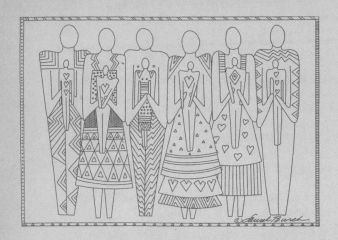

Self-Disclosure

Loving is scary, because when you permit yourself to be known, you expose yourself not only to a lover's balm, but also to a hater's bombs! When he knows you, he knows just where to plant them for maximum effect.

S.M. Jourard

OBJECTIVES

1. Define self-disclosure in the helping relationship.
2. Identify guidelines for appropriate self-disclosure by the nurse.
3. Distinguish between helpful and non-helpful disclosures in selected clinical scenarios.

Self-disclosure is another interpersonal communication behavior that you can use to show your clients and colleagues you understand them. By the end of this chapter you will understand what is meant by self-disclosure and appreciate how this skill can be used to advantage in your relationships with clients and colleagues. You will have a chance to enhance your self-disclosing skills in the exercises at the end of this chapter.

Moments of Connection...
My Mother Had Cancer, Too

"When my mother was terminally ill in a nursing home, I was torn between sympathy for her and embarrassment. As a nurse daughter, my mother's complaints caused me to worry that staff would isolate her. I wished she could be a 'good, compliant patient,' even though I understood her behavior was a reaction to fear. A nurse took me aside, put her hand on my arm and said: 'My mother died of cancer a year ago. Your mother is a lovely lady and we will take good care of her.' That nurse sharing herself helped me to know she understood my pain and my mother's."

SELF-DISCLOSURE IN PERSONAL AND PROFESSIONAL RELATIONSHIPS

Disclose means to "un" close or to open up. To self-disclose, then, means to open up our "self" to others. When we self-disclose, we reveal our thoughts and feelings and make known to others some of our personal experiences. Throughout your life you have used self-disclosure to let others know about you in order to develop a closer relationship.

Self-disclosures can take any number of forms: complaining, boasting, gossiping, expressing political or religious views, and sharing endearments, secrets, or dreams. In social relationships self-disclosures are traded back and forth until the partners establish a mutually agreed upon plateau. Intimate relationships are characterized by more private revelations than those shared between superficial acquaintances. The give-and-take of self-disclosing can occur with or without formal spoken rules. A specific request for deeper closeness, or an observed withdrawal of the usual pattern of sharing, influences the relationship to readjust the established level of intimacy. ". . . Nursing is inherently characterized by the desire to be connected to others at a very basic level of human significance . . . in milestone events of birth, death, illness, and growth in the lives of those for whom we care . . ." (Drew, 1997). Nurses are moved to offer self-disclosure where the need for connectedness "transcends theoretical connections. Sharing . . . for the sake of connection and to give the interaction life, meaning and depth" (Drew, 1997). An example of useful information to share with a client with chronic illness and family members is chronic sorrow. A nurse daughter describes it as ". . . a type of lurking presence that periodically engulfs the life of an individual experiencing chronic illness or disability . . . it is an intermittent, bearable sadness that is interspersed with periods of joy and satisfaction" (Rosenberg, 1998). To understand this experience as distinguished from the acute grief of traumatic injury or the chronic despair with depression can be helpful in listening to clients' shared experience of lifestyle changes.

GUIDELINES FOR SELF-DISCLOSING IN THE HELPING RELATIONSHIP

Client-nurse relationships demand special considerations for the use of self-disclosure. A helping relationship is established for the benefit of the client; in other words, this is a client-centered relationship. It follows that anything you reveal about yourself—your thoughts, feelings, and experiences—should be revealed for the benefit of your clients. You need to consider the why, what, when, and how of self-disclosing with your clients.

Why Nurses Should Use Self-Disclosure With Clients

Whereas in a social relationship you might self-disclose to allow others to understand you better, the opposite is true in the professional client-nurse relationship. Self-disclosure is a skill that you can use to show clients how much you understand them because of your similar thoughts, feelings, or experiences, and to increase their comfort with the interaction. When inquiring about breast self-examination practices, for example, a nurse might remark, "Sometimes, as busy as I am, I have difficulty remembering if I examined my breasts that month. Do you have trouble remembering?" The client then feels free to agree. This allows the nurse to introduce information about self-exam reminder systems. The intent of a self-disclosure is to be empathic—to show that you really understand your clients because you have walked a similar path. An effective self-disclosure can transmit all the benefits of empathic responses outlined in the previous chapter.

Because self-disclosure is a sharing of your personal self with your clients, it can deepen the bond between you. While still within the parameters of a professional helping relationship, your self-disclosure lets your clients know that you are a normal human being.

What Nurses Should Reveal to Clients in Self-Disclosures

As nurses we have to use our judgment about specifically what we will reveal to clients. Two questions to answer before self-disclosing are: "Is what I am planning to reveal likely to demonstrate to my clients that I understand them?" and, "Do I feel comfortable (safe from repercussions and embarrassment; legally and morally secure) about revealing this information to my clients?" Both questions should receive a solid affirmative response before you self-disclose.

When you self-disclose, it is important to set up a client-wins/nurse-wins situation. If your clients win, your self-disclosure makes them feel understood. If you win, you feel good that you have been skillful in making your clients feel better. If your clients lose, it is because your self-disclosure is irrelevant so that they are distracted from their major issue and left feeling misunderstood. If you lose, it is because your self-disclosure leaves you feeling uncomfortably exposed or embarrassed.

When Nurses Should Use Self-Disclosure With Clients

The purpose of a therapeutic self-disclosure is to let your clients know that they have been understood. Self-disclosure augments an empathic reply and deepens the trust between you. When you wish to increase your level of understanding and strengthen that trust, and you feel comfortable revealing the content of your self-disclosure, then self-disclosure would be the right choice.

Bateson, a noted anthropologist, wrote a book of stories of reflections on her experience in many cultures (1994). "Our species thinks in metaphor and learns through stories." Human beings can join and communicate and learn in spite of profound differences. As we meet people we have never met before, in situations we've never faced, as we try to apply communication skills to real people in real crises we must, "improvise responsibly and with love." This "quality of improvisation characterizes more and more lives today, lived in uncertainty, full of the inklings of alternatives." Consider as you struggle to choose communication techniques, to say just the right thing, disclose just the right incident and amount of detail, to be helpful without being self-absorbed. Rarely is it possible to study all the instructions to a game before beginning to play, or to memorize the manual before turning on the computer. We can carry on the process of learning in everything we do. Ambiguity is the warp of life, not something to be eliminated . . . we . . . learn to savor the vertigo of doing without answers or . . . making do . . . as we face difficult situations. We are called to join in a dance whose steps must be learned along the way, so it is important to attend and respond . . . . Even in uncertainty, we are responsible for our steps.

I remember my first communication course in a diploma nursing school, taught from a simplistic text. It all seemed so obvious when I was seventeen. Not until years later did I realize clear communication takes work, and the skills to achieve it are anything but obvious. Take these skills and tools you read about here and practice as much as you can and with serious intent to learn. Communication is a part of your journey and may cause great pain and joy in your personal and professional life as you learn from experience.

How to Self-Disclose in the Helping Relationship

To successfully implement a helpful self-disclosure, you need to follow all the guidelines for conveying empathy outlined in the previous chapter. Here is a concise list of those steps:

1. Clear your head of distracting agendas.
2. Remind yourself to focus on the speaker.
3. Attend to your clients' (and colleagues') verbal and nonverbal messages.
4. Ask yourself: "What does this person want me to hear?"
5. Convey empathy, beginning with an empathic response followed by a self-disclosure. It is usually better to self-disclose after you have conveyed an empathic response. Using an em-

Moments of Connection...
Out of Our Struggle, We Offer Others Our Comfort

"Although I have always known my career was in the Lord's hands, it wasn't until the past 10 years that I realized that my own struggles could help me offer comfort to patients in our chronic pain clinic. My spouse had a kidney transplant and bilateral hip replacements. My mother had fibromyalgia and posttraumatic stress, and had become depressed and inactive. I recently had a herniated disc with two previous epidural steroid injections. My husband is doing fantastic despite his physical trials. My mother is goal-setting and moving off the couch. I am able to calm anxious patients through my experience of epidurals and surgery. I have made a great recovery both spiritually and physically. Through adversity, comfort and connections can heal."

> **Box 10-1**   **Recommendations for Sharing of Self in Geriatric Practice**
>
> - Understand that the connection is dynamic. The client likes and trusts the nurse who shares. The perception of the nurse as a real person helps establish the helping relationship. One nurse shared an interest in pottery with the wife of a resident. This topic provided a nonthreatening common ground that established the foundation for the nurse to help the wife cope and grieve.
> - Remember that nurses control how much information they want to share. Nurses who use this technique learn how to let the client get to know them without the burden of high levels of intimacy.
> - The nurse's sharing of self may help decrease the client's level of anxiety and decrease the stress of illness and treatment.
> - Although an intuitive sharing of self can be useful, consider the value of self-disclosure as a pre-planned intervention chosen with a therapeutic goal in mind.
> - Reminiscence is enhanced in elders when they are encouraged to share about specific events. Nurses can speak of personal holiday traditions and question clients about theirs.

Modified from Nowak KB, Wandel JC: The sharing of self in geriatric clinical practice: case report and analysis, *Geriatr Nurs* 19(1):34-37, 1998.

pathic response first keeps the focus on others before shifting it to yourself. Your self-disclosure enhances and augments your empathic reflection. Beginning with an empathic response and following up with a self-disclosure deepens other people's convictions that they have been understood. As with empathy, the final step is:

6. Check to see if your empathic response and self-disclosure were effective.

In short, the steps for implementing self-disclosure are the following:

1. Listen.
2. Reply with empathy.
3. Self-disclose.
4. Check it out.

You may find you begin to see life as a collection of experiences—your own stories as well as those of others. Listen with the understanding that the experience of clients, family, or staff members may serve you in the future. These moments can enrich your practice of nursing and your life.

Geriatric clinical practice offers rich opportunities for connections made through self-disclosure (Box 10-1).

EXAMPLES OF HELPFUL AND NON-HELPFUL SELF-DISCLOSURES

For the following situation an acceptable empathic reply has been provided. Following this example, several ineffective self-disclosures are provided, with a rationale to explain their limitations. Finally, an acceptable complete response is shown.

Situation 1: With a Client

A client, Mrs. Kern, has just relayed the following information to you: "I was so scared this weekend when I had Jack at home on a pass from the hospital. He started coughing and got all red in the face . . . and then he bent over with this violent chest pain. I thought he was going to die. Luckily his nitroglycerine was right on the window sill. As soon as I gave it to him he calmed down right away. His pain left within minutes, thank goodness!"

1. Listen.

Mrs. Kern wants to hear messages related to the fright she suffered because of her husband's pain and the relief she experienced when he recovered.

2. Reply empathically.

Before using your self-disclosure you would convey an empathic response such as:

"Gosh! I guess you were scared your husband might have a fatal heart attack when he doubled up like that with his chest pain. It was probably twice as frightening because you were at home without the security of all the hospital emergency equipment. What a relief for you when the nitroglycerine worked. . . ."

This satisfactory empathic introduction would be followed up with a self-disclosure.

3. Self-disclose.

The following examples will help you differentiate between satisfactory and unsatisfactory ways of implementing self-disclosure.

Unsatisfactory response 1

"I remember hearing about my grandfather having chest pain, and I recall them saying that my grandmother used to have some hair-raising moments. They lived in the country and even the telephone system was unreliable. . . ."

This attempt at self-disclosure is inadequate because it is not your personal experience and the extra details would likely confuse and distract Mrs. Kern.

Self-disclosure should be brief and used only if your experience is similar. It is better to choose not to use this technique if you have not had the experience. It is also important to remember that no two people experience things in the same way, and that this technique is only one possible way to be supportive.

Unsatisfactory response 2

"Scares like that are really traumatic. I, too, had a frightening situation on the weekend. The fire alarm went off and I was the only nurse on the floor. I almost panicked, but like you, I kept calm and luckily it turned out to be a false alarm."

This response competes with Mrs. Kern's. One important feature of a self-disclosure is that the content must be pertinent to the speaker's situation. If your self-disclosure is beside the point or, worse still, unrelated, then the message Mrs. Kern will get is that you do not really comprehend her situation. This response has little to do with Mrs. Kern's anxious moments with her husband. Shifting gears to talk about your unrelated experience will likely convey the message to Mrs. Kern that you are trying to upstage her. She might be jarred into refocusing on your plight and become the helper instead of the helpee.

Unsatisfactory response 3

"Yes, I sure know how terrible it can be watching someone suffer excruciating chest pain right before your eyes. Last week there was a woman on the unit who suffered an episode of extreme chest pain, and like you,

I was anxious and worried. This lady had three children at home and you really wondered how they would cope if she died. She was a single parent, so they said . . . guess her husband left her years ago . . . a drinker, even abused her I've heard. You know, it makes you wonder. . . ."

This response is far too vague and tangential. The irrelevant material is distracting and detracts from any caring intended by the response. The whole purpose of a self-disclosure is to reassure others that you understand their plight because you have had a similar experience yourself. The self-disclosure should be brief and focused on the important issues pertinent to the situation. For Mrs. Kern, it would be important to relate your understanding of her fear and relief as succinctly as possible. The more focused your self-disclosure, the more clearly your understanding will be transmitted.

Satisfactory response

"My dad had severe angina, too, and I had some pretty anxious times when he would turn ashen and look so tortured when his chest pain got excruciating. When all I could do was just stand by and hope that the nitro' would work, I used to feel so desperate and helpless. Did you feel that way this weekend?"

This response meets one of the criteria for an effective self-disclosure because it empathically demonstrates that you have had a similar personal experience with a loved one; therefore, your revelation is relevant to Mrs. Kern's. This self-disclosure is brief and focused so Mrs. Kern would perceive immediately that you are absolutely tuned in to how she felt about being alone with her ill husband.

4. Check it out.

This response meets an additional criterion for self-disclosure: it is tentative. The question, "Did you feel that way this weekend?" invites Mrs. Kern to talk more about her feelings. It refocuses on her and allows her to confirm or expand on how she felt. A question like this helps you check to see whether your self-disclosure has hit the mark. By inviting Mrs. Kern to comment, you appropriately return the focus to her reactions about her situation.

A complete and fully acceptable self-disclosure to Mrs. Kern could be worded this way:

"Gosh! I guess you were scared your husband might have a fatal heart attack when he doubled up like that with his chest pain. It was probably twice as frightening because you were at home without the security of all the hospital emergency equipment. What a relief for you when the nitroglycerine worked. My dad had severe angina, too, and I had some pretty anxious times when he would turn ashen and look so tortured when his pain got excruciating. When all I could do was just stand by and hope that the nitro' would work, I used to feel so desperate and helpless. Did you feel that way this weekend?"

This response integrates the steps of listening, responding empathically, self-disclosing, and checking it out. It is clear that you have understood Mrs. Kern and are interested in discussing her situation with her.

Situation 2: With a Colleague

A fellow nursing student, Joan, says to you: "I'm just thrilled! I've had the most wonderful day on the neuro unit where I'm doing my practicum. I'd been paying close attention to this young client's pupillary response and blood pressure. I kept checking his vital signs, and I was sure I could detect a rising trend in his blood pressure and some sluggishness in his pupillary reflex. I decided to point out my observations to the neurosurgeon who came by on his rounds. He checked out my concerns and promptly arranged for my client to go to surgery. In the O.R. they removed a life-threatening hematoma. I felt so pleased that my careful attention helped save his life. Days like this make all the hard work and studying worth it."

1. Listen.

The message your classmate wants you to hear is that she is proud of her astuteness and grateful that her diligence helped save her client's life.

2. Reply empathically.

Before self-disclosing, you would convey an empathic response such as:

"Wow! No wonder you're ecstatic! Thanks to your vigilance your client's life was saved. You look thrilled that your astuteness paid off so dramatically. It was life or death, and you're grateful that you picked up on the subtle changes in his vital signs. . . ."

This satisfactory empathic introduction would be followed up with a self-disclosure.

3. Self-disclose.

The following examples will help you differentiate between satisfactory and unsatisfactory ways of implementing self-disclosure.

Unsatisfactory response 1

"My sister had the same experience when she was a student nurse. It was 5 years ago now, but it meant so much to her that she still talks about how excited she felt. She happened by a client's room and saw him choking. She did the Heimlich and of course rescued the man. . . ."

This attempt at self-disclosure is inadequate because it is not your personal experience and does not demonstrate to Joan that you really understand her moment of achievement. Your story about your sister would not convince Joan that you have been where she is, felt what she is feeling, or experienced what she is experiencing. A personal disclosure of your own is the best way to persuade Joan that you understand her. Joan may interpret this response as a competitive remark, a story to upstage her own.

Unsatisfactory response 2

"I know just how you feel. I had a great day, too. I got my whole assignment finished, and all the orders caught up by noon. So, then I was able to take the clients out for a walk. They enjoyed the break and the fresh air, so I, too, feel like I accomplished something today."

Your situation is not one of life or death and does not compare to Joan's. The irrelevance of this response would create a gulf between you and Joan, rather than bring you closer together through understanding. Your feeling of accomplishment is not equivalent to Joan's because she was directly responsible for saving a life.

Your self-disclosure must be relevant to the speaker's situation to show that you completely grasp the significance of her reaction. If your self-disclosure is off the mark, as this response is, it tells Joan that you do not really comprehend what she has told you.

Unsatisfactory response 3

"I know how thrilling it can be to save someone's life. Last summer I saw a boat out on the water in front of our cottage . . . you know the spot right near the small island . . . well, it was there a long time. I could see this person waving both arms overhead back and forth. I remembered that Jan had told us that arm waving like that was the international distress signal. It turned out to be two young girls who were joy riding in their parents' motor boat and had run out of gas. They had no paddles and no life jackets. And one of them was quite sick. She was a diabetic and she'd had some beer and too much sun, and she desperately needed her insulin. We brought them back to shore and got them to safety, so I know what it's like to have saved someone's life."

Instead of feeling understood with this response, Joan would likely feel bored and irritated. It can be exasperating to wade through unimportant details and sift through irrelevant recollections. It is considerate to word your self-disclosure as briefly and clearly as you can. Succinctness will cause your speaker to understand your message sooner, not later or never, as in the example above.

Satisfactory response

"I've had that proud feeling of knowing that if it hadn't been for me my client might not have lived. When I was on floor 4J, I discovered a client having a myocardial infarct. I called the code and started CPR . . . and he lived! Isn't it reassuring to know that you can remember what you've studied and apply it correctly in the real world?"

This response meets the criteria for an effective self-disclosure because the similarity of your experience makes it relevant. It is brief and focused so that your colleague Joan immediately receives your message that you have understood her.

4. Check it out.

The tentative question at the end is an effective technique for checking out with Joan if your self-disclosure corresponds with her experience. Your question returns the attention to Joan, where it should be. Joan has the chance to elaborate further on how she is feeling. This response does not upstage her excitement but adds to it. By sharing your relevant experience you have made her feel understood.

A complete and accurate self-disclosure that includes the four steps could be phrased like this one:

"Wow! No wonder you're ecstatic! Thanks to your vigilance, your client's life was saved. You look thrilled that your astuteness paid off so dramatically. It was life or death and you're pleased that you picked up on the subtle changes in his vital signs. I've had that proud feeling of knowing that if it weren't for me my client might not have lived. When I was on floor 4J I discovered a client having a myocardial infarct. I called the code and started CPR . . . and he lived! Isn't it reassuring to know that you can remember what you've studied and apply it correctly in the real world?"

This response combines the steps of listening, responding empathically, self-disclosing, and checking. Your clients or colleagues will feel heard, understood, and respected when you actively listen with empathy and self-disclosure, and then close by turning the conversation back to them.

It is responsible to self-disclose because you bring your own relevant experiences to the interaction. When you self-disclose you are assertively safeguarding others' rights to be understood and preserving your right to communicate in a caring way.

Wit and Wisdom

Self-Disclosure

As I grow older,
Crises I master.
Lessons I've learned.
Growth comes faster.

From my experience
I may offer reflection.
It's not up to me
To offer direction.

When you feel pain
I think I've seen
I can share a few words.
On me you can lean.

I share my path. Was that your view?
I want to understand.
Was it like that for you?

Think About It...
What, So What, and Now What?

Consider what you read about what it means to share your experience with clients and families. How has this technique worked for you in the past? Has sharing information ever caused a problem for you? Self-disclosure is a communication skill that takes understanding, experience, and purpose.

What? . . . Write one thing you learned from this chapter.

So what? . . . How will this impact your nursing practice?

Now what? . . . How will you implement this new knowledge or skill?

THINK ABOUT IT

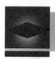

Practicing Self-Disclosure

Exercise 1

During the next few days, note when people self-disclose with you. Are these self-disclosures relevant, brief, and personal? Are they conveyed to make you feel understood? Note your reactions to these self-disclosures from colleagues, sales people, teachers, or friends. Consider what characteristics of their self-disclosures led you to feel cared for and what features jarred you and made you question the genuine interest of the self-disclosure.

After you have done this exercise individually, get together as a class and compare your findings about the communication behavior of self-disclosure.

Exercise 2

This time observe your own self-disclosures with others. Note your intentions when you self-disclose to people you contact. Is it for their benefit or yours? Remark on the characteristics of your self-disclosures. Are they your own personal experiences? Are your self-disclosures brief and focused? Do you end them with a tentative question?

From your observations, assess your ability to effectively self-disclose. Where are you doing well and what improvements could you strive for in your use of self-disclosure?

Exercise 3

For this exercise work in groups of three. One of you will be the speaker, another the listener, and the third the observer. Speakers should choose a topic with which their listeners are familiar. This way it is more likely that they will have had similar experiences so that they can realistically make a self-disclosure.

As speaker your task is to talk for 5 minutes about this topic, conveying your thoughts, feelings, and reactions. The listener's task is to attempt to implement a self-disclosure at every appropriate opportunity. The observer will make note of the listener's self-disclosures and give feedback about how the self-disclosures meet the following criteria.

Criteria for a Complete Self-Disclosure

- Empathic response: Was an empathic response included before the self-disclosure?
- Self-disclosure: Was the self-disclosure personal? Was it brief, focused, and relevant?
- Checking: Did the listener complete the self-disclosure with a tentative question as a way of validating with the speaker?

After 5 minutes stop and debrief with these questions:

As Listener: How did you feel using the skill of self-disclosure? What aspects were awkward and which went smoothly for you?

As Speaker: How did the listener's self-disclosures make you feel? From your point of view, is there anything the listener might have done differently to make you feel more understood?

As Observer: What aspects of the listener's self-disclosures were done well? What suggestions can you make for improvement?

Continued

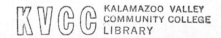

Practicing Self-Disclosure—cont'd

Rotate roles so that each of you has a chance to be speaker, listener, and observer.

This exercise gives you a chance to think about self-disclosures from many different angles. What has your contemplation taught you about the important communication behavior of self-disclosure? Compare your thoughts with those of your colleagues.

Exercise 4

Like any new skill we learn, whether typing, tennis, or dancing, the most progress is made when we practice. To improve your ability to self-disclose, attempt to include a self-disclosure wherever appropriate in your day-to-day encounters with others.

Take the opportunity to evaluate yourself. Critique your self-disclosures using the criteria outlined in Exercise 3. Also make note of the response you receive from your speaker. Did your self-disclosure result in your clients or colleagues opening up more about their experiences? Did your speaker look pleased and convinced that you understood?

Remember to congratulate yourself on your successes. Be clear about how you want to improve and visualize yourself successfully meeting your goal.

Exercise 5

Select a nurse faculty member or a colleague and ask if this person would be willing to share a life story that has increased personal understanding of the patient or family experience. As we share our own stories we increase our understanding of the value of self-disclosure and its effects on others.

References

Bateson MC: *Peripheral visions: learning along the way,* New York, 1994, Harper Collins.

Drew N: Expanding self-awareness through exploration of meaningful experience, *J Holistic Nurs* 15(4):406, Dec 1997.

Nowak KB, Wandel JC: The sharing of self in geriatric clinical practice: case report and analysis, *Geriatr Nurs* 19(1):34, Feb 1998.

Rosenberg CJ: Faculty-student mentoring: a father's chronic sorrow: a daughter's perspective, *J Holistic Nurs* 16(3):399, Sept 1998.

Suggestions for Further Reading

Benner P: *From the novice to expert: excellence and power in clinical nursing practice,* Menlo Park, Calif, 1984, Addison-Wesley.

A classic book that details the use of intuition as part of expert practice.

Buckman R: *How to break bad news: a guide for health care professionals,* Baltimore, 1992, The Johns Hopkins University Press.

Coates C: Let them see the scars, *Am J Nurs* 93(9):17, 1993.

Derlaga VJ, Metts S, Margulis ST: *Self-disclosure,* Newbury Park, Calif, 1993, Sage Publications.

Eakes GG: Chronic sorrow: a response to living with cancer, *Oncol Nurs Forum* 20:1327, 1993.

Eakes GG: Theory: middle-range theory of chronic sorrow. In Burke ML, Hainsworth MA: *Image* 30(2):179, 1998.

Kusserow S: The guide for true education: life experience, *Revolution* p. 24, Summer 1994.

Long L: *Understanding/responding: a communication manual for nurses,* Boston, 1992, Jones & Bartlett.

Morse JM: Negotiating commitment and involvement in the nurse-patient relationship, *J Adv Nurs* 16:455, 1991.

Moore BG: Reminiscing therapy: a CNS intervention, *Clin Nurse Spec* 6:170, 1992.

Pagano MP, Ragan SL, Booten S: *Communications skills for professional nurses,* Newburg Park, Calif, 1992, Sage Publications.

Stewart J: *Bridges, not walls: a book about interpersonal communication,* ed 2, Reading, Mass, 1977, Addison-Wesley Publishing.

In Section VI, Stewart includes two papers by Sidney M. Jourard and John Powell. These essays are beautifully written and open up readers' awareness of the significance of self-disclosure. These readings provide nurses with the philosophical aspects to the issue of self-disclosing in interpersonal relationships.

Teel CS: Chronic sorrow: analysis of the concept, *J Adv Nurs* 16:1211, 1991.

Thompson GJ: *Verbal judo: the gentle art of persuasion,* New York, 1993, William Morrow.

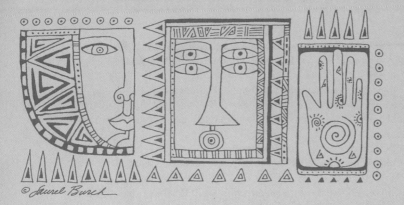

11

Specificity

If no thought your mind does visit, make your speech not too explicit.

Source unknown

OBJECTIVES

1. Define specificity.
2. Identify the usefulness of specificity and its effect on communication behavior.
3. Identify strategies to communicate with specificity.

WHEN SPECIFICITY IS USEFUL

Being specific means being detailed and clear in the content of our speech. It means being concrete, so that our communication is focused and logical. In contrast, vagueness can be frustrating, and lack of clarity creates distance between people who are trying to communicate. As well as clarifying our own speech, the technique of specificity involves assisting clients (or colleagues) to move from broad, elusive areas of discussion to narrower, more pinpointed areas of concern.

Using concrete communication is especially advantageous in certain interpersonal situations. It is important to be specific when we are:

- Explaining our thoughts and feelings
- Reflecting others' thoughts and feelings
- Asking questions
- Giving information or feedback
- Evaluating

This list covers situations that nurses repeatedly encounter with clients and colleagues. Specificity benefits communication in three ways:

- The process of communicating is more satisfying when we are "on the same wavelength" as those with whom we are communicating.
- Communicators achieve clearer comprehension of their own thoughts and full understanding of others' thoughts.
- The foundation for problem solving is complete and accurate, enhancing the success of further communications in our relationships with clients and colleagues (Arnold and Boggs, 1995).

Wit and Wisdom

On Specificity

Details do matter.
Please listen with care.
The facts that you gather
May show something rare.

Please make no assumptions.
Ask 'til you're certain.
Look, learn, and listen.
You'll find out what's hurtin'.

These poems go on.
Read them. Don't wait.
You never know when
You'll find one that's great.

To learn can be fun.
Life itself, quite amusing.
The attitude you take
Is yours for the choosing.

Copyright 1995 Julia W. Balzer Riley.

BEING SPECIFIC WHEN EXPLAINING YOUR THOUGHTS AND FEELINGS

There are gradients to any emotion, and it is important to choose the one that says exactly what you want to convey to your listener. In the anger category, for example, you might be feeling enraged, frustrated, furious, annoyed, or irritated. Each subtle variation conveys a slightly different mood. Hitting the mark by expressing exactly the right flavor of emotion ensures that your meaning is crystal clear.

If you tell clients that you are enraged with them for being late for their clinic appointments, when you are really only mildly irritated, you may create a gulf between the two of you by overstating your case.

With the emotion of sadness, you might feel "blue," depressed, hopeless, or discouraged. If you tell your co-workers that you are merely out of sorts, when you are really in despair because your child support check has not arrived and your taxes are due, such minimizing of your feelings risks diminishing the intimacy and trust between you.

When we are not specific about describing our thoughts and feelings, we invite misunderstanding. Since the purpose of communicating is to enhance the understanding between two people, being indirect or unclear is unproductive.

In addition to hitting the mark about the quality of emotion, saying specifically what makes you feel a certain way clarifies your feelings further. For example, you are happy that your client has initiated a reduced-calorie diet and has begun to walk two miles a day. You convey your pleasure by saying:

"Mr. Weller, I'm pleased that you are working to improve your health with diet and exercise. I know it can be a challenge, but you will find you have more energy when you take time for yourself."

Being specific by adding a rationale for your feelings enhances the sincerity of your message. Your explanation has built-in rewards for Mr. Weller. Such a response would make a lot more sense to him than:

"That's great, Mr. Weller. Glad to see you are doing well."

In this example it is unclear why you are pleased: because he is a dutiful client? because you will not have to spend time reminding him to eat well and exercise?

Here is another example from the workplace. You are grateful that your colleague on the night shift has highlighted all abnormal lab results and displayed them clearly for your inspection when you arrive for the day shift. You tell her:

"I'm thrilled with this chart you prepared, Jo, and grateful for the time it'll save us on the day shift. Your highlighting will streamline our alerting the physicians and indicate at a glance which patients need temperatures done or repeat laboratory work. Thank you."

This specific articulation about why you feel grateful adds depth and conviction to your feelings. It respectfully conveys your appreciation, more than a glib "Great" or "Thanks" would have.

Some nurses, clients, families, and colleagues prefer logical, rational thinking processes; they are proficient at appreciating, and being specific about, facts. They may not readily consider feelings, or be comfortable dealing with them (Myers, 1980). Since their strength lies in logical, objective thinking, they may lack the vocabulary to be specific when discussing feelings. Those who prefer thinking over feeling tend to decide things impersonally, are more analytical, and will respond more easily to others' thoughts (Myers, 1980). Nurses, clients, families, and colleagues who prefer to make decisions on the basis of personal feelings and human values are more attuned to others' feelings and likely have more vocabulary and the comfort to talk about feelings (Lawrence, 1982; Myers, 1980). They tend to be more concerned about the human feelings and values in communication than the factual, objective information.

You can learn more about specificity in relation to expressing your thoughts and feelings in Chapter 10.

BEING SPECIFIC WHEN REFLECTING OTHERS' THOUGHTS AND FEELINGS

Listening is not a silent pastime. It is active and vocal. Through your warmth and respect you can show you are attending to what your clients or colleagues are saying. By being specific, you can convince them that you have heard and understood the meaning of their dialogue.

When you reflect others' thoughts and feelings, you are like a recording, giving them a chance to hear what they are really saying. When helpers respond with clear, concise, detailed statements about others' concerns, it helps the people with problems clarify them.

For example, one of your clients has given you a lengthy description of her son's epilepsy:

Mrs. Cant: "I'm so frightened he'll forget to take his medication that I often call the school nurse to check that he's taken it. And when he's late getting home from school, I worry to death that he's lying on a sidewalk somewhere having a seizure. When he plays soccer I'm right there on the sidelines—not so much cheering as praying that all that running won't fire off a seizure. My Lord, will it always be like this?"

Here is an example of a specific reflection:

Specific you: "You're wondering if your son will be able to live a normal life, and whether you'll ever be free from worrying about his health and safety."

You can pinpoint the essence of other people's meanings by being specific when they get engrossed in relating their thoughts and feelings. This tactic helps them grasp more fully both the sense and the significance of what they are saying.

Contrast the clarity of this response with these nonspecific alternatives:

Nonspecific you: "You must be very tense fretting about your son," or, "It sounds like you spend a lot of time worrying."

Neither of these statements captures the exact meaning that Mrs. Cant was trying to convey. Replying accurately and specifically demonstrates that you fully understand your listener. Chapter 9 discussed more about the communication behavior of reflecting others' thoughts and feelings in a concrete way.

BEING SPECIFIC WHEN ASKING QUESTIONS

As an interviewer, there are times when you might wish to purposefully not be specific so that the interviewee takes the lead. This open-ended strategy usually occurs at the beginning of an interview ("How may I be of help to you?" or "What is the pain like?"), or at a point in an interview when you want more information ("Could you tell me more about your family?" or "your exercise habits?").

As clinicians, we often want specific information from our clients. To get exactly what we want, we must specifically ask for it. You may wish to know more about a client's family health history, for example. If you ask: "Tell me more about your family health," you might get everything from "It's fine!" to "Well, let me see, in 1901 my great-grandfather was ill on his sailing venture." A brief response provides you with no information, and a lengthy response requires sifting through to glean the essential details. Occasionally clients' historical recountings may be jumbled or confused, either because they are unsure of dates and details or because their emotional reactions to their changed health status are interfering with their clarity. When this occurs, it's helpful to stop undirected digressions, backtrack, and reestablish specific points. This process helps clients' thinking to become clearer and more focused.

It is likely that you will need specific aspects of your clients' family history: history of cancer, history of cardiovascular diseases, and so on. Getting to the point and asking for specific information simplifies for your clients what you want and increases your chances of getting it. Using the skill of specificity, you can prevent frustration or fruitlessness in the communication encounter. As nurses, if we fail to achieve clarity, our clients may be left feeling confused and may even doubt our ability to contribute to the interaction. Phrases like, "I'm not sure I understand that," or, "Would you go over that again?," let our clients know we are interested and that we need help in understanding what they want us to know (Sundeen et al, 1998). Several health and physical assessment guidelines provide systematic questionnaires for clarifying clients' symptoms. The symptom analysis in Bower and Thompson's *Clinical Manual of Health Assessment* (1992) is an excellent reference for pinpointing essential data about changes in clients' health status.

BEING SPECIFIC WHEN GIVING INFORMATION OR FEEDBACK

As nurses, we are often involved in teaching clients about their treatments, tests, medications, and health behaviors. To provide clients with material that is new to them and avoid the disrespect of boring them, it is important to focus on the aspects that they particularly want to know. A good general screening question for clients is, "What would you like to know about your treatment (test, medication, diet)?" Posed in an inviting way, this question will make your clients delineate the most important areas for them. Jumping right in with a complete and chronological explanation wastes time, might be irrelevant, and may even focus on material that is too frightening.

The same approach can be used with clients or colleagues who want feedback from you. Clarifying the nature of their request at the outset ensures that your feedback will be focused on the area that is important to them.

Imagine a situation, for example, in which a newly hired nurse with 6 months postgraduate experience asks you for feedback on her performance as a team leader during the past five shifts. At this point you could enthusiastically jump in with praise and advice, but you pause before bombarding her. Instead you respond to her request for feedback with, "I'd love to comment on your

Moments of Connection...
Never Assume; Clarify!

"I was working with a 16-year-old young man with Hodgkin's disease who had just been told by his doctor that he would be 'infertile.' After the doctor left the room, the look on his face told me he was devastated. I asked if he knew what the word *infertile* meant, and he replied, 'I won't be able to have sex.' I was able to clarify what the term meant and put his mind somewhat at ease. He did well, had a complete remission, and went off to college. We need to be specific in the use of language."

Moments of Connection...
To Reduce Anxiety, Provide Information

"One of my patients had been having extreme pain from postherpetic neuralgia and was not able to sit or lie still at all for about 6 weeks. She was exhausted and scared. I went to see her 4 days in a row to explain how epidurals are done and how they can help to control pain. She said she finally understood, believed it would help, and agreed to have the medication. About 5 minutes after the medication was injected, she fell asleep. When she awoke, she said she had never slept so deeply, hugged me, and thanked me for making a difference in the quality of her life. She received two injections and needed no more."

team leadership abilities. What specific areas would you like me to focus on?" This approach allows her to clarify that her abilities to delegate and to handle unforeseen crises are what she wants you to address. Requesting specificity allows you to focus your feedback so that it is helpful to the other person.

BEING SPECIFIC WHEN EVALUATING

After you have implemented any nursing action, it is important to evaluate its success. Whether you have led a training session or carried out a treatment, it is important to find out if you have accomplished your goals. Your evaluation questions can be phrased specifically. Instead of asking a vague question like, "How was that?" or "Have you got the hang of it now?," you can phrase your questions to reflect the objectives that necessitated your nursing action.

For example, you could ask your colleague who wants feedback on her team leadership: "Has my feedback on your abilities to delegate and to handle crises been helpful to you?" To the client who wants to know what would be facing him in the week after surgery, you could say: "Did I cover all the points you wanted to know about the recovery phase after your open-heart surgery?"

You could ask the first-time father who feels awkward and nervous about bathing his baby: "Has my demonstration on how to bathe your son helped your confidence?" These specifically focused questions help nurses evaluate whether they have been helpful. Asking these follow-up questions completes the nursing process.

PROVIDING SPECIFIC DOCUMENTATION

Employing specificity to collect information from clients needs to be complemented by systematically recording the data. Clear documentation increases the likelihood that clients will receive the best care. Today, when the courts are holding nurses liable for their own actions, as many as one out of four malpractice suits are decided from nursing documentation in clients' charts. Obviously, good care and avoidance of a malpractice suit are two solid reasons for completing the nursing record in a clear and logical manner (Edelstein, 1990). Your nursing records should follow the care plans and indicate that the care you provided responded to specific client needs and was appropriate for specific nursing and medical diagnoses. Where nursing documentation is written with specific problems and outcomes in mind, the nurses' notes provide a concise, chronological, factual, and easy-to-audit record of clients' progress (Edelstein, 1990). Careful documentation impacts the ability of a health care agency to be reimbursed for services. Greater precision and detail are being demanded to offer legal protection (Krantz, 1998). There is an old adage, "If it isn't documented, it wasn't done." Although this may not be literally true, an agency's documentation procedures must be followed to ensure a compete representation of the care given and assessments completed. Review documentation procedures of the organization where you work to make sure you are being as specific as is required.

Philpott (1985) outlines 22 reasonable and prudent nursing recording policies, practices, and systems. Following are a few of Philpott's key points pertinent to the skill of specificity.

- The complexity of the health problems and the level of risk posed by clients themselves, their condition, or by the use of medical, nursing, or other therapies dictate the detail and frequency of documentation.
- The higher the risk to which a particular client is exposed, the more comprehensive, in-depth, and frequent should be the nursing recordings.
- Effective nursing recording is factual, honest, and based on accurate data taken directly from visual, verbal, and/or olfactory cues and palpation.
- Effective recording shuns bias, avoiding tendencies to prejudge or label patients.
- Effective documentation tends toward quantitative expression, avoiding vague generalizations. For example, with a client who is experiencing a sleeping problem, nursing recording such as "usual night" or "fair night" offers no useful understanding, waste charting space and nursing time, and may mask a serious problem. Specific documentation, such as "slept from 0200 hours to 0300 and states she slept soundly and feels refreshed," provides a clear, accurate, and concise picture of the client's situation; it also enhances credibility for the nurse writer.

Professional care is reflected by proficient charting, which not only proves what nurses have done, but effectively communicates clients' status and progress, saving time for everyone on the health care team.

Think About It...
What, So What, and Now What?

Consider what you read about being specific in communication with clients, families, and colleagues. Clarity and accuracy in communication are necessary for successful relationships.

What? ... Write one thing you learned from this chapter.

So what? ... How will this impact your nursing practice?

Now what? ... How will you implement this new knowledge or skill?

THINK ABOUT IT

Practicing Specificity

One way to really understand the benefits of an interpersonal skill is to experience the negative reactions in a situation when the skill is not being used. The first phase of each of the following exercises provides that opportunity.

Exercise 1

Find a partner with whom to work. One of you will role-play a nurse, the other a client. As the client, you want specific information from the nurse. Decide in advance exactly what information you want and for what reason you want it. During the interview, attempt to be as specific as you can. As the nurse in this role-play, you will not make any efforts to determine the exact nature of what the client wants to know or why she wants the information; also, you will be unfocused, vague, and unclear. Proceed with a discussion for 4 minutes, and then pause to debrief with these questions as guidelines:

As the client: How did you feel when the nurse neglected to determine what you specifically wanted to know or the reasons you had for wanting the information?

As the nurse: How did you feel when you neglected to determine what your client wanted?

Switch roles so that each of you has the chance to give and receive vague, unspecific communication.

Continued

Practicing Specificity—cont'd

Exercise 2

Find a partner with whom to role-play. One of you will be a home health nurse, the other a physician. The nurse telephones the physician to obtain orders for a client. The nurse uses vague language when describing the client's condition. The physician must either ask many questions or risk making a decision based on inadequate data. After a 4-minute discussion, debrief using these questions as guidelines:

As the physician: What thoughts were you having about the nurse and her skills? How did this affect the way you responded to this nurse's questions?

As the nurse: How effective were you at getting what you needed for the client?

Replay the exercise with the nurse giving the physician clear, specific information. After a 4-minute discussion, debrief using these questions as guidelines:

As the physician: What thoughts did you have about the nurse's skills? How did this affect the way you responded to the nurse?

As the nurse: How effective were you at getting what you needed for the client?

Exercise 3

Find a partner to do this exercise. In this role-play you will be nurse colleagues on a unit. One will be the speaker and the other the listener. As speaker, you wish to discuss with the listener a problem you are having on the unit. In relating your situation, you will be unspecific, unclear, and vague. As the listener, you will use the skill of specificity to try to determine the nature of the speaker's problem situation. After a 4-minute discussion, debrief using these questions as guidelines:

As the listener: How did it feel to receive unspecific, vague communication from the speaker?

As the speaker: How did it feel to receive specific, focused communication from the listener? Did the speaker's use of specificity lead to any changes in your communication?

With the entire class, examine what you have learned about the importance of specificity by employing it and by being vague.

Exercise 4

Choose a partner in the class. One of you will role-play a client who wants some information about his or her illness and the tests he or she is undergoing. The other will role-play the nurse who employs the skill of specificity. Engage in a discussion for 5 minutes and then debrief using these questions as guidelines:

As the client: How did it feel when the nurse made an effort to find out what you needed to know and tried to be clear and focused in her explanation?

As the nurse: What was it like to use the skill of specificity when determining the client's request, giving him information and determining if you had been helpful?

After debriefing, switch roles so that each of you will have the opportunity to practice and receive specificity.

With the whole class, discuss what using specificity correctly has taught you about that particular skill.

References

Arnold E, Boggs K: *Interpersonal relationships: professional communication for nurses,* Philadelphia, 1995, WB Saunders.

Bowers AC, Thompson JM: *Clinical manual of health assessment,* ed 3, St. Louis, 1992, Mosby.

Reimbursement: be prepared, *Contemp Long-Term Care* 20(8):56, August 1997.

Edelstein J: A study of nursing documentation, *Nurs Manag* 21(11):40, 1990.

Krantz J: Taming the new E & M guidelines; *Physician's Manag* 38(3):41, 1998.

Lawrence G: *People types and tiger stripes: a practical guide for learning styles,* ed 2, Gainesville, Fla, 1982, Center for Applications of Psychological Type.

Murray RB, Zentner JP: *Nursing concepts for health promotion,* ed 3, Englewood Cliffs, NJ, 1985, Prentice-Hall.

Myers IB: *Gifts differing,* Palo Alto, Calif, 1980, Consulting Psychologists Press.

Philpott M: *Legal liability and the nursing process,* Philadelphia, 1985, WB Saunders.

Reiley PJ, Stengrevics SS: Change of shift report: put it in writing!, *Nurs Manag* 20(9):54, 1989.

Sundeen SJ et al: *Nurse-client interaction: implementing the nursing process,* St Louis, 1998, Mosby.

Suggestions for Further Reading

Baron R: *What type am I? discover who you really are,* New York, 1998, Penguin Books.

Hirsch S, Kummerow JM: *Life types,* New York, 1989, Warner Books.
> Readable book on the personal application of personality types delineated by the M.B.T.I.

Hirsch SK, Kummerow JM: *Introduction to type in organizations,* Palo Alto, Calif, 1993, Consulting Psychologists Press.
> Useful for the application of psychological type to organizations.

Miller P, Pastorino C: Daily nursing documentation can be quick and thorough! *Nurs Manag* 47, Nov 1990.

Scheet N: Medicare surveys: don't panic! get ready! *Home Health Focus* (4):6, 1994.

Schmidt D et al: Charting for accountability, *Nurs Manag* 21(11):50, 1990.

Stemple J: Asking the right questions, *Home Health Focus* 1(4):5, 1994.
> Timely information about the field of home health care, where specific communication is crucial for outcome measurement and for full reimbursement for services and survival of the agency.

Tidall JA: *Peer power: strategies for the professional leader: becoming an effective peer helper and conflict mediator,* Muncie, Ind, 1994, Accelerated Development.

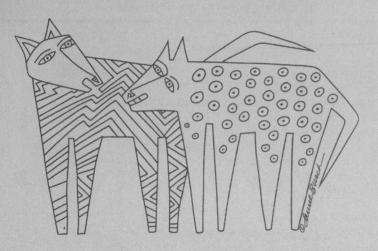

12

Asking Questions

A fool may ask more questions in an hour than a wise man can answer in seven years.

English proverb

OBJECTIVES

1. Discuss the importance of effective skill in asking questions.
2. Identify six points to keep in mind when asking questions.
3. Identify common errors in asking questions and strategies to avoid them.
4. Participate in exercises to assess and build skills for asking questions

THE IMPORTANCE OF ASKING QUESTIONS EFFECTIVELY IN NURSING

Asking questions is fundamental to nursing assessment and to building the helping relationship. Consider as you make initial contacts with clients that they are performing their own assessments to see if you measure up to their expectations (Sundeen et al, 1998). As a professional nurse, you will spend about half of your working time asking questions of clients and colleagues. Pay careful attention to building this skill, remembering to listen for what is said and what is left unspoken.

Moments of Connection...
Questions to Help Move Beyond the Obvious

"I was working with a 31-year-old woman with myelitis who was in tremendous pain. As I was doing the morning assessment and we were discussing her pain, she began to cry. Upon further exploration, the client revealed it was not the pain that was her worst concern. With support, she began to tell me about her grandfather who was dying and her grandmother whose cancer was no longer in remission. She was afraid she would never see her grandfather again to be able to tell him what he had meant to her. She touched me deeply because I had a similar experience. To help her regain some control of her situation, I helped her place a call to her grandfather and she was able to find closure.

Adeptness at asking questions is a fundamental requirement for competent and considerate nurses. The more effective you can be in asking questions, the more time you will save yourself and others, the more pertinent and useful the information you will collect, and the more effective your interviewing experience. Effective questioning will ensure that you collect the data you need to provide quality nursing service.

From the time your clients enter your care until the completion of your helping relationship, you will be asking them questions. You will ask them about the nature of their concerns so that you can agree on a nursing diagnosis. Finding out what they hope to achieve with the help of your nursing services requires effective questioning. You will discover their preferences for a treatment plan and frequently check with them about its effectiveness. Determining their readiness for termination of your relationship, and their readiness to take care of their own health concerns after discharge demands that your questioning skills be clear and focused.

You might be thinking that the client-nurse relationship is composed primarily of questioning. Well, to a great extent it is. Therefore, it is crucial that you attain proficiency in this fundamental nursing communication behavior.

In your role as a nurse, the main reasons for asking questions are to secure data that are essential to providing quality care to your clients. Six questions need to be answered to ensure you secure the facts you need.

THE WHY, WHAT, HOW, WHO, WHEN, AND WHERE OF ASKING QUESTIONS

If it is important for you to find out the information you want, then it is worthwhile to spend the time planning the strategy that is most likely to secure these facts.

The Why of Asking Questions

Before you make any inquiries at all, you should be sure about why you need the information. If your questions are rooted in personal curiosity or uncertainty (you decide to ask everything you can think of with the hope that what you need will be included), then you are unlikely to get what you want—or know you have it when you get it—and in the process you may offend your clients. Before you speak, silently answer this question: "How will the information I am seeking direct me in helping my clients?" If you can justify the question, then ask it!

If there is any doubt that your clients may not understand your reasons for asking, then explain those reasons in advance. For example:

In your investigations of your client's fall off a ladder, you want to learn about his safety habits in general to determine if he is in danger of future home accidents. Before barraging him with what might seem to be unrelated or even nosy questions, it would clarify your objective to say something like:

"I'd like to ask you some questions about your safety precautions with the ladder and about your home safety measures in general. About 80% of accidents occur in the home; my questions might trigger some ideas that could make your home a safer place to work and live. Are you agreeable to exploring this area with me?"

Here is another example:

Within the past year, your 79-year-old client has been brought to the emergency department three times after fainting. The cause of the fainting has not been discovered, and your observations about her thinness and lack of vitality make you wonder whether inadequate nutrition might be at the root of her fainting. The following statement would clarify the purpose of your questions:

"We still don't know what is causing your fainting, Mrs. Jones, and we want to investigate every likely source. One possible cause could be a lack of the nutrients essential to keep you going. I'd like to ask you some questions about your diet to find out whether you are getting all you need from the foods you eat. Is that okay with you?"

Both these examples illustrate how you can prepare your clients for your line of questioning. When clients understand your purpose, they are more likely to be open and reveal information, in contrast to being guarded because they are uneasy about your intentions.

The What and How of Asking Questions

What you will ask and how you will ask it are the next considerations in your strategy. When you have determined why you require the information, then you must plan what to ask to ensure you are clear in your intentions and know how to phrase your question in a way that invites your client to respond.

What you say must be phrased clearly, and a logical progression to your questions is helpful. They should be phrased in a way that shows your respect for your clients' privacy and personal information. Any judgments you have about the responses should not be spoken.

For example, imagine that you require some information about a client's overall activity level and day-to-day schedule in order to help him fit in his colostomy hygienic care. Having explained your purpose and secured his permission, your next step is to proceed with your inquiry. You choose to proceed in a systematic order with:

"Let's begin with your mornings. Could you outline what you do, hour by hour, on a typical weekday morning, from the time you get up until lunch time?"

This question outlines for your client exactly what you want to know. He can focus on the mornings, and it is apparent that you will proceed to other times in his weekly schedule.

Consider another example:

You are completing a health history on a client who has just arrived in an outpatient surgical center. He will be having an anesthetic, and you need information about his past health status, past illnesses, and family health history. Your facility employs a concise preoperative assessment tool to efficiently obtain this extensive material from clients. Having secured your client's permission, after explaining the purpose of your line of questioning, you proceed with:

"As you know, this is a lot of material to cover. To streamline things I'm going to use this guideline our unit has developed. It's a good checklist to ensure that we cover everything. Please ask me if there's anything I say that isn't clear to you. Beginning with your childhood, did you ever have diphtheria? . . . or whooping cough? . . . or rheumatic fever?"

Explaining your format helps clients accept what might otherwise seem like a barrage of unrelated questions.

Any material that clients provide is of a personal nature, and some areas are more sensitive than others. For some clients, talking about sexual activity or birth control practices may be difficult. For others, talking about personal hygiene or alcohol consumption may be embarrassing. Some clients do not feel comfortable revealing their self-care practices; others hesitate to reveal family issues or job-related information. You cannot know in advance which topics might be difficult for your clients, so you must keep in mind that any information clients reveal about themselves, their significant others, or their health care practices might be sensitive for them.

As a nurse you can take certain steps to put your clients at ease and to make them feel more comfortable in revealing this information. One thing you can do is reassure them about the confidentiality of your relationship. This step should be taken right at the beginning of an interview or at the earliest point possible in your relationship. By waiting until later you may have lost opportunities for uncovering important information.

Confidentiality has a wide range of meanings, and you must be honest and clear with all your clients so that they understand exactly what the parameters are. Does confidentiality mean that you will not repeat what your clients have said? Does it mean that you will verbally pass the information along to a trustworthy colleague but not put it in writing? Does it mean that you will convey information to team colleagues at client-care conferences? Or does it mean that confidential information will be written on a chart for other team members to read and be aware of? Exactly what your clients may reveal will likely be determined by what you intend to do with the information they contemplate telling you.

It is essential that you and your clients have an identical understanding of the meaning of confidentiality. Sundeen et al (1994) remind us that clients may feel betrayed if they have been under the impression that client-nurse relationships are confidential, and then discover that you have revealed what they consider personal information to another health team member or have written it on their chart.

Another way you can increase your clients' comfort is to treat all areas you discuss respectfully and professionally. Making the effort to ensure that your clients have privacy and the time to respond unhurriedly will facilitate their replying openly and fully. Being equally relaxed and straightforward, whether discussing sexual matters, family health history, bowel habits, or exercise patterns, will contribute to putting your clients at ease. If you flush, wriggle in your chair, lose eye contact, or lower your voice, your clients will quickly get the message that this topic is a sensitive one for you and they may feel even more embarrassed. To improve your ability to be at ease when asking questions in a variety of areas, you will find rehearsal with friends or colleagues helpful.

The Who of Asking Questions

Who to ask is another important consideration. If your clients are able to speak for themselves, then they are the ones to approach. Occasions may arise, however, when you need information that your clients might not be able to provide. There are times when the observations of significant others can shed light on a client's situation, and this perspective is also valuable to have. For example, if your client has been on a mood-elevating medication, you may wish to have his wife's observations of any changes, in addition to your client's sense of the effectiveness of the drug. Or on one of your home health visits to a client with multiple sclerosis, you may wish to get family members' perspectives of the client's abilities to manage at home. Whenever you consult family members or friends, it is courteous and respectful if you do so with the knowledge, and when possible in the presence, of your client. In some agencies it is the policy to secure written consent from clients before questioning significant others and previous or concurrent health care providers. To respect client confidentiality and protect the legality of your actions, it is important that you make yourself aware of such policies.

There are times when clients cannot answer questions. For example, unconscious, aphasic, or psychotic clients are not able to provide information that might be important in their recovery. In these instances you will have to do some detective work to discover the essential people from whom to get this information.

The When and Where of Asking Questions

When and where to carry out your questioning is your next consideration. The physical setup of many hospitals and clinics makes it difficult to secure a completely private place to interview your client. You should make every effort, however, to arrange for a time and place where you will not be interrupted by phone calls, noise, other clients, agency activity, or visitors. Arranging such a time and place may require patience, since both you and your client have days filled with scheduled and unscheduled activities. It does not usually pay to rush an interview or talk about sensitive issues in an open ward area. Clients have every right to privacy and a sense of unhurried attention from you.

Keeping in mind these six aspects of asking questions will improve your effectiveness by making you a systematic and sensitive interviewer.

COMMON TACTICAL ERRORS IN ASKING QUESTIONS AND WHAT TO DO ABOUT THEM

The broad strategies outlined in the preceding section will be valuable in guiding your inquiries in a general way. When it comes to the nitty-gritty of speaking, you will find the following suggestions about avoiding or overcoming poor techniques a helpful reference.

The Long-Winded Buildup

In efforts to explain the purpose of our line of questioning to our clients and colleagues, we sometimes go overboard. When we provide a rambling, detailed introduction, we run the risk of confusing or boring the other person. When providing an explanation of the rationale for our questions, the KISS principle is best: Keep It Short and Simple!

Wrong way:

Long-winded you: "Mr. Haddon, I'd like to ask you some questions about your allergies so that we can eventually work out a lifestyle plan that will allow you to avoid or minimize the stressful reactions you suffer from the various things that irritate you. As you know, repeated allergic reactions can be stressful for the body when it has to constantly fight to return bodily functions to normal. When you are in an allergic reactive state, your body is in the alarm phase and is working overtime trying to return things to normal. When you feel miserable because of the allergies, you also feel tense and anxious, and maybe even at times frightened that your allergic reactions will get out of control. It's only when we have all the information that we can help you plan the best ways to avoid your irritants. Shall we begin?"

A long-winded buildup like the one above can put off the client who understands the purpose and wants to get down to business of the task. Openers that are redundant, wordy, and too detailed are diversions that detract from the task.

Right way:

Focused you: "Mr. Haddon, I'd like to ask you some questions about your allergies so we can eventually work out a lifestyle plan that will allow you to avoid or minimize your stressful reactions to the various things that irritate you. Your chart indicates you have both food and environmental allergies. To begin, could you tell me to which foods you are allergic?"

This concise opening spells out your purpose and how and why you will be asking this client your particular questions. The clarity and brevity of this statement will not bore, frighten, insult, or confuse him.

The Thunder Stealer

Our questions sometimes take the form of asking clients their opinions about the cause of their health problems, their preferences for effective treatment, or what degree of cure or alleviation of the problem they think should be sought. It is respectful to give our clients the opportunity to offer their ideas, especially when we have requested their perspective. In our enthusiasm we sometimes jump in with our views and opinions before giving our clients a chance to speak. This zealousness on our part can be intimidating for clients and prevent them from expressing their real views. Jumping in and upstaging clients can anger some of them. Many clients feel hurt that we would barge ahead, expounding our beliefs, without having the courtesy to hear their point of view about their own health care situation.

Wrong way:

Upstaging you: "Well, Miss Ricco, together we have agreed upon six possible steps you could take to minimize your facial blemishes. I am interested in knowing what you think of each of these options. I know which I would recommend. Definitely get rid of any oil-based skin care products you have and start using oil-free products. Don't you agree that this change would prevent your pores from clogging up? And you'd likely agree you should buy the special soap Dr. Best recommended, wouldn't you? I think you should go for our second option too. . . ."

Miss Ricco soon would have the message that you are not in any way interested in her views. Usurping every chance for your client to speak is frustrating and demeaning. Stealing our clients' thunder gives them the message that we think what we have to say is more important and that they should depend on us for direction. This picture is out of line with today's well-informed health consumer and a health care system that is striving to get people to take charge of their health care responsibilities.

Right way:

Considerate you: "Well, Miss Ricco, together we have agreed upon six possible steps you could take to minimize your facial blemishes. I am interested in knowing what you think of each of the options we've talked about."

The nurse who is genuinely interested in discovering what Miss Ricco really thinks about the treatment options would stop here and let the client proceed. Clients have preferences that motivate them to choose certain health behaviors, as well as barriers—like cost and time—that mitigate against other treatment choices. Clients have a responsibility for their own health care, and as nurses we can encourage their participation by giving them a chance to speak and listening to them when they answer our questions.

The Multiple Choice Mix-up

As interviewers we sometimes get carried away and assault our clients with a barrage of questions. After receiving a string of questions, our clients become confused and do not know what information we are looking for or where to begin answering.

Wrong way:

Bombarding you: "Mrs. Parker, there are some things we need to know to help you through your labor, delivery, and your postpartum stay. Have you discussed what kind of delivery you prefer? Have you and your husband met with your physician and gone over all the options? What I mean is, have you decided on whether you will receive analgesics and/or any type of anesthetic during labor? Do you know the various types: general, spinal, perineal block? And next we need to know your plans for breast-feeding. Have you decided on that yet?"

Whew! Mrs. Parker's head would be spinning as she tried to keep pace with this bombardment. Just as she would have formulated a response to one question, you were off to the next, probably making her feel distracted, confused, and irritated.

Right way:

Clear you: "Mrs. Parker, there are some things we need to know to help you through your labor, delivery, and your stay afterwards. I'd like to review your plans for pain management during labor and for feeding your baby. Are you comfortable enough to go over these two areas now?" You pause to check out her readiness. "First, are you planning to use any type of pain medication during your labor and delivery?"

Mrs. Parker has been given one question to answer in this example. She knows there are more questions forthcoming, but she knows exactly what you are seeking when a single, clearly worded question is posed.

Incomprehensible Cryptic Codes

As nurses, we become accustomed to medical terminology and develop our own shorthand to abbreviate long, unwieldy medical terms. Using this jargon among professionals is fine, but using it with clients only adds to their confusion. Clients have a right to receive questions that are worded clearly in language they can understand.

Wrong way:

Cryptic you: "I've come with your digoxin, Mr. Winters. Before I give it I need to check out your apical and radial pulses and estimate your edema. Have you had any angina, palpitations, or SOB this morning? We want to prevent chemotoxicity."

Mr. Winters would almost need a medical dictionary or decoder to decipher your questions! Using medical jargon might make him feel stupid or uncomfortable. And just as bad, you might receive incorrect information from clients who give answers to questions they do not understand because they are embarrassed or confused.

Right way:

Clear you: "Mr. Winters, I've come with your heart medication—digoxin. Before I give it I need to check your heart rate over your heart with my stethoscope and at your wrist. Have you had any chest pain this morning?" After pausing for an answer, you ask: "Have you noticed any fluttering or fast beating of your heart this morning?" After receiving his answer, you ask: "Have you had any shortness of breath at any time this morning?"

Asking questions in plain English increases the probability that clients will understand what you are asking and, in turn, give appropriate responses.

The Offensive Misuse of "Why"

As nurses we do a lot of detective work trying to determine why our clients are sick, why they are upset, why they do not follow their treatment regimen, and so on. These "whys" are all legitimate questions, but when it comes to asking, it is usually best to refrain from using "why" too frequently with clients because it tends to make them feel threatened. To avoid such an aggressive tactic, it is better to rephrase the question so it is softer and more receivable.

Wrong way:

Threatening you: A client is slamming his pillow against his bed frame: "Why are you doing that, Mr. Kent?"
A teenager is using his crutches incorrectly: "Why aren't you weight bearing more?"
A diabetic woman is having three toes on her left foot amputated: "Why don't you take better care of your feet?"
An elderly widower is sad: "Why are you letting life slip by you instead of getting back into things?"

Each of these "why" questions is aggressive and blunt. Each one might force the client to be defensive, curt, or, in some other way, protective. Withdrawal or hostility diminishes the chances for an open and honest response.

Right way:

Gentle you: To the client who is slamming his pillow against his bed frame: "Will you tell me what's wrong, Mr. Kent?"
To the teenager who is using his crutches incorrectly: "What is it that prevents you from weight bearing more?"
To the diabetic woman who is having three toes on her left foot amputated: "What factors make it difficult for you to take better care of your feet?"

To the elderly widower who is sad: "What are some of the things that keep you sad and prevent you from getting involved in things you used to enjoy?"

Each of these questions seeks the same information as the questions above, but they are less aggressively phrased. These questions do not put the client on the spot; rather, they invite the client to respond.

Open and Closed Questions

Closed questions are focused and posed to elicit specific and brief responses from clients. Open questions invite respondents to elaborate in whatever direction they choose. Skilled interviewers know when to use each type of question.

Wrong way:

Closed you: A client has just returned from the x-ray department where he underwent a barium enema, a procedure he was dreading. You ask: "Did your barium enema procedure go okay?"

This question only requires a "yes" or "no" and does not invite your client to elaborate further about his experience.

In an initial health history you ask your client: "Do you eat a well-balanced diet?"

The "yes" or "no" response to this type of question would tell you little about his nutritional intake.

Your 63-year-old client is going to be transferred to an extended care facility. You ask: "Are you looking forward to going to Haven's Point?"

This approach gives your client little choice about how to answer.

Right way:

Interested you: A client has just returned from the x-ray department where he underwent a barium enema, a procedure he was dreading. You say: "Tell me how the procedure went for you."

In an initial health history you ask your client: "What did you eat for breakfast today?"

Your 63-year-old client is going to a long-term care facility. You ask: "How do you feel about leaving here and going to live at Haven's Point?"

These three examples are open-ended questions that would require your client's elaboration. The information obtained by these questions would give you fuller comprehension of your client's perspective.

In nursing practice, we err more frequently on the side of posing closed questions where open-ended ones would provide more useful information. However, we are sometimes too general when we should be more focused in our question asking. Therefore, it is worthwhile to examine your question-asking practices to see if there are times when you might make your questions more focused.

The Mystery Interview

When we ask questions of our clients, they respond with the belief that as skilled clinicians we are sorting, sifting, and analyzing their data in order to contribute to their nursing care plan. It makes our clients feel connected and respected when we give them feedback on our problem-solving process.

   Wrong way:

Abrupt you: You have been doing an initial health assessment with a client admitted for extreme and rapid weight loss. The time allotted for the interview is over and you say to your client: "I've got to go now. I'll see you later and we can continue our interview then."

   Clients feel left out when we end an interview without giving them any indication of our assessment.

   Right way:

Clear you: If it is necessary to end an interview before you can complete your assessment, you can say something like: "We've talked about your weight loss problem a fair amount today. In order to know all the factors that might be contributing to your weight loss, I need to get some more information from you at our next interview. Until we meet again this afternoon, could you be thinking about anything you can recall, anything unusual that happened to you at the time you first started losing weight?"

Wit and Wisdom

All These Questions . . .

Questions come easy
To some folks, I'm told.
For others, the questions
They may seem too bold.

These guidelines will help you
To know how to ask
The facts that you need
To complete your tasks.

The questions you pose
Show that you care.
To feel really heard
Is just all too rare.

Remember each person
Has his or her story.
The essence of nursing,
This is its glory.

Copyright 1995 Julia W. Balzer Riley. Used with permission.

Even though this closing remark does not offer a definite summary, it does show that you are up-to-date with your clinical assessment of the problem. Informing our clients of what is happening, including our plans and what they can expect next, provides helpful transitions so that they can map their progress, feel included, and minimize worrying about erroneous assumptions.

If you use the suggestions in this chapter, your question asking will be assertive and responsible. You will respect your right to secure the information you need to complete the nursing process yet maintain the dignity of your clients.

Think About It...
What, So What, and Now What?

Consider what you read about asking questions and the importance of these skills. Consider how asking questions in a professional relationship is different from asking questions in a personal relationship.

What? . . . Write one thing you learned from this chapter.

So what? . . . How will this impact your nursing practice?

Now what? . . . How will you implement this new knowledge or skill?

THINK ABOUT IT

Practicing Asking Questions

Exercise 1

For this exercise you get to watch TV or listen to the radio. Over the next week or so, observe the skills of TV and radio interviewers. Make note of what interviewers do well and where you think they could improve.

- Are their introductions long-winded or focused?
- Do they give interviewees a chance to express their opinions before jumping in with their views?
- Are their questions succinct and clear or are they a barrage of seemingly unrelated topics?
- Do they phrase their questions in clear English or do they use technical jargon that might confuse the interviewee?
- Are "why" questions used aggressively or is the interviewer nonthreatening?
- Are open-ended questions used appropriately?

At the end of the week, compare what you have learned about effective ways to ask questions with your colleagues.

Exercise 2

For this exercise work in threes. One person will be the interviewer, one the interviewee, and one the observer. The interviewee will choose to be interviewed about anything; for example, an interest in music, windsurfing, or skiing, the latest paper he or she is writing for a course, or a new product he or she is planning to buy. The interviewee must let the interviewer know what the topic is before the interview begins.

For 8 minutes the interviewer will ask questions about the topic the interviewee has chosen. During the exchange the observer will make note of how effectively the interviewer asks questions. At the end of 8 minutes the observer will have feedback on the strengths of the interviewer and where the interviewer could improve.

The questions in Exercise 1 can be used as guidelines for giving feedback. Tape recording this exercise will give you a chance to review your work more thoroughly.

The group of three should change roles so that each gets the chance to try all roles.

What has this exercise taught you about the skill of asking questions?

Exercise 3

Client-nurse situations are not the only occasions when we ask questions. We can learn a lot about our question-asking skills from how we interact with friends, family, and colleagues at work. Over the next week or so, make notes on the effectiveness of your question asking. What do you like about your approach to asking questions of your friends and family and peers? What are some changes you could make to improve your competence?

Observe how others ask questions of you and notice what is effective and what is unclear or uncomfortable.

Continued

Practicing Asking Questions—cont'd

Exercise 4

As you go into your clinical units, take some extra time to assess your skill level in asking questions of your clients. Prepare for your interviews by paying attention to the why, what, how, who, when, and where of asking questions. As soon as possible after an interview with a client, stop and reflect on how effective you were. Review the common mistakes and make note of areas where you excelled and where you need to improve.

If possible, tape record an interview with one of your clients and critique your question-asking ability afterward. Having the verbatim account of your question asking is the most ideal learning situation. You must have your client's total agreement to record an interview, including permission about who can listen to the tape. Some clients prefer to review a tape-recorded interview before releasing it to nurses. Some agencies require nurses to obtain written consent before tape recording an interview with a client. It is important to erase the tape after you have critiqued your interviewing skills and to follow through by informing your client that you have done so.

Exercise 5

As a nurse working on an orthopedic unit, you are nursing a newly admitted, elderly female client, Mrs. Haley, diagnosed with Alzheimer's disease and a broken left hip. This evening her son and daughter-in-law and her frail elderly husband, with whom she lived before her recent admission, have come to the unit to visit your client. It is your responsibility to investigate how your client fell and broke her hip.

Working on your own, choose and write down what your first three questions would be. Be able to defend

- Why you chose to ask those questions
- What exactly you would ask
- How you would ask the questions
- Whom you would ask
- When you would pose your questions
- Where you would ask your questions

When you have finished writing down your three questions on your own, compare the similarities and differences in your approaches as a class. This exercise focuses on your question-asking and problem-solving skills. What has this exercise taught you about the relationship between question-asking and problem solving?

Reference

Sundeen et al: *Nurse-client interaction: implementing the nursing process,* St Louis, 1998, Mosby.

 ## Suggestions for Further Reading

Copp LA: The spectrum of suffering, *Am J Nurs* 90(8):35, 1990.

This humbling article reminds nurses about one question to ask our clients who have pain: what have they found helpful to ease their pain? Often this simple question is not asked, and valuable information about client coping, as well as an opportunity to acknowledge client responsibility for successful problem solving, is overlooked.

Harvey K: The power of positive questioning, *Nurs Manag* 21(5):94, 1990.

This intriguing article proposes that nurses risk asking questions in ways that promote affirmative responses and agreement in certain situations.

High DM: Truth telling, confidentiality, and the dying patient: new dilemmas for the nurse, *Nurs Forum* 24(1):5, 1989.

This excellent article challenges nurses to reevaluate their concept of confidentiality in relation to the privilege of nursing terminally ill clients. Balancing clients' need to talk intimately is their right to privacy and respect. High poses this question for nurses: "What do you let your patients tell you?" The relevance of this query has implications for the art of question asking in nursing.

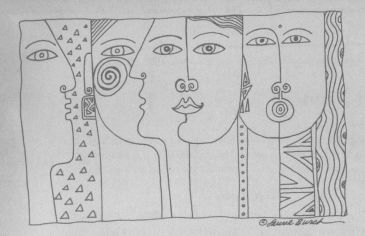

Expressing Opinions

Boldness, without the rules of propriety, becomes insubordination.

Confucius

THE DIFFERENCE BETWEEN GIVING ADVICE AND EXPRESSING OPINIONS

Expressing opinions as a nurse refers to the act of disclosing what you think or feel about health care situations affecting your clients or colleagues. Expressing opinions or offering recommendations is an assertive behavior. In a professional setting, your opinions are offered as additional information for your clients' (and colleagues') problem-solving and decision-making process. In contrast, giving advice is a unilateral process of solving problems or making decisions for others. Offering advice prevents clients from becoming independent and gives colleagues the idea that you might think they are incapable of self-direction.

Expressing opinions can be part of providing clients with a fuller picture to make choices about their health and treatment plans. Clients have a moral right to information and "if they exercise that right by asking questions or seeking information, there is a duty to provide that information" (Freel, 1994). Expressing opinions is not telling others what to do, but giving them the benefit of your point of view. It assists clients in their health decision making and avoids both the dependency of clients relying on their nurses and the anger and blame when the nurses' advice is rejected at some point.

WHEN TO EXPRESS YOUR OPINIONS AS A NURSE

Clients and colleagues may seek your nursing counsel when they are at a point where they must make a decision about any of the following.

Whether to Provide or Withhold Information: For example, clients may wonder whether they should expose information about their condition to a physician or another family member. Colleagues may be in a quandary about whether to reveal information to clients and/or their family, or to colleagues or supervisors. Fellow students may be undecided about whether to confide in their nursing instructor about personal problems.

Whether to Comply With a Treatment Plan or Resist It: Some clients may have conflicting doubts and hopes about their health problem and might be unsettled about whether to follow a treatment plan or attempt to survive without it. Fellow nurses may have mixed feelings about adhering to restrictions imposed on tasks they can perform while making a home visit. Student colleagues may have a dilemma about whether to report an honors violation.

Which Strategies to Implement in Order to Get the Desired Outcomes: Clients who know what expected health status they are aiming for may not be able to decide which treatment plan to follow. Colleagues at work may know exactly what outcomes they want but need help in deciding what actions they can take that will most likely ensure that they reach their goal. Classmates may be lost about what approach to take to ensure that they receive a high grade on their next assignment.

Your views may be sought by clients or colleagues at any one of these decision points. Your opinions provide others with information that can be incorporated into their decision making.

Although they are referring to the psychotherapeutic helping relationship, Jensen, Josephson, and Frey (1989) have several pointers about sharing information with clients that also apply to the client-nurse helping relationship. Nurses might share their opinions about any of the preceding situations when there is uncertainty about outcome, both negative and positive effects of the options, or when one course is not necessarily superior to the other (Jensen, Josephson, and Frey,

1989). Providing your opinions as a nurse can create a situation for discussing any one of these decision points and provides an opportunity to collaborate about the health care of your clients. Both of these mutual acts will strengthen your relationship.

Your Feelings About Expressing Opinions

Before proceeding any further, take a pencil and jot down your responses to these questions:

- How do you feel when others express their opinions to you without your seeking them?
- How do you feel when others refrain from giving you their opinions when you have sought their counsel?

After you have expressed your feelings about these questions, compare your reactions with those of colleagues in your class.

Many of us feel differently about opinions we have sought versus viewpoints we did not seek. In our culture, where we place a high value on liberty and the freedom to act as we choose within the limits of the law, it is likely that many of us feel some resentment when others take it upon themselves to try to influence us without our consent. We are usually more willing to consider opinions that we have agreed to receive. This knowledge of our nature suggests a principle for expressing opinions: whenever possible, find out if your opinion is wanted. You may have strong opinions about what decision a person should make, but you are wasting your time and may be jeopardizing a relationship if you persist without their consent.

Many of you will have indicated that you expect to be given opinions from someone whose counsel you have sought and that you feel cheated when denied. When we ask lawyers, physicians, and teachers for their professional opinions, we expect them to provide us with guidance. So it is with our clients and colleagues who seek our points of view in our professional capacity as nurses. Remember that people sometimes have the right to learn from their own mistakes. It could be possible that your answer is not the best one for them anyway. When others make their own decisions, the blame or the glory is their own.

Wit and Wisdom

Sometimes not to decide is to decide.

Author unknown

Here are two more questions about expressing opinions.

- How do you feel when clients (or friends, family members, or work colleagues) who have asked for your opinion do not act on the views you express?
- How do you feel when clients (or friends, family members, or work colleagues) incorporate your opinions into their actions?

You may have no strong feelings about whether other people act on your opinions. On the other hand, you may experience pride or relief that others act on your counsel, or may feel hurt or disappointment when they do not. The strength of your feelings may be related to how much you derive a sense of power or control over other people's actions. Consider to what extent your self-esteem as a nurse depends on your clients or colleagues doing things your way versus knowing you offered them your wisest counsel so that they had adequate information on which to base their decision?

The degree to which we allow others the freedom to make their own decisions depends on whether we care more for their autonomy and well-being than whether our opinions are revered. As nurses, we must keep in mind what expectations regarding seeking opinions our clients come with and, more importantly, what agendas we carry around about offering others our viewpoint.

HOW TO EXPRESS YOUR OPINIONS IN AN ASSERTIVE WAY

As a nurse you will be called upon to express health care opinions in your professional life by your clients and colleagues, and in your personal life by friends, family, and even perfect strangers. Because you are an educated, professional nurse, there will be innumerable times when you will be tempted to express opinions to clients and friends or family about their health care. You will feel more confident about handling these situations if you have worked out some principles to stand by for expressing opinions. Here are some guidelines:

Get the Consent of Your Receiver Before Expressing Your Opinions

To avoid generating feelings of hostility or resentment in your clients or colleagues, ask if they are interested in hearing your viewpoint. Here are several phrases you can use to complete this courteous step that can flow naturally into your conversation:

"A former client told me a good way to get around a situation like yours. Would you like to hear that suggestion?"

"I've just read an article that had some excellent ideas on how to solve your problem. Do you want to hear what it had to say?"

"Last year I had the same difficulties you are now having. By trial and error, I learned some great ways to get rid of the problem. Would you be interested in hearing how I worked things out?"

"I've seen many people with a similar problem to yours. I have some recommendations for you that have come from those experiences. Would you like to hear them?"

"I've thought about this issue for a long time, and I have some opinions I'd like to express to the team if you'd like to hear them."

Although you think may have helpful information, the other person may not necessarily want to hear it. As one friend of a psychiatric nurse once remarked, "If you know of any other developmental crisis I'm about due for, just keep it to yourself!"

Clients or colleagues from whom you are requesting permission to proceed will let you know whether they want to hear your ideas. Those who are verbal and direct will reply with a definite "yes" or "no." Those who are less direct will send you nonverbal signals that will tell you whether to proceed or refrain from sharing your conclusions. If they look away, change the subject, or argue that their situation is unique, they are warning you to back off and keep your opinions to yourself. If they give interested gestures, that is your cue to continue.

Make Allowances for the Uniqueness of Your Client or Colleague

We give opinions based on the knowledge that our ideas have worked in similar situations with like people and circumstances. However, it is impossible for us to know all the circumstances and personal factors that affect everyone we deal with. Consequently, we should avoid being dogmatic when expressing our opinions. We should be tentative about offering our persuasions in order to show our consideration of others' special circumstances.

Avoiding strong phrases like, "I really think you should," "You really ought to," or "It should be clear to you that this is the direction to take," will make your views more receivable so that they can be incorporated into other people's problem-solving processes.

When offering your opinion, you can include one of the following phrases, which will give others a fair chance to accept or reject your ideas:

"Do you think this idea will help in your situation?"
"What do you think about these recommendations?"
"How do you think this suggestion will fit your lifestyle?"
"How does my slant on your situation strike you?"
"Can you adapt any of these ideas to your situation?"

Include the Rationale for Your Viewpoint

Your clients and colleagues expect you to have opinions about health care and work- or school-related issues. Giving your rationale is a responsible way to defend your position. It ensures that sufficient information is available for clients and colleagues to make the final decision.

Moments of Connection...
"If It Were Me . . ."

"As a hospice inpatient supervisor, I had an end-stage cardiac client come in who was dying. He was having great difficulty breathing and wanted to sit up in a chair at all times. The staff was upset, because they were afraid he was going to die in the chair. I approached the physician, whose idea of pain management was Tylenol or Darvocet, and asked him for IV morphine. He asked me why. I looked at him and said, "If it were me, struggling to breathe and dying, I would want someone to put an IV in me to give me morphine and help me to breathe." He reluctantly agreed. The gentleman was started on IV morphine and was able to rest. He died later that night in peace." *Author's note:* We all understand a reluctance to administer morphine because we are taught it can depress respirations. This pain management nurse expressed her opinion as an expert who understood that morphine can decrease air hunger. Her willingness to express her opinion helped the physician in their mutual goal of comfort and care for the client.

Here are some phrases that you might use to include your rationale with your opinions to clients:

"In my view, options 2 and 4 would be the most likely to get the results you are looking for. Which options do you favor?"

"If you have the money, I think going to the clinic in Healthtown is the best resource for you. If finances are strained, you might wish to consider one of the self-help groups here in town. What do you think?"

"If I were feeling as desperate as you seem to be, I think I would go for the quick-start option rather than the slower one. After you get some relief from your symptoms, you could shift over to the regular stream. How does that plan sound to you?"

"I hesitate to suggest plan A because all your social supports and family are out of town. Plan B would ensure that you get some regular supervision while you are learning the technique. What are your preferences?"

"In my clinical experience, using the prepared formula has proven to be more successful than the one clients have to mix from scratch. That's my recommendation. Does that help you make a decision?"

"I really don't know which way would be better for you. In my experience, there have been clients that have been happy with both treatment choices. The final choice gets down to personal preference since both options are solid in every respect. So my advice is 'choose the one you like!'"

In all these examples the nurse has offered a reason to defend his or her preferences and turned the final decision back to the client. If we want clients to take charge of their own health care, we can offer them our professional opinions yet make it clear that the final responsibility is theirs.

With your colleagues on the health care team, you might include your rationale in the following ways:

"Mrs. Jones is beginning to improve, so I think it would be a mistake for us to transfer her just now. Maybe Mrs. Hanes could be moved first so that Mrs. Jones would have an extra week of physical therapy. What do you think?"

"Our Kardex system is outdated. I think we should adopt the system written about in the latest issue of the *American Journal of Nursing*. It describes how to keep all the pertinent information updated and right at your fingertips. I'll bring the article in so that you can see how useful it might be for us."

"I think we should ask the instructor to go over the section on neuroanatomy one more time before the exam. It's worth 40%, and she only spent one lecture period on it. What do you think?"

"I think we should consider purchasing computers to enter data on the home health clients since proper documentation affects reimbursement. Do you think administration would agree?"

"We have nursing students from two different universities on this unit this month. Even though they are on different shifts, the patients are having to answer the same questions and have commented about it. Do you see this as a problem?"

"I think we should have a first-year student representative on the faculty curriculum committee in addition to the second-year rep. We need a student there to get our perspective across to the faculty, don't you think?"

"Since you ask, Dr. Kenson, I have been Mr. Jones' nurse for the last week and a half, and I feel strongly that he could be discharged sooner than you are recommending. His condition is stabilized and the home care nurses could see him daily for his injection and dressing change. He is very anxious to get back to his own surroundings and begin to take up his life again, especially to start a bit of writing on his home computer. What do you think?"

"Thanks for the chance to give my input to the safety committee. In the 3 months I've been here, there has not been a fire drill, and I notice that the two exit lights on our unit aren't lit. I think we could all benefit from regular fire drills and scheduled inspection of the equipment. Would you agree?"

These examples demonstrate how to give your opinions assertively and still consider your colleagues' viewpoint. Giving your opinions does not mean coercing your colleagues to adopt your ideas. Providing a rationale for your point of view and inviting others' opinions makes the decision-making a collaborative process.

It is possible that the decision-making climate set by nurse managers influences the style of decision making used by staff nurses with their clients. In a study of nurse problem solving, Schmieding (1990) reports that the majority of head nurse actions do not involve staff nurses in any way. Nurses who are committed to a mutual problem-solving approach with clients want the same kind of respect and collegiality as in a participative management climate. Nurses can influence how decisions are made by keeping alert and assertively making and taking opportunities to express their opinions as another source of information for the workplace decision-making process. Bushy and Smith (1990) encourage nurses to become politically proactive and lobby for changes they would like to see in the health care system. Developing political savvy is an extension of being assertive.

Expressing your opinions is also assertive and responsible. It protects your right to have your point of view included in the decision making and respects others' rights to know what you are thinking. By including your views you are ensuring that another piece of information is available to the decision makers.

HOW TO SHARE YOUR POSITIVE REGARD FOR OTHERS

You may notice a particular behavior of a client, family member, or colleague that, in your opinion, is noteworthy. Giving specific positive feedback is another form of expressing your opinions that can demonstrate your assertive communication style. Berent and Evans (1992) give examples of how to compliment and commend people for their actions:

"You're always willing to help."
"You're always open to new ideas."
"I see improvement in . . . ."
"It took a lot of courage for you to . . . ."

Contribute your opinion of shared good work:

"We've worked hard on this."
"We came up with some good ideas."

In work groups or other successful collaborations, humorous positive comments create energy and goodwill:

"Are we a great team or what?"
"We are so wonderful, I can hardly stand it."
"We want a prize . . . we did so well."
"Just call us terrific!"

Sharing positive opinions sets the stage for others to feel comfortable in loosening up a bit and sharing their ideas in a friendly, accepting environment. This promotes creativity and teamwork . . . a non-evasive, cost-effective tool! In a climate of professional and personal change coming at an unprecedented rate, rewarding colleagues with praise or by other methods becomes important.

THE ART OF NOT EXPRESSING YOUR OPINIONS

Some of us do not need any help expressing our opinions, but rather need an awareness of knowing when *not* to share and having the strength *not* to be right. When someone tells a story in which the details are not absolutely correct, consider whether the accuracy is crucial. You hear someone say it was "100 degrees" yesterday, but you heard on the weather report that there was "a high of 99 degrees." Is your usual response to correct the person? Consider the results. This is experienced as a "put-down" comment, which does not build relationships. This is a startling concept to some of us. Just give it some thought. Exercise 7 (near the end of this chapter) will help you explore this further.

HOW TO EMPOWER YOURSELF THROUGH EXPRESSING OPINIONS

At times in your career you may feel powerless in the face of decisions that are made without your input or with which you will disagree. You can make a choice about when to share your disagreement even if you see no choice but to comply with the decision. For example, if a new policy is to be implemented that seems unreasonable to you, but not unsafe, you can say:

"I understand that this new policy is in place. I will comply with it, but I do want to voice my disagreement for the following reasons . . . I will try it this way and see how it goes, but I'll get back to you with any problems we encounter."

A teenage patient with asthma has chosen to smoke cigarettes. You might say,

"John, of course, your choice to smoke is your decision, but I want to express my concern for how this can affect your health. I can tell you more about how that can happen if you are willing to hear, but I can't in good conscience avoid opening up the discussion."

Wit and Wisdom

To Share or Not to Share . . .

Expressing opinions
Is not hard for me.
I have one on everything.
Just wait and see.

Opinions are precious.
We each have our own.
Discretion will tell us
Which ones to loan.

Copyright 1995 Julia W. Balzer Riley.

Sometimes just being able to voice your disagreement makes you feel more authentic, more assertive. Assertiveness is a matter of choice and not necessary or appropriate in every situation. You may have a strong sense of fairness, but if another customer who is obviously belligerent and inebriated cuts in front of you in line at the grocery store, you would probably make a choice not to share your opinion about fairness. This does not mean you are nonassertive but that you have good judgment. You make decisions about what opinions to share, with whom, and when. Some of these decisions are based on unpleasant results from past experience. Try to remember that everyone has to learn some things the hard way. As you learn when to take appropriate risks to express your opinion and earn the respect of clients and colleagues, you may find your input is requested as you are viewed as an authentic person who is willing to take a stand.

Think About It...
What, So What, and Now What?

Consider what you read about expressing opinions. Think about your own experiences in health care and how asking questions makes a difference.

What? . . . Write one thing you learned from this chapter.

So what? . . . How will this impact your nursing practice?

Now what? . . . How will you implement this new knowledge or skill?

THINK ABOUT IT

Practicing Expressing Opinions

Exercise 1

For this exercise you will work in groups of three. One of you will role-play a client with a problem about which she is seeking the nurse's opinion. Another will role-play the nurse in this interaction. The third will be the observer and will give feedback.

For 4 minutes the "client" will make clear her request for the nurse's opinions and the nurse will attempt to express her views assertively. Debrief with the following questions:

As the observer: Did the nurse gain the client's permission to express her opinions? Did the nurse take into account the client's unique circumstances when she expressed her opinions? Did the nurse provide a rationale to defend her opinions? Overall, how assertive was the nurse in expressing her opinions to her client?

As the client: How did you react to the nurse's offering of her opinions? What did you like about the nurse's approach to sharing her views? What suggestions for improvement would you make?

As the nurse: What is your assessment of your ability to assertively express your opinions from your participation in this exercise? What did you like about how you expressed your opinions? What suggestions for improvement would you make?

Alternate roles so that each of you has a chance to be client, nurse, and observer.

Exercise 2

Repeat Exercise 1, but this time one of you will role-play a colleague (nurse, physical therapist, physician, clergy), rather than a client, who wants the nurse's opinions on an issue. Proceed as outlined in Exercise 1.

After completing both exercises, discuss your feelings about expressing your opinions to colleagues and clients. What similarities and differences are there for you? What accounts for any differences you notice?

Exercise 3

Over the next few days, note the way others express their opinions to you. Check out if they ask your permission and consider your particular situation, how tentative they are, and whether they provide a rationale. Your reactions to receiving advice from a variety of people will tell you a lot about how to effectively express your opinions.

As a class, compare and contrast your observations and conclusions about expressing opinions.

Exercise 4

Over the next few days, observe how you express your opinions to others in your day-to-day encounters. Assess the assertiveness of your approach. Congratulate yourself on your effectiveness, and make note of where you need to improve.

Continued

Practicing Expressing Opinions—cont'd

Exercise 5

For one day, observe opportunities to express your positive opinions of others. Take the plunge and give one compliment that you would ordinarily not share. How did the person respond? Commit yourself to giving one compliment each day for a week and ask one colleague to try the experiment, too. Arrange for a specific time to sit down and share your experiences. This kind of positive energy can do wonders for the profession. Imagine if every nurse gave one compliment each day!

Exercise 6

This exercise requires no action on your part. For one week, just be aware of any decisions that affect you with which you disagree. Make a mental note of whether it is the right time or situation to share your opinion. The purpose of this exercise is only to increase your awareness, not to stir you to action.

Exercise 7

Practice *not* sharing your opinion. Do you ever feel the need to correct someone whose facts in your opinion are not accurate? For one week, note when this happens. Ask yourself if it is important that you correct the person. If it is not a life and death matter, try resisting the impulse to be right. This may well be a stress-reducing activity for you and others—the area of letting it go!

References

Berent IM, Evans RL: *The right words: the 350 best things to say to get along with people,* New York, 1992, Warner.

Bushy A, Smith TO: Lobbying: the hows and wherefores, *Nurs Manag* 21(4):39, 1990.

Freel MI: Truth telling. In McCloskey JC, Grace HK, editors: *Current issues in nursing,* ed 4, St Louis, 1994, Mosby.

Jensen PS, Josephson AM, Frey J: Informed consent as a framework for treatment: ethical and therapeutic considerations, *Am J Psychother* 43(3):378, 1989.

Nelson B: *1001 ways to reward employees,* New York, 1994, Workman Publishing.

Schmieding NJ: Do head nurses include staff nurses in problem-solving?, *Nurs Manag* 21(3):58, 1990.

Suggestion for Further Reading

American Nurses Association: Maximize involvement in workplace decision making. In American Nurses Association: *Survival skills in the workplace: what every nurse should know,* Kansas City, Mo, 1990, The Association.

This chapter expands nurses' awareness of the larger organizational structure in the workplace and provides practical suggestions for strengthening their professional influence.

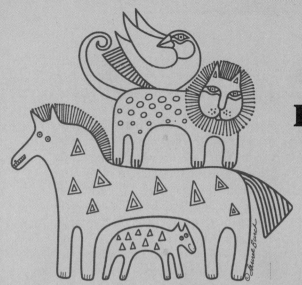

14

Humor

Humor is a prelude to faith and laughter is the beginning of prayer.

Reinhold Niebuhr

OBJECTIVES

1. Define humor as it is used in health care.
2. Distinguish between positive and negative humor.
3. Identify three criteria for the appropriate use of humor in health care.
4. Discuss the functions of humor in health care.
5. Identify strategies to implement humor in health care.
6. Discuss the use of a humor kit in health care.
7. Identify three ways humor can be used to promote positive communication in health care.
8. Discuss creative ways to add humor and play to relieve stress and build relationships.

A DEFINITION OF HUMOR

As we begin to discuss humor, remember that the best advice is to follow the client's lead and try a "toe in the water" to see if humor fits the occasion (McGhee, 1998). Broadly defined, humor is "an exceptional frame of mind, a way of perceiving and experiencing life" (Kipplinger, 1987). Humor adds a perspective that frees us from conformity and puts us in touch with our authentic, spontaneous self (Kipplinger, 1987). To be able to laugh at yourself in uncomfortable situations, in the face of life's incongruities, is essential to good mental health. Former Chrysler Chairman Lee Iacoca would often exchange jokes with members of the press and with stockholders. His humor put people at ease and built upon his image as a leader who had high esteem and control of situations (Green, 1993). Nurses can use positive humor with the same effect. ". . . Humor is not only the telling of jokes to patients. It is the attitude, the relaxation and the smile that really make the difference" (Bakerman, H, 1998, p. 6). Remember to be yourself. Often it is the immediacy of a genuine, light response that makes the connection (Fonnesbeck, 1998). Patti Davis, daughter of former President Ronald Reagan writes, humor is "a tonic . . . and a life raft . . . Humor dulls the edges, makes life smoother, lets it go down easier" (Davis, 1995, p. 18).

To be able to laugh at a tough situation provides temporary relief from fear and worry. This changes the perception of a stressful event and adds a sense of control, the power to choose your own attitude or response. A nurse who has experienced the challenges of menopause, for example, may use her own humorous perspective to reframe, or alter the view, of the situation for her client. Hot flashes become "power surges." This can lead to a discussion of the positive side of the middle years.

Humor can also help nurses build relationships with clients and colleagues. After all, it is hard not to like a person who makes you laugh (McGhee, 1989).

Humor
- Invites interaction
- Puts others at ease
- Wins affection
- Helps us cope with stress and fear (Green, 1993)

Wit and Wisdom

A person without a sense of humor is like a wagon without springs— jolted by every pebble in the road.

Henry Ward Beecher

If you can laugh at your own shortcomings and learn from your mistakes, you are freed to be creative. Being creative means taking the risk to fail. Nurse managers who can tolerate personal mistakes create a safe environment where staff can dare to be innovative.

POSITIVE VERSUS NEGATIVE HUMOR

It is important to distinguish between positive and negative humor. Positive humor, "constructive, empathic humor" (Fry and Salameh, 1987), is associated with love, hope, joy, creativity, or a gentle sense of playfulness. Its intent is to bring people closer together. Negative humor puts people on the defensive, makes them feel put down, and may be sarcastic, racist, sexist, or ageist. It reinforces negative stereotypes about different cultures, age groups, or conditions. Negative humor isolates you and alienates people (Box 14-1).

Positive humor communicates that the human condition is shared, that we all have problems, and that no one is perfect. The highest form of humor is the ability to laugh at ourselves. Follow this adage: "Take your work seriously, but yourself lightly." One nurse who volunteers as a clown in her hospice work relates an example of humor with an elderly man whose movements have slowed with his illness. The nurse and the client often joke about this because she admits to being slow in the mornings too. The nurse gave her client a button that showed a turtle saying, "I may be slow, but I won the race." The client loved the gift and wears it whenever the nurse visits. Positive humor adds to your relationships with clients, families, and colleagues by eliciting cooperation (Box 14-2).

Your response to another person's humor says something about who you are. To reinforce positive humor by laughing and sharing your own humorous perspective, but to refuse to laugh at or participate in demeaning humor by remaining quiet or gently commenting, "I don't think that is funny," is an assertive statement of one's belief system. Although it may be difficult, it is a responsible way to deal with demeaning humor and does not encourage or reinforce put-down humor as does nervous laughter. Recognize, however, that humor serves to relieve tension, and neg-

---

Box 14-1   Negative Humor Can Build Barriers Between People

Avoid
- Racist humor
- Sexist humor
- Ageist humor
- Sarcasm
- Put-downs

Box 14-2   Positive Humor Can Build Bridges Between People

- Laugh at yourself.
- Follow the patient's lead.
- Remark on humorous cards.
- Share cartoons.
- Share jokes.
- Use gentle banter: "Our gowns aren't skimpy; they're air-conditioned!"

ative humor may be a coping mechanism in tough situations. The "medical" humor, or gallows humor, that staff use to cope is appropriate when kept among staff because it permits shared frustration and promotes group cohesion (Simon, 1988).

Negative humor may serve to relieve tension for the sender of the communication, but it can demean others and undermine your credibility if shared inappropriately. When information about AIDS first became public, several radio stations aired macabre jokes about the illness. It was not uncommon to hear people repeat these jokes. People often make jokes about subjects that cause anxiety such as sexuality, relationships, and death. AIDS is one issue that touches all three.

National tragedies, such as the space shuttle disaster, can also be the source of jokes. Humor is often used as a catharsis to provide relief. In a study of such jokes, it was found that this humor served as an "antidote to personal tension and pain" and helped "neutralize the pain of a nation" (Green, 1993).

Humor is highly individualized. People find different things funny. Pay attention to the subjects of your clients' jokes or humorous comments. This will give you a clue about their topics of concern. If a preoperative patient lightly says, "Well, I won't die from it," it is likely he would benefit from a little extra time to talk about these fears. Be alert for what seems like inappropriate humor in timing or subject. This is a clue that clients or colleagues may benefit from more serious discussion of the issue. Allow your clients the right to hostile or macabre humor, but do not participate in it yourself. To listen without using off-putting body language shows your ability to allow for individual coping responses. To build on this negative humor may create problems. Consider a time when you are upset with a relative or close friend. You make negative comments or jokes to relieve tension. If a friend or spouse joins in, you may be offended; it's OK for me to joke about my mother, but not for you!

In humor workshops held for clients who are HIV-positive, participants suggest that nurses "allow us our own form of humor. We know it is black humor. Don't take offense at it and please, touch us more, don't act as if you can't wait to get out of the room." Although this may be seen as negative humor by nurses, it is initiated by clients as a way of coping with anxiety. Coping styles vary. What people find funny varies. What is constant is your clients' need to feel that someone understands and accepts them wherever they are along their own journey of coping with illness.

Wit and Wisdom

What I can laugh at, I can cope with.

Julia W. Balzer Riley

If humor should become offensive, you can change the subject or tell your clients that you appreciate their need to use humor but that you are embarrassed.

CRITERIA FOR THE APPROPRIATE USE OF HUMOR

Have you heard the adage, "There is a time and place for everything"? Pay attention to timing, receptivity, and content (Leiber, 1986) in the use of intentional humor as an intervention.

Timing: When patients are admitted to an acute setting such as the emergency room, they and their family want efficient, caring attention and treatment. Humor may be inappropriate unless initiated by patients or family members. You will be able to distinguish between banter among clients and family members to ease tension, and the put-down humor or sarcasm that needs intervention. In chronic illness, humor may be a much-needed coping technique. One woman with arthritis refers to her condition as "Old Arthur."

Receptivity: Some people have been raised to believe that humor is frivolous; thus a humorous intervention would not be appreciated. If you try to use humor and it offends, apologize and explain that your intentions were to be helpful.

Content: Avoid sexist, racist, or sarcastic humor. Remember, just because someone makes light of an issue such as obesity does not give you permission to joke about these personal issues. Your efforts might be interpreted as ridicule.

Nurse-client relationships may provide occasions for humor that seem to be taken out of context when retold. Trust your own judgment when relating a story. Observe a colleague whose sense of humor you admire. If you have an idea about how to use humor and question its appropriateness, check it out with a co-worker.

FUNCTIONS OF HUMOR IN HEALTH CARE

Robinson (1990) examines the functions of humor used in the hospital setting by studying jokes told, finding that humor serves both social and psychological functions.

Social functions include the following:

1. Coping with disruptive acts of hospital custom. Consider the banter about "air-conditioned" hospital gowns.
2. Establishing relationships. Clients who are disfigured may have a series of one-liners they use to break the ice when someone seems shocked by their appearance.
3. Coping with social conflict. One nurse who has good rapport with a physician was surprised by his irritability one day. Realizing that he was having a bad day but was unaware of the effect of his behavior, she retorted, "Dr. Smith, did you have nails for breakfast this morning?" He laughed and apologized.
4. Promoting group solidarity. Two teams of nurses with separate medication carts competed to dress a stuffed animal attached to their carts with a different costume for every holiday.

Psychological functions include the following:

1. Relief of tension. One supervisor of a telemetry unit puts on oversized, clown sunglasses and strolls down the hall when staff members are irritable.
2. Release of hostility and anger. A Nerf basketball and hoop or a Koosh ball to toss in the staff lounge are helpful.
3. Denial of reality. Humor in the operating room that would seem offensive elsewhere helps staff diffuse tension.
4. Coping with disability and death. HIV-positive individuals practice their "death rattle" and laugh about it.

In a study of registered nurses in a graduate nursing program, five themes emerged from an analysis of the use of humor in health care:

- Helped nurses to manage difficult situations and difficult clients
- Helped build cohesiveness in nurse-client and nurse-colleague relationships
- Helped intervene with clients' anxiety, depression, and embarrassment
- Could be part of the routine or spontaneous
- Produced positive effects beyond the moment of humor (Beck, 1997)

A review of literature on the research of caring revealed that humor was a part of the emotional care of clients (Watson, 1988, in Sherwood, 1997).

Nursing Practice Confirms the Research

The use of humor in health care settings can be simple interventions that serve these functions. A nurse in a veteran's hospital, for example, says, "G.I. issue comes in two sizes, too big and too small; welcome back to the military!" Pediatric staff wear customized buttons with teddy bears in addition to formal name pins. A nurse in a heart center wears a button that says, "Speak slowly, I'm a natural blonde." This pin consistently breaks the ice with patients. Computer-generated certificates or banners can be used for clients to illustrate a shared funny experience, such as "Best Dressed" for clients with an elaborate cast. "Happy Birthday" banners can make a client feel more like a real person, not just a collection of symptoms.

When asked how they think humor works in health care, nurses reply:

- Humor shows you care.
- Nurses are accepted better when they have a sense of humor.
- Humor shows you your clients' personality with their defenses down.
- Humor reduces tension and helps you get on with work.
- Humor makes us equals, because we all laugh at the same things.

Clients will initiate humor that shows creative coping skills. An 83-year-old woman in a rehabilitation unit of a nursing home, for example, takes great delight in wearing large, colorful earrings. She lives in southern Florida and wears her "resort" jewelry when she goes to physical therapy. Now her therapist has begun wearing wild earrings, and a nurse has gotten in on the act by presenting a pair of earrings to the client to fuel the competition. This same woman has also been given a pair of purple high-top basketball sneakers by her daughter. The client has been asked to wear shoes that help her navigate better in her wheelchair since she has weakness on one side. At the nurse's encouragement, the daughter has glued jewels to the purple sneakers. Her mother is thrilled and calls people to her room to see them. This woman clearly has a rich sense of humor that she has passed on to her daughter. Walking down the hall, you can hear them laughing and talking. The physical therapist and nurse see the use of humor and playful attitude as positive coping strategies in this family and build upon it. This strengthens their working relationships and creates an environment where the patient can talk about serious concerns with people who understand her.

To teach humor as a coping strategy, consider children's books. An especially useful book is *The Jester Has Lost His Jingle* (Salzman, 1995). This book was written and illustrated by a young man who died at 23 years old of Hodgkin's disease. His mother published the book and donates copies to children's hospitals.

HUMOR STRATEGIES

Try Gentle Banter

"A light touch may be the right touch" (Green, 1993). Humor provides comic relief from tension and worry. For example:

A client rushing onto a gynecology unit for an early morning admission was greeted by a nurse who said, "Congratulations! You win. You're the first one here." The client laughed and talked about how "wild" her morning had been trying to get there on time.

A client was wearing a large fabric protective shoe after foot surgery. One nurse said, "I hope you got that in some glamorous way . . . maybe skiing in Aspen?" The client laughed and shared her story.

A home health nurse reported working with an elderly couple while giving insulin injections to the wife. They had a running joke about how the client could make healthy food choices at the fast-food restaurant the couple went to each day. When the nurse would leave she would tell the wife, "No sausage biscuit today, OK?" They shared many good laughs over this. The nurse talked with pride about this couple's mobility well into their 80s. She uses humor to try to teach, yet recognizes that these trips to the restaurant are the highlight of this couple's days.

Let Humor Take the Lead

Green (1993) calls this the "art of putting things lightly." Observe what is happening to your clients and see how you can add a light touch. Try using the "good news, bad news" approach.

"The bad news is you have to leave your room for a test. The good news is we can have a fascinating conversation on the way."

Green (1993) offers some examples of putting things lightly:

The doctor says, "Well, Mr Saunders, you'll be able to resume your normal activities soon, but you may not be able to play shortshop for the Detroit Tigers this season."

"This injection will make you feel like a kid again—getting your first bee sting."

Being able to laugh at yourself may provide some great material. Consider all those embarrassing moments that you can use to make a real connection with a client. A hospital chaplain relates a story of another chaplain new to the hospital who was shy about approaching clients for fear of disturbing them. One day, after trying to visit a client several times, the chaplain entered the room, tripped, grabbed onto the curtains to keep from falling, swung widely and landed face-down in the bed beside the client. The chaplain looked up and said, "This certainly is an icebreaker, isn't it?" The client laughed and was able to initiate a conversation about her own discomfort at being in the hospital and how hard it was for her to talk; this was the beginning of a very human relationship!

Wit and Wisdom

There is nothing left to you at this moment but to have a good laugh.

Zen master

Look for the Positive

Take the initiative to encourage a positive attitude. Ask your clients what is going well for them today. Share your own positive moments.

"I saw the first rose in my garden today."
  "My grandson is visiting and watched me shave this morning. His father uses an electric razor, and my grandson asked, 'Grandpa, why do you put whipped cream on your face?'"(Green, 1993).
  "There was a rainbow after the storm today."
  "I saw a hot air balloon on my way to work this morning."

Encourage clients and staff to share their own stories. Listening for clues about your clients' interests suggests positive conversation ideas. Asking about children or grandchildren may be well received too.

Be Creative

Each of us has different talents. Often we separate our personal selves from our professional selves. Consider people who love and raise animals. One director of a human resource department brought his eight Dalmatian puppies for a visit to work one day. Never has staff from that department been so united in their delight on any one subject! One home health agency was forced to require a family to contain its dog before a home visit, because the nurse had once been bitten and was afraid of dogs. The family sent the dog to obedience school and mailed the diploma to the agency. Grateful, the nurse delivered a bone as a graduation present for the dog.

Staff and volunteers who are clowns can share their talents by visiting pediatric or geriatric facilities. Staff who play musical instruments or sing can perform for other staff members on special occasions.

One hospital has a plant-filled atrium in its central hall. The staff in plant facilities keep a large rubber lizard among the plants and reposition him frequently. He gets a bow for special occasions. This little bit of humor provides visible relief for people who linger a moment to see something of beauty in a hospital.

To contribute to the morale of staff and clients, consider how you can use your own talents and ideas to add a little joy to your workplace (Box 14-3). Box 14-4 lists strategies listed by nurses using humor, joy, and play to build positive communication.

| **Box 14-3** | **Get Creative** |

- Celebrate holidays; decorate your unit or office. One intensive care unit staff hung handmade paper snowflakes from the ceiling at Christmas.
- Enlarge and post cartoons on the ceiling over examining tables or on walls in examining rooms.
- Use cartoons or funny clip art in client teaching materials or newsletters.
- Give stickers to adults and children after a procedure; the stickers given when people donate blood are popular.
- Use crafts. One examining table has crocheted "booties" on the stirrups. Wear holiday accessories, a crocheted pumpkin pin, festive earrings.

| **Box 14-4** | **Humor Strategies** |

Following are ideas collected from nurses at various humor workshops:
- Put cartoons on bulletin boards.
- Collect cartoons in a photo album and share book with patients as needed.
- Sing at holidays, for clients' birthdays, or just when the mood strikes.
- Wear a funny hat on Halloween (full costume may be inappropriate).
- Share jokes.
- Stage silly puppet shows.
- Use light banter (e.g., when strapping a client onto a stretcher, say "Time to fasten your seat belt!").
- Use pet therapy.
- Keep Silly Putty or Koosh balls on hand for tension relief.
- Blow bubbles.
- Keep the television tuned to comedy shows.
- Play humorous audio tapes.
- Stage theme days for dress (e.g., Western Day).
- Wear a clown nose.
- Smile!
- Keep a positive attitude.

Use Toys and Props

A humor kit in a colorful basket can be useful to add a light touch. A clown doll that laughs can be used when staff is tense. Wearing a clown nose adds a bit of comic relief.

Green (1993) shares the story of wearing funny glasses while visiting her father in the hospital. He loved them and used them to greet his physicians. Some hospitals have humor carts or humor rooms equipped with items to pass the time or get a good laugh. Box 14-5 gives suggestions for building your own humor kit.

Box 14-5	**Building and Using Your Humor Kit**

These items can be used with patients and staff. Let your imagination, a bit of whimsy, and your good judgment be your guide!

Supplies	Uses
Magic wand	"ABRACADABRA . . . now you will have a better day." At a health fair with long lines, try "ABRACADABRA, you'll be finished soon!"
Whistles	Start off an in-service or staff meeting to grab their attention and inspire creativity
Bubbles	Lighten up a tough time
Joke books	Amuse a discouraged client
Koosh ball	Toss around to aid in brainstorming sessions or just to get a smile
Games such as cards, checkers, chess	Offer these to clients to help pass the time
Clown nose	Carry for emergencies

Copyright 1995 Julia.W. Balzer-Riley.

Moments of Connection...
A Touch of Magic

A nurse received a magic wand at a workshop given by the author. She wrote to tell a story of its use. When visiting a friend who had just had a mastectomy, she took her several gifts including the magic wand. The friend inquired about the use of the wand and the nurse replied it was so she would always have a nurse when necessary. About this time, the door to the room opened and in came a nurse asking if the client needed anything. The friends looked at each other and burst into laughter. Later, the door opened and another nurse entered asking if the client had called. Now they were true believers. As they talked, the friend was able to share her fears and joked that the surgeon had also taken a few nips and tucks for figure improvement. The wand had been an icebreaker, and laughing together had set the stage for comfort in sharing concerns (Balzer Riley, 1999).

HOW HUMOR WORKS TO PROMOTE POSITIVE COMMUNICATION

Humor works in three ways:

Prevention: Using humor strategies before a crisis occurs in a work environment makes staff more willing to work together when tension can be great. Have a baby picture contest for staff. Provide a candy jar labeled "Grump Beans" for a grumpy day. Get involved in a community project where people can work together in an informal setting. Organize a

Box 14-6	Humor Goes to School

- Design games to review medical terminology. "The Gastric Voyage" . . . burp . . . go back 2 spaces. Use a television game show format such as Jeopardy.
- In fire safety classes, distribute "Fire Ball" candy. Play songs with the word "fire" in them. Dress as a fireman. In electrical safety training, try a tombstone with the words, "She was the ground."
- To limit negative comments, take a roll of pennies to class. Give each person 2 pennies. They can make a comment but must pay 1 cent each time. When they have put their "2 cents worth" in, they cannot complain again.
- When teaching a controversial topic, put a bullseye on your chest or wear a construction hard hat to break the ice.
- Begin the class with something funny so participants know it is safe to laugh.
- Make a list of quotes by funny people and add quotes frequently used by participants.
- Slip in unknown abbreviations. TSWNE is "this shift will never end." RP is a "real person."

Ideas compiled from the Carolina Society of Health Education and Training conference, 3/26/98, Myrtle Beach, SC, conducted by the author.

community project for colleagues that could be done in conjunction with the traditional Christmas party.

Perception: Injecting humor into a situation changes the perception that the situation is so terrible that it cannot be handled. Keep a magic wand at the desk. When the pace is hectic, grab the wand and make a promise that the end of the day is in sight!

Perspective: Humor helps us to keep the big picture in view and not to take ourselves too seriously. Make light of your own idiosyncrasies. Get people to laugh *with* you (Balzer, 1994).

Consider that "Humor endears the person who is engaged in it to others; such an individual can enjoy a sense of the outrageous as well as the sublime. The ability to play defuses anger, disarms grief . . . Mirth often derives from a joint recognition of the ridiculousness of life" (van Wormer and Boes, 1997, p. 87).

HUMOR IN HEALTH CARE EDUCATION

Humor can create a climate of trust in the classroom and can engage the learner in the process of learning (Box 14-6).

HE WHO LAUGHS, LASTS

R. Dale Liechty (1987) delivered an address, "Humor and the Surgeon," in which he concluded:

. . . Humor is an innate but fragile part of human life . . . and this scary world can sometimes erode it. To hold on to this gift of laughter, we must develop two faculties. The first is perspective, knowing that we exist somewhere between the tiniest and the infinite mysteries. Perspective is indeed the secret of philosophy. The second is a humorous outlook . . . that senses 'the world is mad' . . . but also understands that human vanities and pretenses have made it that way. It tells us, from time to time at least, to stand back and smile or laugh at them.

Wit and Wisdom

Life must be lived as play.

Plato

Practicing Using Humor

Exercise 1

"An average 6-year-old laughs 300 times each day. How often does a typical adult laugh?"
  What is your guess?
  Answer: 15-1000 times per day (*USA Today,* 1998). Discuss your ideas about these statistics.

Exercise 2

  Recall an incident when you were the recipient of negative humor. Describe how you felt.

Exercise 3

Identify someone with a rich, positive sense of humor. Describe how you feel when you are with this person.

Exercise 4

Keep a log for one week of your clients' use of humor. Do your clients tell jokes? What are the subjects of the jokes? Do the clients use humor to introduce topics of concern? Do you see this humor as positive or negative? Describe your comfort level. Remember that people might disagree as to whether humor is positive or negative. Ask yourself what purpose the humor serves. Does it distance you or elicit your support?

Exercise 5

For this exercise, select a small group of students. Each student is to briefly interview a nurse who uses humor in a positive way in the clinical setting. Ask for examples of situations where humor worked with a client. Share the results of these interviews, compile a list of interventions, and share with the class.

Exercise 6

A noted comedian, Steve Allen, says there is no need to construct jokes; life is funny enough! In small groups, share stories of embarrassing moments. Solicit a volunteer to share an especially funny story with the whole class.

Discuss the changes in the mood and behavior of the class before the exercise and during it. (You might note increased volume, movement, laughter, and more energy; humor creates energy.)

Exercise 7

Work in groups of three or four and share "embarrassing moment" stories. Pay attention to the changes you observe as a group of people laughs together.

Exercise 8

Bring the comic strips from several newspapers to class. Share your favorites and discuss what is funny. Comment about why certain individual comics are funny and compare your favorite comic strips to see differences in humor styles.

Exercise 9

This is just a test: read the following quotes and see for yourself if a little comic relief works.

- Warning: Humor may be hazardous to your illness.
- Sometimes you just need to look reality in the eye, and deny it (Garrison Keillor).
- At my age it's nice to have birthday parties. All my friends can stand around the cake and keep warm (George Burns).
- There are two things that everyone must face sooner or later: a camera and reality. A smile is a big help in both instances (source unknown).
- On his death bed, Oscar Wilde looked around the room and said: "This wallpaper is terrible. One of us has to go" (Wooten, 1994).
- A sign on a pastor's door reads: "Don't feel totally, absolutely, personally responsible for everything. That's my job—signed God" (Dunn, 1994).

Think About It...
What, So What, and Now What?

Consider what you read about the use of humor and how you already use humor. Can you comfortably add humor to your skills for relating to clients and colleagues?

What? . . .   Write one thing you learned from this chapter

So what? . . .   How will this impact your nursing practice?

Now what? . . .   How will you implement this new knowledge or skill?

—— **THINK ABOUT IT** ——

References

Balzer JW: Creating energy through humor and other humor workshops, 1994.

Balzer Riley J: Add a light touch to your patient education, *Patient Education Newsletter,* 4:4, 1995.

Balzer Riley, J: *From the heart to the hands: keys to successful healthcaring connections,* Ellicott City, Md, 1999, Integrated Management and Publishing Systems, Inc.

Bakerman H: Nursing humor: a perspective, *Therapeutic Humor* XII(3):6, 1998.

Beck CT: Humor in nursing practice: a phenomenological study, *Int J Nurs Stud* 34(5):346, 1997.

Davis P: *My father's gift of faith,* New York, 1995, Harper Collins.

Dunn JR, editor: *Humor & Health Letter* 3(5):1, 1994.

Fonnesbecl BG: Are you kidding? *Nursing '98* 28(3):64, 1998.

Fry WF Jr., Salameh WA, editors: *Handbook of humor and psychotherapy: advances in the clinical use of humor,* Sarasota, Fla, 1987, Professional Resource Exchange.

Green L: *Making sense of humor: how to add joy to your life,* Manchester, Conn, 1993, KIT Publisher.

How in the world, *USA Today,* July 29, 1998, p. B-1.

Kipplinger B: Humor in psychotherapy: a shift to a new perspective. In Fry WF Jr., Salameh WA, editors: *Handbook of humor and psychotherapy: advances in the clinical use of humor,* Sarasota, Fla, 1987, Professional Resource Exchange.

Leiber DB: Laughter and humor in critical care, *Dimens Crit Care* 5(3):162, 1986.

Leichty RD: Humor and the surgeon, *Arch Surg* 122:519, 1987.

McGhee PE: *Humor and children's development,* New York, 1989, Haworth Press.

McGhee PE: *The laughter remedy: health, healing, and the amuse system.* Available from: The Laughter Remedy, 380 Claremeont Avenue, #8, Montclair, NJ 07042, 1991.

McGhee P: RX: Laughter, *RN* 28(7):50, 1998.

Robinson VM: *Humor and the health professions,* Thorofare, NJ, 1990, Charles B. Slack.

Saltzman D: *The jester has lost his jingle,* Palos Verdes Estates, Calif, The Jester Co, Inc. (1-800-9-jester).

Sherwood GD: Meta-synthesis of qualitative analyses of caring: defining a therapeutic model of nursing, *Adv Nurs Pract Q* 3(1):32, 1997.

Simon JM: Therapeutic humor: who's fooling who? *J Psychosoc Nurs* 26(4):9, 1988.

Van Wormer K, Boes M, Humor in the emergency room: a social work perspective, *Health Social Work* 22(2):87, May 1997.

Wooten P: Jest for the health of it, Seminar handouts, Davis, Calif, 1993.

Wooten P: Heart humor and healing, Mt. Shasta, Calif, 1994, Commune-a-key.

Suggestions for Further Reading

Abramis DJ: Humor in healthy organizations, *Human Resources* 37(8):72, 1992.

The American Association for Therapeutic Humor, 222 S. Meramec, Suite 303, St Louis, Mo 63105, (314-0863-6232). Website: www.aath.org (Membership includes a newsletter and bibliographies).

Balzer JW: Humor adds the creative touch in CQI teams, *J Nurs Care Qual* 8(4):13, 1994.

Balzer Riley J: *Customer service from A to Z: making the connection,* Albuquerque, NM, 1999, Hartman Publishers, Inc.
  Contains activities using humor and creativity to teach customer service to healthcare givers.

Balzer Riley J: *Humor and health,* revised 1998, Home Study, A.K.H. Consultant, 1532 Kingsley Ave, Suite 115, Orange Park, FL 32073 (904-264-0674).

Balzer Riley J: *Humor in the workplace,* Cumming, Ga: 1996, CSP.

Balzer Riley J: *Instant tools for healthcare teams,* St Louis, 1997, Mosby.
  Has activities using humor and creativity as meeting icebreakers, to teach team dynamics, and to teach quality improvement tools.

Barreca R: *They used to call me snow white. . . . but I drifted: women's strategic use of humor,* New York, 1991, Penguin.

Berk LS: New discoveries in psychoneuroimmunology: an interview with Dr. Lee S. Berk, *Humor Health Letter* 3(6):1, Nov/Dec 1994.

Bombeck E: *I want to grow hair, I want to go to Boise, I want to grow up,* New York, 1989, Harper & Row.

Brausa R: The comedy club, *Psychosoc Rehabil J* 17(2):189, 1993.
  Report of a study of a humor group in a day treatment program in a VA medical center. Humor helped members take a break from their focus on problems and helped to decrease stress.

Brilliant A: *All I want is a warm bed and a kind word and unlimited power,* Santa Barbara, Calif, 1985, Woodbridge Press.
  One of a collection of books of cartoons and one-liners that add perspective, wit, and wisdom. Highly recommended. Another title to look for: *I may not be totally perfect, but parts of me are excellent.*

Buxman K: Make room for laughter, *Am J Nurs* Dec:46-50, 1991.

Buxman K: Humor in therapy for the mentally ill, *J Psychosoc Nurs* 29(12):15, 1991.

Cousins N: *Anatomy of an illness: as perceived by the patient,* New York, 1983, WW Norton.
  The author's well-known account of his use of humor in triumphing over illness.

Daubman KA, Nowicki GP: Positive affect facilitates creative problem solving, *J Personality Social Psychol* 52:1122, 1987.
  Studies demonstrating the creativity-inducing characteristics of laughter.

Feingold A, Mazzella R: Preliminary validation of a multidimensional model of wittiness, *J Personality* 61(3):439, 1993.

The authors conclude that the ability to produce and comprehend humor is related to verbal ability and creativity.

Fry WF Jr.: Homeodynamics: a lesson of laughter, *Humor Health Letter* 3(5):1, 1994.

Griffiths J: Mind, the mirthful brain: where the belly laugh begins, *Omni* Aug: 18, 1992.

A summary of the work of Dr. Peter Derks, who studied humor appreciation in stroke victims. He uses 21-electrode EEG typographical brain mapping to study brain activity related to humor.

Herth KA: Laughter: a nursing Rx, *Am J Nurs* 84(980):991, 1984.

Kenefick C, Young AY: *The best of nursing humor: a collection of articles, essays, and poetry published in the nursing literature,* Philadelphia, 1993, Hanley & Belfus.

Klein A: *Healing power of humor,* Los Angeles, Calif, 1989, Tarcher.

Allen Klein's work began with the positive use of humor with his terminally ill wife.

Leap TL, Smeltzer LR: Racial remarks in the workplace: humor or harassment? In *Differences that work: organizational excellence through diversity,* Boston, 1994, A Harvard Business Review Book.

In a diverse workplace, negative humor becomes a sensitive issue and a legal one.

Matz A, Brown ST: Humor and pain management, *J Holistic Nurs* 16(1):68, March 1998.

Miller DA: Laughter in leadership: bringing out your lighter side, *Creative Nurs* 3(2):6, March 1997.

Orig E: Humor and suppression of sentiment, *Int J Humor Stud* 7(1):7, 1994.

Expands on Freud's view that humor is an expression of unacceptable sexual and aggressive impulses.

Paulson TL: *Making humor work: take your job seriously and yourself lightly,* Los Altos, Calif, 1989, Crisp Publications.

Rosenberg L: Clinical articles: a qualitative investigation of the use of humor by emergency personnel as a strategy for coping with stress, *J Emerg Nurs* 17:4, 1991.

Schmitt N: Patients' perception of laughter in a rehabilitation hospital, *Rehabil Nurs* 15:143, 1990.

Seuss, Dr.: *You're only old once: a book for obsolete children,* New York, 1986, Random House.

Simon JM: Humor and its relationship to perceived health, life satisfaction, and morale in older adults, *Iss Mental Health Nurs* 11(1):17, 1990.

Simon JM: Humor and the older adult: implications for nursing, *J Adv Nurs* 14:441, 1988.

Swift AT, Swift B: Humor experts jazz up the workplace, *Human Resources* 39(5):72, 1994.

Time and humor help shield physicians from lawsuits, *Med Pract Commun* 5(2):7, 1998.

Traynor D: Laugh it off, *American Fitness* 15(3):56, May/June 1997.

Weinstein M: *Managing to have fun,* New York, 1996, Simon & Schuster.

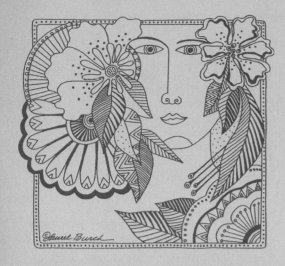

15

Spirituality

Courage is fear that has said its prayers.

Italian proverb

OBJECTIVES

1. Discuss themes of spirituality.
2. Discuss strategies to nurture the spirit.
3. Identify nursing interventions to meet spiritual needs of the client and family.
4. Describe behaviors that the nurse can use to have a hopeful perspective and offer hope.
5. Review a spiritual assessment tool for use in a clinical settting.
6. Discuss the role of the nurse in helping the client find meaning in illness.

A DEFINITION OF SPIRITUALITY

The concept of spirituality is elusive. Donnelly and Cook (1989) reflect that "to be spiritual is to be connected—to the inner self, to others, or to a transcendent being or energy." Spirituality in practice is "to demonstrate a unique capacity for love, joy, caring, compassion, and for finding meaning in life's difficult experience." Nurses' spiritual interventions "reflect the human traits of caring, love, honesty, wisdom, and imagination . . . a belief in a higher power, higher existence, or a guiding spirit . . . something outside the self and beyond the individual nurse or patient" (Dossey, June 1998, p. 47).

Spirituality is good science. . . Over 250 studies now show that religious practice—the specific religion doesn't seem to matter—is correlated with greater health and increased longevity . . . some say that clinicians have no business taking on the role of spiritual guide . . . but we are not being asked to become spiritual counselors. We're being asked to integrate a holistic approach and extend love, compassion, and empathy . . . the bedrock upon which nursing has always rested. (Dossey, August 1998, p. 37)

Spirituality has been part of the vision of nursing since the time of Florence Nightingale in *Suggestions for Thought* (Schette, 1998).

In this chapter you will explore the concept of spirituality, a notion that may be feared or ignored by health care professionals, perhaps because it reminds us of the fallibility of science in healing (Donnelly and Cook, 1989). It is this spiritual connection that is the essence of being present with clients in moments of tragedy where the seeds of personal triumph are planted. This discussion is not based on religious denomination, but on the spiritual path to find personal meaning and to help the patient and family find meaning in illness and suffering (Travelbee, 1970). This chapter will help you recognize opportunities to introduce the idea to clients and families that we learn lessons from life's difficulties, and show you how to give them a chance to value this knowledge through sharing it.

THEMES OF SPIRITUALITY

Nagai-Jacobson and Burkhardt (1989) review general themes that emerge in the literature that broaden the concept of spirituality. They found that spirituality:

- Is a broader concept than religion
- Involves a personal quest for meaning and purpose in life
- Relates to the inner essence of a person
- Is a sense of harmonious interconnectedness with self, others, nature and an Ultimate Other
- Is the integrating factor of the human person

Discussions of spirituality in nursing suggest that interactions between nurses and their clients involve the spirituality of both and that this relationship can transform them all in the search for meaning in life. The nature of such nurse-client relationships is sacred. It is a walk on holy ground as two people meet at what Newman (1989) calls choice points presented by health crises; these events are "opportunities to experience more fully the reality of the patterns of our lives." These are times when former ways of coping and relating to life no longer work. When a person is confronted with disability, new ways of existing, of behaving, of finding meaning are necessary. A woman whose husband was experiencing the deterioration of Alzheimer's disease, for example, found her own health affected by the strain of being a caregiver. Unable to drive or visit with friends, she befriended a wild, stray cat who was reluctant to make physical contact. Over time, the mother cat brought her kittens to the woman. Feeding these kittens and playing with them gave this woman's life purpose and some joy in the midst of the suffering she was sharing with her husband. "God sent me this cat," she said. "We needed each other." She slowed down and stayed focused in the present.

THE NURSE AS A SPIRITUAL PERSON AND CAREGIVER

Life is a journey. Peck (1993) suggests that we must appreciate the fact that life is complex. This means to "abandon the urge to simplify everything, to look for easy answers, and to begin to think multi-dimensionally, to stay in the mystery and paradoxes of life." Those who would simplify nursing practice would teach students how to do "things"—treatments, techniques, procedures. How easy it would be if the quality of nursing care could be quantified by how accurately or quickly procedures could be performed. Consider that "the essence of nursing is not doing . . . but being open to whatever arises in the interaction with the client. It is being fully present with an un-conditional acceptance of the client's experience" (Newman,1989). Perhaps we can think of life not as a series of problems to be solved but rather as a mystery to unravel.

To facilitate your clients' growth and coping, you must be open to your own life experiences, continue on your own journey to make sense of life, and nurture your own spirit. Your own un-met needs can get in the way of being able to be fully present with your clients and their family.

Spiritual Care Begins With the Nurse

To be a nurse is a sacred trust. Clients and families come to us fearfully in their darkest hours, in the face of their own mortality or, at the time of childbirth, in the face of the wonder of creation. Burkhardt and Nagai-Jacobson speak of "reawakening spirit in nursing practice" (1994). To have the ability to stay connected to the experience of another, you must pay attention to nurturing your own spirit. Moore (1992) speaks of living artfully as a necessity for the care of the soul or spirit. To do so, he suggests:

- Pause—the opposite of busyness—stop, reflect, savor the moment, experience wonder at the things around you, be still.
- Take time for self, people, relationships, and things—living creatures, too! To take time for relationships, even difficult ones, deepens understanding and appreciation.
- Be mindful of, or pay attention to, what is happening all around you so that you recognize the need to stop and focus on this moment rather than thinking about the past or the future.

But how can you slow down, considering the demands of nursing? Other chapters in this text address methods such as relaxation techniques and meditation. Practicing these techniques helps you to be in touch with your own spirit, helps you to be centered. The process of centering helps you focus on this moment. Remember the value of rest, of time to do nothing, and of playful leisure time. Focusing on the moment can mean slowing down to really enjoy the taste and texture and smells of the food you eat; taking time to stroke the fur of a cat or dog; listening to the sound of birds singing; enjoying music rather than using it for background noise; stroking the hair of a child; listening to another person without offering an opinion; hugging a friend; listening to laughter, and joining in. In a series of community classes for cancer patients and their families, one man said cancer had changed his focus from "working for a living to the art of living." These simple suggestions are mindful activities. They are what clients tell us they do to stay connected to life in tough times; for them, these are the things that make life worthwhile. Perhaps these activities can replenish your energy to do your life's work.

Communication is more than verbal and nonverbal behavior. The ability to stay present in the moment requires conscious effort, which is sometimes a struggle. When you feel overwhelmed, take time to return to being still and paying attention to the gifts of the senses.

Spiritual Care of the Client and Family Attitude

Spiritual care is not separate from all other aspects of nursing care. Spiritual care is how you do what you do. It is an attitude and an openness to the shared experience of the human condition. When you assist a patient with morning care, when you offer a bedpan or a urinal, when you take a temperature, when you bathe a person who has soiled himself, these ordinary tasks, when done mindfully, provide spiritual care. In a book on spiritual fulfillment in everyday life, Fields et al (1984) talk about simple daily tasks as a way to get in touch with the natural cycles of life and death.

Being Fully Present

The daily routine of nurses is not routine to clients. One reason it takes courage to be fully present with clients is that to be present is to understand their fear and pain. Words and procedures you will come to see as commonplace strike fear in the hearts of company presidents who find themselves in a setting they cannot control. Do not be fooled by clients who seem to be calm and confident. Assume that your clients and their family see you as a lifeline, and work from there.

Being present means listening empathically and connecting what you are hearing to your own life experience. McKivergin and Daubenmire (1994) define therapeutic presence as "a conscious act of being fully present—body, mind, emotions, and spirit—to another person." In the following box, one nurse is fully present with a novice nurse and her patient, sharing her own convictions.

She responded "as whole being to whole being, using all of her . . . resources of body, mind, emotions, and spirit" (McKivergin and Daubenmire, 1994). This response was brief. Spiritual care does not take extra time. It is a part of all you do.

Moments of Connection...
Where Can I Begin?

The foundation began in my first year of nursing, at age 21, when an experienced nurse noticed my confusion and helplessness in dealing with a dying patient one evening. I didn't ask for help; I never did. The patient had no family present, so it really was up to me. This nurse took me in the room and said, 'Hello. We're with you. You are not alone.' She was speaking to the patient and to me. It was years before I finally believed what she said. By the grace of God I know that we are never alone, and I can share this belief now with conviction."

Being Silent

Being still, being comfortable with silence, understanding that it is acceptable not to have answers—or even words—may come naturally to the introvert, a person who thinks to talk. For the extrovert, a person who talks to think, it may be growth. One therapist, who is an extreme extrovert, said the only way he could still his mind and his mouth was to learn to meditate. Yes, it is acceptable and even therapeutic to be quiet, just to be, not to do all the time. Thirty years ago, a nursing instructor said, "If you don't know what to say, just be quiet and stay there. Try saying, 'I don't have any words to help, but I will stay with you a while.'" These words are still good counsel.

A psychologist, when talking about her experience as a patient, said, "I want the nurse to understand that I am not myself when I am ill. I'm not the person I present to the outside world. I appreciate your understanding this and not judging me or my behavior. I don't want you to try to fix my problems. All I want is for you to acknowledge my pain, even by just a kind look when you stop in to check on me."

Silence means acceptance. There are no expectations that clients or nurses must have all the answers. There is no right thing to say or perfect nursing care plan to write that can make things all better for clients. Part of the challenge for all nurses is to live with this ambiguity.

Moments of Connection

Martin Buber (1958) distinguishes between two types of relationships, the I-It and the I-Thou. The I-It relationship can be experienced as nurses do the work of patient care. Teaching and caring can become routine and, although excellent in form, may lack substance or a real connection with the patient. The I-It is the world of "experiencing and using . . . a typical subject-object relationship" (Friedman, 1966). The I-Thou relationship can only be spoken with the whole being. The I-Thou is "characterized by mutuality, directness, presentness, intensity" (Friedman, 1966). "The It is the eternal chrysalis, the Thou, the eternal butterfly" (Buber, 1958).

Just as the world of the nurse provides potential for a genuine relation with the patient, the I-It can become the I-Thou in special moments of connection to the patient or to a family member, within the potential crisis situation of surgery and illness.

A nurse's personal or family experience with surgery and/or illness can contribute to a deeper understanding of patient and family needs. Nursing is a sacred trust wherein the patient and family agree to give up conventional constraints on behavior in exchange for acceptance of their personal response to the traumatic experience of surgery. The nurse's ability to stay connected to the pain of the human condition is one ingredient that can create I-Thou relationships. These moments of connection, however brief, sustain the patient and family throughout the crisis and provide the meaning the nurse so badly needs to revitalize in the nursing practice.

Nearing Death

As clients near death, nurses work as part of a team to provide spiritual care. When is the right time? Nurses learn to trust their intuition about the right time to talk about the client's concerns. Nurses offer nurturing touch, silent presence, a prayer, or if the client prefers, a chance to speak to a member of the clergy. Nurses create a climate for hope to grow and flourish (Box 15-1). The nurse can ask clients to consider special messages or special mementos for which they want to make arrangements (Piemme, 1998).

Box 15-1   Notes on Hope

Hope is trust and confidence. Hope is patient. Hope brings enthusiasm and adds animation. Hope is a fuel to keep us going, a tonic to energize, a driving force that keeps us going, daily bread to feed the soul. Hope is in contrast to expectation that takes us from the present to a focus on the future which can bring disappointment when things do not go as we planned (Brussat and Brussat, 1996). "Hope is the belief . . . that one can have a *life* in the midst of trauma and suffering. Hope that you will be able to cope with the suffering, hope that something good will come from it, hope for remission—if not a cure, hope for an extension of time, hope for the future welfare of your family, hope to keep your dignity, hope for life after life" (Hampton, 1998).

   To bring hope you must have hope. To keep a hopeful countenance, learn to forgive yourself your mistakes so you can take the risk of opportunities of the future, to leave room for future, love yourself, laugh and keep a sense of humor, trust in God, celebrate your imagination, cherish your dreams, create visions, set goals. In the face of difficulties, remember: Within every problem there is a lesson. Embrace the lesson and release the problem. To face the uncertainty of life, consider this notion: I am uncertain about the future, but I am certain it will be positive.

   To instill hope you show it in your face; your kind positive words; your ability to truly face someone . . . to look into the eyes; your presence not avoidance; your presence in the face of suffering; your openness to hear hopeless words; an offered prayer; music and flowers; cards and photographs displayed.

Moments of Connection...
Having the Courage to Share a Prayer

A patient who had been on the Acute Pain Service three previous times during the same admission was received in the PACU after an exploration of the abdomen and was in a great deal of pain as I started her patient-controlled analgesia (PCA). I told her I would stay with her until the pain was controlled. For the next two hours I gave her multiple boluses, but her pain was not relieved satisfactorily. During this time I patted her forehead and moistened her lips. When I asked her what else I could do for her, she asked if I would pray with her. We were still in the PACU, and I was aware that several other nurses were rolling their eyes. We said the Lord's Prayer. She soon relaxed and appeared more comfortable.

   Several Moments of Connection help illustrate the different forms communication may take as nurses support clients and families in these intimate times.

Finding Meaning

Understanding that meaning can come from suffering, you will be alert to times when clients or family members want to share what they have learned. Clients may give you clues that they want to talk further. Here are some things your clients might say and possible interventions to help them share their understanding of what has happened.

Moments of Connection...
Wishes and Dreams

It was springtime, and she was a young leukemia patient who would probably not leave the hospital before a 'celestial discharge.' We had chatted for days about her wishes and dreams. She had never gone to a circus, seen a bluebird, or been to Disneyland. Several nurses got together. Mickey Mouse appeared in her room. I came as a clown with my 'trick' dog bringing a video of the circus. A pet shop owner brought in two blue birds to spend the afternoon. She was laughing and crying. She said she didn't know nurses did all these things. I asked her if she was happy and content. She replied, 'The only thing I haven't seen is God, and I'll see Him soon, but I know I've seen the angels.'

Moments of Connection...
I Clearly Felt Her Presence

I was working as a hospice nurse with a very independent client who always wanted to be in control, up in the chair each day. As her pain increased and my visits became more frequent, I took on more of a nurturing role. I am also a massage therapist, and when she became bedridden, I would frequently give her a massage. She asked to purchase a gift certificate for a massage for her sister. On the day she passed, I went into her room where her body lay, cold and still. I thanked her for the opportunity to be her friend and nurse. I clearly felt her presence and love. A month later, her sister came for a massage after having been very distraught over her loss. It was a marvelous experience for both of us. She still returns monthly for massage, and each time we remember her sister and her gift.

Client: "So much has happened in such a short time. I never knew I could handle so many things."
Nurse: "You've been thinking about all the things you've been through. Tell me about it."
Client: "Having AIDS makes me value life more."
Nurse: "Can you share how you see life now?"
Client: "When you lose a child, your other children become all the more precious."
Nurse: "How do you think things will change between you and your children?"

Hannaford and Popkin report things that people have learned from loss, as listed in Box 15-2. Their book *Windows* is used as a text for a grief class that is taught to caregivers who may support clients and families during loss. Hannaford and Popkin suggest questions and statements that may "encourage the griever as he turns loss into meaningful experience" (1992) (Box 15-3). They also include statements that might block the struggle to find meaning in loss (Box 15-4).

Box 15-2 Possible Meanings

I have learned . . .
- That I can love.
- That loving hurts.
- That I can survive.
- That healing occurs.
- That I have grown.
- That I can forgive.
- That I can forgive myself.
- That you taught me much.
- That I can be a receiver.
- That change is a necessary part of life.
- That I am grateful for the many things you gave me.
- That I wouldn't miss you if you hadn't been so important to me.
- That I cannot control everything.
- That I can care.
- That I can become involved.
- That I need a significant other.
- That I can reevaluate myself.
- That a new page of my life is being written.
- That I will have to change.
- That I can start again.
- That I am wiser.
- That I have discovered a new level of courage.
- That I am more open.
- That I can make new contacts on my own.
- That I can ask for support.
- That I am stronger, more independent, more joyful, happier.
- That I have choices.
- That I am really never alone.
- The value and importance of the present.
- To fill my days in new ways.
- To appreciate this disruption in my life as motivation to grow.
- To enjoy aloneness.
- To appreciate life more.

Reprinted from Hannaford MJ, Popkin MH: *Windows: healing and helping through loss,* Atlanta, 1992, Active Parenting Publishers, pp. 77-78.

| **Box 15-3** | **One of These Questions or Statements Might Help** |

As you look at this experience, is it possible that you have found new meaning in relationships that you were not aware of before?

- Have you considered your growth during this time, the changes in you which this loss seem to have brought?
- How has the experience changed your life?
- How has it influenced your life purpose and belief system?
- What positive action have you taken or might you take as a result of this lesson?
- You seem to have learned that there are a lot of things over which we have no control.
- You have gained a lot of self-confidence in your ability to handle a crisis.
- You seem to feel that with all the loss, you are gaining a kind of independence that you never knew you could enjoy.
- I like to hear you laugh; it seems that you are more able to express your feelings since your recent experience.

Reprinted from Hannaford MJ, Popkin MH: *Windows: healing and helping through loss,* Atlanta, 1992, Active Parenting Publishers, pp. 129-130.

| **Box 15-4** | **Comments Such as These May Do More Harm Than Good** |

- As you look at this, you have no doubt learned never to do it again.
- Life's lessons are hard, and you have certainly made this one into a hard one.
- When you make mistakes, you always have to pay.
- If you had kept in touch, you wouldn't feel so bad.
- You'll learn from this one to be kind from now on.
- I do hope you've learned your lesson.
- Everything will be all right.

Reprinted from Hannaford MJ, Popkin MH: *Windows: healing and helping through loss,* Atlanta, 1992, Active Parenting Publishers, pp. 129-130.

Wit and Wisdom

He who knocks at the door will not go without an answer.

African proverb

THE SPIRITUAL CONNECTION

We come full circle. Spiritual care begins and ends with the caregiver. You nurture your own spirit, thus becoming open to your clients' experiences in a genuine, holistic way. Your experience with your clients nourishes your spirit and offers renewal. "Presence becomes a gift to ourselves and others in the shared moment of the present and enhances the fullness of our being, filling our cups to overflowing" (McKivergin and Daubenmire, 1994).

Think About It...
What, So What, and Now What?

Consider what you read about spirituality. How do you see your own spirituality? What spiritual interventions are you already using? Write the answers to the following questions.

What? . . . Write one thing you learned from this chapter.

So what? . . . How will this impact your nursing practice?

Now what? . . . How will you implement this new knowledge or skill?

THINK ABOUT IT

Practicing Spirituality

Exercise 1

Answer for yourself these questions that are a sample of those used in a two-day course taught to nurses on the subject of presence (McKivergin and Daubenmire, 1994).
1. "What are characteristics or qualities of presence?"
2. "What does it mean to be fully present to another?"
3. "How can I become more aware of opportunities to be present to others?"

Exercise 2

Identify and share a situation in which someone was fully present with you. Describe your feelings about this interaction. Contrast this with a time in which you talked with someone and did not believe this person was fully present.

Exercise 3

Keep a journal for a day.
1. Choose a clinical day and be aware of how you can live artfully in an ordinary day, not just on vacation.
2. Pay attention to your senses. Record pleasurable moments.
3. Consciously take time to pause and reflect on your thoughts, feelings, and actions. Record these.
4. Take at least 15 minutes in the day for yourself. Surely you can take that time even if you must study for a test. In fact, that is a great time to do this to build your energy and stimulate your creativity.
5. Be mindful of your clients' experiences and pay special attention to understanding their perspective. Consider ways in which these experiences relate to any of your own and how they may have affected your life. Record these thoughts.

Exercise 4

Ask yourself this important question, "How do I experience the sacred?" People have a variety of ways of nourishing the spirit (Burkhardt and Nagai-Jacobson, 1994). Share your answers with at least three other students or peers. If you don't understand the question or can't think of an answer, discuss that instead. It will stimulate your thinking.

Exercise 5

Examine the Spiritual Assessment Tool (Box 15-5). This tool has been published in a number of sources and includes different ways of looking at the concept of spirituality. Read and reflect on the tool and put a check by the questions you would be comfortable asking a client. Share your responses with several other students. Talk about how you can use this tool or parts of it in your current clinical setting. File this tool for future use.

Box 15-5 Spiritual Assessment Tool

The following reflective questions may assist you in assessing, evaluating, and increasing awareness of spirituality in yourself and others.

Meaning and Purpose

These questions assess a person's ability to seek meaning and fulfillment in life, manifest hope, and accept ambiguity and uncertainty.

- What gives your life meaning?
- Do you have a sense of purpose in life?
- Does your illness interfere with your life goals?
- Why do you want to get well?
- How hopeful are you about obtaining a better degree of health?
- Do you feel that you have a responsibility in maintaining your health?
- Will you be able to make changes in your life to maintain your health?
- Are you motivated to get well?
- What is the most important or powerful thing in your life?

Inner Strengths

These questions assess a person's ability to manifest joy and recognize strengths, choices, goals, and faith.

- What brings you joy and peace in your life?
- What can you do to feel alive and full of spirit?
- What traits do you like about yourself?
- What are your personal strengths?
- What choices are available to you to enhance your healing?
- What life goals have you set for yourself?
- Do you think that stress in any way caused your illness?
- How aware were you of your body before you became sick?
- What do you believe in?
- Is faith important in your life? ·
- How has your illness influenced your faith?
- Does faith play a role in recognizing your health?

Interconnections

These questions assess a person's positive self-concept, self-esteem, and sense of self; sense of belonging in the world with others; capacity to pursue personal interests; and ability to demonstrate love of self and self-forgiveness.

- How do you feel about yourself right now?
- How do you feel when you have a true sense of yourself?
- Do you pursue things of personal interest?
- What do you do to show love for yourself?

- Can you forgive yourself?
- What do you do to heal your spirit?

These questions assess a person's ability to connect in life-giving ways with family, friends, and social groups and to engage in the forgiveness of others.

- Who are the significant people in your life?
- Do you have friends or family in town who are available to help you?
- Who are the people to whom you are closest?
- Do you belong to any groups?
- Can you ask people for help when you need it?
- Can you share your feelings with others?
- What are some of the most loving things that others have done for you?
- What are the loving things that you do for other people?
- Are you able to forgive others?

These questions assess a person's capacity for finding meaning in worship or religious activities, and a connectedness with a divinity.

- Is worship important to you?
- What do you consider the most significant act of worship in your life?
- Do you participate in any religious activities?
- Do you believe in God or a higher power?
- Do you think that prayer is powerful?
- Have you ever tried to empty your mind of all thoughts to see what the experience might be?
- Do you use relaxation or imagery skills?
- Do you meditate?
- Do you pray?
- What is your prayer?
- How are your prayers answered?
- Do you have a sense of belonging in this world?

These questions assess a person's ability to experience a sense of connection with life and nature, an awareness of the effects of the environment on life and well-being, and a capacity or concern for the health of the environment.

- Do you ever feel a connection with the world or universe?
- How does your environment have an impact on your state of well-being?
- What are your environmental stressors at work and at home?
- What strategies reduce your environmental stressors?
- Do you have any concerns for the state of your immediate environment?
- Are you involved with environmental issues such as recycling environmental resources at home, work, or in your community?
- Are you concerned about the survival of the planet?

From Dossey BM: Holistic modalities and healing moments, *Am J Nurs* 6:44, 1998. Sources: Burkhardt MA: Spirituality: an analysis of the concept, *Holist Nurs Pract 3*(3):69, May 1989; Dossey BM et al., editors: *Holistic nursing: a handbook for practice,* ed 2, Gaithersburg, Md, 1995, Aspen.

References

Brussat F, Brussat MA: *Spiritual literacy: reading the sacred in everyday life,* New York, 1996, Scribner.

Buber M: *I and thou,* New York, 1958, Charles Scribner's Sons.

Claibourne C: Hope in healthcare today, *Creative Nurs* 3(4):13, 1997.

Donnelly GF, Cook DC: From the editors, *Holistic Nurs Pract* 3(3):vi, 1989.

Dossey B: Attending to holistic care, *Am J Nurs* 98(8):35, 1998.

Dossey, B: Holistic modalities and healing moments, *Am J Nurs* 98(6):44, 1998.

Fields RT et al: *Chop wood carry water; a guide to finding spiritual fulfillment in everyday life,* Los Angeles, 1984, Jeremy P. Tarcler.

Friedman MS: *The life of dialogue,* New York, 1966, Harper & Row.

Hampton C: Hope and healing after traumatic illness. Presentation, Case Management Society of America, Georgia Chapter, September 26, 1998.

Hannaford M, Popkin M: *Windows: healing and helping through loss,* Atlanta, 1992, Active Parenting, Inc.

McKivergin MJ, Daubenmire MJ: The healing process of presence, *J Holistic Nurs* 21(1):65, 1994.

Moore T: *Care of the soul,* New York, 1992, Harper Collins.

Nagai-Jacobson MG, Burkhardt MA: Spirituality: cornerstone of holistic nursing practice, *Holistic Nurs Pract* 3(3):18, 1989.

Newman MA: The spirit of nursing, *Holistic Nurs Pract* 3:3:1, May 1989.

Nightingale F: Suggestions for thought, selections and commentaries, Philadelphia, 1994, University of Pennsylvania Press; edited by MD Calabria and JA Macrae.

Peck MS: *Further along the road less traveled: the unending journey toward spiritual growth,* New York, 1993, Simon & Schuster.

Piemme JA: Discussing end-of-life decisions, *Innovations in Breast Cancer Care* 4(1):31, November 1998.

Schettle S: A nurse's reflection: Nursing in the '90s—old hats, new ways, *Am J Nurs* 98(5):16j, 1998.

Travelbee J: Interventions in psychiatric nursing, Philadelphia, 1970, FA Davis.

 # Suggestions for Further Reading

Balzer Riley J: When the patient is my mother: creating I-Thou relationships in surgical nursing practice, *Point of View* 32(1):6, April 1995.

Byock I: *Dying well,* New York, 1997, Riverhead Books.

Bernard JS, Schneider M: *The true work of dying,* New York, 1996, Avon.

Burkhardt MA: Spirituality: an analysis of the concept, *Holistic Nurs Pract* 3(3):69, 1989.

Burkhardt MA, Nagai-Jacobson MG: Reawakening spirit in clinical practice, *J Holistic Nurs* 12(1):8, March 1994.

Burton LA: The spiritual dimension of palliative care, *Semin Oncol Nurs* 14(2):121, May 1998.

Carpenito LJ: Nursing diagnosis: application to clinical practice, Philadelphia, 1989, JB Lippincott.

Cerrato, PL: Spirituality and healing, *RN* 61(2):49, February 1998.

Christy JH: Prayer as medicine, *Forbes* March 23, 1998.

Davis BH: Disability and grief, *Social Casework: J Contemp Social Work,* June 1987, pp. 352-357.

De Hennezel M: *Intimate death,* Janeway, NY, 1997, Alfred A. Knopf

Dossey BM et al: *Holistic nursing: a handbook for practice,* Gaithersburg, Md, 1995, Aspen.

Dossey LD: *Healing words: the power of prayer and the practice of medicine,* San Francisco, 1993, Harper Collins.

Fahey C: Elderly residents as spiritual beings, *Nursing Homes* 46(10):39, 1997.

    National Hospice Organization website: www.nho.org.

Kaiser L: The hospital is a healing place, *Healthcare Forum J* pp. 38-39, Sept/Oct 1994.

    National Institute of Health's Office of Alternative Medicine website: www.altmed.od.nih.

Rew L: Intuition: nursing knowledge and the spiritual dimension of persons, *Holistic Nurs Pract* 3(3):56, 1989.

Sach R: *Perfect endings,* Rochester, Vt, 1998, Healing Arts Press.

Seidl LG: The value of spiritual health: spirituality and medicine must find common ground in the new healthcare era, *Health Progress* pp. 48-50, Sept 1993.

Stoddard A: *Living beautifully together: how to live graciously in a hectic world by finding time to love your family, your friends, and yourself,* New York, 1989, Avon.

Stuart EM, Deckro JP, Mandle CL: Spirituality in health and healing: a clinical program, *Holistic Nurs Pract* 3(3):35, 1989.

Sumner CH: Recognizing and responding to spiritual distress, *Am J Nurs* 98(1):26, 1998.

Wright KB: Professional, ethical, and legal implications for spiritual care in nursing, *Image J Nurs Scholar* 30(1):81, 1998.

Young-Mason J: *The patient's voice: experiences of illness,* Philadelphia, 1997, FA Davis.

Part III

Meeting Challenges

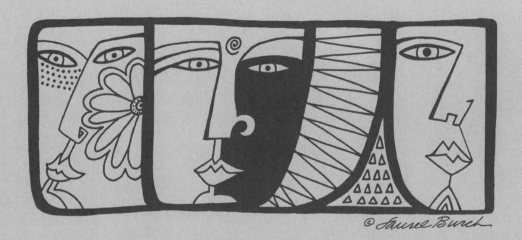

This section helps you to build on your assertive communication skills to refuse unreasonable requests. You will examine assertive communication in difficult situations with clients, families, and colleagues.

Assertive communication is more complex in its application than it seems when selecting responses to exercises in a text. Pay attention to the exercises as you examine what is responsible, assertive communication. Remember that you have assertive rights, and clients, families, and colleagues do, too. Here is your chance to think about your role as an advocate for yourself and for others.

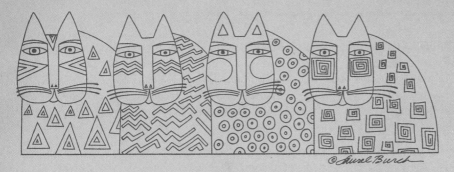

Confrontation

The lessons along your path are God's invitation to grow.

Susan L. Taylor

OBJECTIVES

1. Identify the benefits of confrontation skills.
2. Discuss the steps of the C.A.R.E. model of confrontation.
3. Identify the relationship between confrontation skills and empowerment.
4. Practice confrontation in selected exercises to build confidence in the skills.

DIFFERENT KINDS OF CONFRONTATION

Confrontation skill "is being able to identify and to respond—communicate—provide feedback—regarding those discrepancies in another person's behavior in such a manner that the other person can grow" (Tindall, 1994). An example of one type of confrontation is a nurse's deliberate invitation for clients and colleagues to examine incongruities or distortions between feelings, beliefs, attitudes, and behavior (Egan, 1977; McMahon, 1992; Stuart, Sundeen, 1995). This type of confrontation, designed to make others aware of incongruence, can be offered by nurses when, for example, clients or colleagues are saying one thing and doing another, or obviously feeling one way and exhibiting the opposite emotions. Pointing out these discrepancies can be an invitation to expand their self-awareness. This dimension of confrontation is a gift of feedback, which is covered in Chapter 24.

Here is an example of a confrontation to expand self-awareness:

John tells you he only smokes a few cigarettes a day. He has yellow stains on the fingers of his left hand, he smells of smoke, and wheezes upon inspiration. His wife says he smokes two packs a day.

Nurse: "John, I am concerned about conflicting information concerning your smoking. The stains on your fingers, the smell of smoke on your clothes, and the sound of your breathing indicate that you smoke more than a few cigarettes a day."

Confrontation that involves an explicit request for a behavior change along with feedback is the focus of this chapter.

WHEN CONFRONTATION IS APPROPRIATE

Confrontation has two parts: the first is making others aware of the destructiveness or lack of productiveness of their behavior, and the second is making a suggestion about how they could behave in a more constructive or productive way. Two situations warrant confronting clients or colleagues: when their behavior is unproductive or destructive to them, and when their behavior invades our rights or the rights of others. In confronting others, we are attempting to get them to change in a way that protects their self-interests or is more considerate of others. One note of warning: consider that the problem belongs to the other person and it is not our role to "fix" other people to meet our standards of behavior (Cox, 1998).

Some nurses shudder at the thought of confronting another person. It conjures up images of a heated argument. For most nurses, verbal attacks conflict with their image of themselves as level-headed professionals.

To avoid being labeled aggressive, many times we refrain from saying anything about others' unproductive or destructive behavior. Later, we watch our clients or colleagues get into trouble

Moments of Connection...
A Caring Confrontation

During a series of electrical treatments for myofacial pain, the client and I had an opportunity to talk. She was concerned about her diabetic husband who refused to eat properly, exercise, or take care of his health in any way. She tried hard to prepare the right foods and motivate him, but his health was deteriorating rapidly. Based on my own experience, I suggested to her she might need to focus on herself, developing friendships and work on improving the quality of her own life. We talked about her getting her finances and other business in the best of order in preparation for the time when her husband might not be there. She was silent and thoughtful. On her next appointment, she thanked me for my insight and said she knew she had done all she could for him, that it was time to help herself.

because of their misdirected actions and then we feel guilty and regret that we did not take the opportunity to speak up. In other situations we fume because we do not quite know how to confront those who have violated our rights or the rights of others and we stew in frustrated helplessness. The next time you hesitate to confront others when you believe it needs to be done, remember this: short-term gain, long-term pain. Being nonassertive may get you off the hook for now, but in the long run the problem will only escalate.

Neither of these two extremes—aggression or nonassertion—is acceptable to nurses who want to feel confident and act competently. There is a way, however, to confront others that makes you feel like you are effectively doing something about troublesome behavior. It is possible to confront people in such a way that they are unlikely to be offended. Moreover, they may appreciate your perspective and opinions.

THE C.A.R.E. CONFRONTATION

When confronting your clients or colleagues it is important to do so in a caring way that shows concern for both your feelings and theirs. Outlined below is a caring way to confront others. (The format for this comprehensive confrontation is adapted from Bower and Bower, 1991.)

Clarify the behavior that is problematic. Be specific about the aspect of your clients' or colleagues' behavior that is self-destructive or destructive to others. The behavior to be changed should be the focus so that it is clear you are attaching no hurtful labels to others.

Articulate why their behavior is a problem. Your articulation may include how their behavior is likely to hinder them or irritate others or how it makes you feel.

Request a change in your clients' or colleagues' behavior. Your suggestions should be offered tentatively and respectfully.

Encourage your clients or colleagues to change by emphasizing the positive consequences of changing or the negative implications if no change occurs.

Remember, too, not to expect a negative response; to use neutral words without blame; and to stay open to the responses, not jump to conclusions (Ryan et al, 1996). It is important to respect that the client's values maybe different than yours and to be careful not to take a lecturing tone when you confront (London, 1998).

Examples of C.A.R.E. Confrontations

The two situations outlined below demonstrate how you can confront someone in an assertive way without being aggressive.

Situation One

Your roommate is untidy. He leaves his clothes strewn around the bedroom you share, and the bathroom looks like a pharmacy. Frequently his notes and textbooks arc laid out all over the apartment. Although he does a major clean-up about every 2 weeks, he slides back into his messy ways and you have to put up with his disarray for the rest of the time. Not only is this mess aesthetically displeasing to you, it makes you hesitant to invite friends over. You confront your roommate with:

Clarify

"John, you have your clothes spread out over the bedroom and all your notes and articles for your paper are strewn around the living room and on the kitchen table."

Articulate

"I'm feeling annoyed that you are messing up the shared space in our apartment."

Request

"I'd like you to keep your personal belongings in your area of our den."

Encourage

"That way it'll be more spacious for both of us in the apartment and I'll feel free to invite friends over without worrying whether the place is a mess."

Presented with this respectful and assertive confrontation, John will most likely comply and change his behavior. If such a confrontation does not result in the desired behavior change, you have the option of indicating a negative consequence such as, "If you don't become neater, I will . . ." (and give a possible consequence, such as hire a maid and charge you, find another roommate, or move out).

Situation Two

Your colleague Janet is upset. She has been trying to lose weight for the past 6 months. You notice that she has a pattern of starting off successfully on Mondays, and by the end of the week she has gorged herself on her favorite fattening foods. Afterwards she fasts for several days and then overeats again. You think that these feasts and famines are not helpful for Janet and that it would be better if she distributed her calories more evenly.

After you have asked her permission to express your views, you confront Janet about her unproductive behavior in this way:

Clarify

"Janet, I notice you do well on your diet at the beginning of the week and then you have ups and downs of eating more than you want to or eating so little that you are starving."

Articulate

"I think one reason you are unsuccessful in losing weight is because you don't have an adequate intake of calories on a consistent basis."

Request

"Perhaps if you figured out a daily calorie intake that would make you feel satisfied and give you the energy you need, you may not binge as often."

Encourage

"If you weren't so hungry you might stop overeating and be more likely to lose weight. If you can cut out the overeating you won't feel guilty and have to starve yourself. What do you think?"

The respectful and clear way this confrontation is delivered is likely to invite Janet to consider your idea and possibly implement it. An accusatory confrontation would only be ignored.

CONFRONTING CLIENTS OR COLLEAGUES

We can often see how another person's behavior is not safe or in keeping with their goals. Each of us has blind spots about how some of what we say or do is predisposing us to emotional or physical harm, or is incongruent with our professed values or attitudes. As nurses we can offer an objective perspective on how others can change and act in a way that will serve their best interests. The following examples use C.A.R.E. confrontations to offer clients and colleagues ways to enhance their goals and avoid emotional or physical dangers.

Situations in Which Your Client's Behavior Is Self-Destructive or Unproductive

Mr. Jones, a finance officer for a large corporation, is a 35-year-old client who has suffered a massive myocardial infarction. Yesterday he was moved from ICU to the cardiac step-down unit. You overhear him asking his secretary to come to the unit to bring his portable computer so he can keep up with his electronic mail.

Your nursing knowledge warns you that Mr. Jones is escalating his work schedule too quickly and that his workaholic habits may detract from his heart's healing, or even put him at risk for another heart attack. You want him to slow down his reentry into the business world and gradually build up his stamina. You strongly believe that a gradual increase in his workload will augment his chances for a successful recovery. You confront Mr. Jones this way:

"Mr. Jones, I overheard you making arrangements for your secretary to bring your computer to the hospital. I can imagine that you must be eager to keep up with things at work. However, jumping in too quickly and taking on too much responsibility at this point in your recovery will likely make you tense, and the stress on your heart may increase. Your chances for a successful and complete recovery will be better if you ease back into work more slowly. I suggest that you put off asking for your computer and limit your work with your secretary to 15 minutes a day by phone for this week and then gradually increase. If you build up your stamina slowly you'll reduce the risk of another heart attack. What do you think?"

John, an 18-year-old client, has just had a torn Achilles tendon repaired. After his lesson using crutches, you notice that John is bearing too much weight on his affected leg. In doing so he is increasing the chance of his sutures weakening and putting strain on his tendon, thus preventing healing. You confront John with:

"When you put any weight on your injured leg, you are risking further injury to your tendon. If you weaken your tendon you may not recover full use of your leg. I'd like you to practice using your crutches so that you only place weight on your good leg. That way you'll ensure maximum healing of your injury. Will you try that please, John?"

Situations in Which Your Colleague's Behavior Is Self-Destructive or Unproductive

On the medical unit in your hospital, you and Judy have been working together on the evening shift for the past three evenings. Judy has been complaining of a strained back, which she has attributed to turning, positioning, and transferring the heavy clients on the unit. You have noticed that Judy takes few or no precautions to protect her back. After you have received her permission to express your views, you decide to confront her about her negligence in the following way:

"Judy, it sounds like your back is bothering you quite a bit. I've noticed that when you are turning our heavy patients, you tend to take the clients' full weight on your own without help from one of us or the Hoyer lift. I think you could save your back from a lot of discomfort and injury if you took the precautions of getting help and using protective devices. What do you think?"

Note the different order of this C.A.R.E. confrontation. The reordering makes it sound more natural in this case, yet it still contains the essential elements.

Your classmate, Toni, has not been achieving the grades to which she has been accustomed on her nursing exams. Toni is complaining about the severity of the exams and the tough grading of her instructors. You are aware that Toni has not been studying as much since she began dating two men at the same time and going out almost every night. She asks you what she should do. You decide to confront her about her recent unproductive behavior:

"Toni, I know you always do well even if the teachers are tough. It's just since you've been dating on weeknights that your grades have been less than what you used to receive. I'd have the same problem if I couldn't have extra time to review my class notes. It's a tough call. You know when we go over the notes several times we see a difference in the test grades. Maybe if you took a few minutes after classes to review you'd see a difference, but that is not easy to do when it's tempting to go out. What do you think?"

In each of these four situations the client or colleague has been confronted about something he or she is doing or not doing that is causing physical or emotional problems. The confrontation points out the specific behavior that is problematic and proposes a clear alternative, which is checked out with the client or colleague.

Let us examine some situations in which you use the skill of confrontation to deal with behavior that violates your rights or the rights of others.

Situations in Which Your Client's Behavior Is Bothersome to You or Others

Mr. Wars is a 53-year-old cardiac client who has been aggressive in the 3 days he has been on the unit. He has complained about the food, the room, and the other clients, and today he has been angry and abusive with you in the corridor. He complains that you are the slowest nurse he has ever encountered and that you don't know what you are doing. He has picked on your appearance, questioned your credentials, and repeatedly insulted your nursing care. His aggressiveness is embarrassing, time consuming, and unpleasant for you. You recognize that he is feeling out of control and assess that a referral to the psychiatric clinical nurse specialist might be of help to you and to him. You confront him when you are in the privacy of his room:

"Mr. Wars, we need to talk about how things are going for you. I know you are not happy with your care and I want to talk about what we can do. I would like to help you be as comfortable as possible during these tough times for you. It upsets me to be unable to make things better for you. We have a nurse whom we can call whose job it is to evaluate such situations. She could spend some time with you to help you sort things out. I hope you are willing to let me call her so we can work together to turn things around for the better. How does that sound to you?"

Miss Debris is a colleague with whom you share an office. She often moves your paperwork and leaves the desk in disorder. Yesterday you could not find any pens or the stapler. Today Miss

Debris has left a dirty coffee cup and the wrapper from her sandwich on the desk. She is about to leave without cleaning it up when you confront her:

"When you leave the desk we share cluttered I have to search for the things I need to do my work. I know you get busy, but this time I see trash, too. If we both are aware of keeping the work space clear, it will be ready when each of us needs it. How about taking a few seconds to dump the trash and make sure the papers and supplies are handy? It would make it easier to for me to face my work and I would appreciate it. Does that sound fair?"

Wit and Wisdom

One finger cannot lift a pebble.

Hopi Indian proverb

Situations in Which Your Colleague's Behavior Is Unpleasant for You or Others

You have been working the night shift for the past five nights. In the three previous mornings your nurse relief has been about 15 to 25 minutes late. You are not free to leave the unit until she arrives because there is only one nurse on duty. Her tardiness puts your own personal schedule off by making you late getting home to see your family before they head off to school and work. You decide to confront her:

"Rena, I want to speak to you about your coming in 15 to 25 minutes late in the mornings. It puts my whole routine out of whack because I've been getting home too late in the mornings to see my family. I would like you to arrange to be here at 0730 from now on so that I can give you the report without being too rushed and still get home on time. Can you do that?"

Margaret is a new graduate working on a psychiatric unit with you. You notice that each time Margaret has an interview with a client she goes into the session with coffee only for herself and then puts her feet up on the desk. You know this casual behavior makes clients feel insulted and not respected and gives them the impression that Margaret is less than interested in their case. Since the clients have not had the nerve to challenge Margaret, you decide to say something to her about her behavior.

Wit and Wisdom

Unless you stop the crack you will rebuild the wall.

African proverb

"Margaret, I couldn't help notice that when you interview some of the clients you have a very casual style, with a coffee cup in your hand and your feet up on the desk. I think your manner may give the impression to some clients that you aren't taking them seriously. We don't wear uniforms, so it is important that our behavior sends a clear message that we are caring professionals. Since I know you are interested in your work and like to do a good job, I thought you'd want to know if your behavior might be misinterpreted. (Await approval from Margaret before continuing.) Perhaps if you offered your clients a cup of coffee, too, and didn't put your feet up you would show your clients your real interest in them. What do you think?"

The C.A.R.E. confrontation provides a way of approaching others when either their best interests or yours are threatened. C.A.R.E. confrontations allow you to take action in a calm, controlled, assertive way. They prevent you from being immobilized in a situation where you want to be confrontive but not aggressive.

THE MAGIC OF A LITTLE WORD

Try using the word "and" instead of "but" when offering criticism or differing opinion. The word "but" may put the person on the defensive. Berent and Evans (1992) give some examples when offering advice or criticism:

- "I appreciate the intensity of your feelings about this, and I think if you were to hear my side of it you might feel differently."
- "I can understand your reasons, and I think my reasons for doing it differently are also understandable."
- "That's an interesting idea, and here's another way to think about it."

CONFRONTATION IS ONE PART OF EMPOWERMENT

Confrontation is an important skill to learn and is one aspect of many that you will use as you move forward as an empowered professional nurse. (Did you notice the use of "and" rather than "but"? Using "but" would have diminished the importance of the skill of confrontation.) As you feel more confident with your own nursing skills, the necessity for the skills of confrontation will be more obvious. Murphy (1994) admonishes nurses not to be doormats, but discusses the personal responsibility of nurses who want to be more effective in conflict resolution. Nurses need to:

- Make self-improvement a priority.
- Pay attention to feelings of anger and fear as signals to deal with a situation.
- Speak up respectfully and before an angry blowup occurs.
- Commit to treating others respectfully.
- Be honest and confront colleagues when friction first occurs rather than let it escalate.
- Practice self-care skills such as exercise, relaxation, and recreation.

Later chapters talk about self-care skills that help you to be responsive to colleagues and clients, rather than reactive. This means being able to take time to sort out which situations require confrontation and which can be tolerated or are simply an overreaction due to fatigue or personal stress. Noddings (1994) concludes that "everywhere—in personal, social, political, and even professional life—people misunderstand one another." Confrontation takes thought, energy, and a caring attitude. In nursing . . . "in the caring orientation, we are more concerned with connecting, feeling—with responding positively to expressed needs, and understanding ourselves well enough to be able to summon the attitude of caring" (Noddings, 1994).

Wit and Wisdom

The best remedy for a dispute is to discuss it.

African proverb

Think About It...
What, So What, and Now What?

Consider your own experiences with confrontation and how they affect your willingness to try on these new behaviors.

What? . . . Write one thing you learned from this chapter.

So what? . . . How will this impact your nursing practice?

Now what? . . . How will you implement this new knowledge or skill?

THINK ABOUT IT

Practicing Confrontation

Exercise 1

For each situation below attempt a C.A.R.E. confrontation. After you have prepared a response, get together as a class and discuss your different approaches. Compare your suggestions with those at the end of this exercise.

1. Mr. Steiger, your 38-year-old client, suffers chronic bronchitis. You have noticed him smoking in the patients' lounge and as you enter his room you can smell cigarette smoke coming from the bathroom. Your nursing knowledge tells you that his smoking is self-destructive. How would you confront him?
2. Your client, 60-year-old Mrs. Cantor, has severe pitting edema of the ankles. She has been taught to raise her legs on a chair when sitting, and to wear elastic stockings from toe to midthigh. You have observed that Mrs. Cantor is not wearing her stockings and each time you have seen her in the chair her feet have been on the floor. How would you confront her about her self-destructive behavior?
3. You and Jane started working in an emergency center 6 months ago, after your graduation from nursing. Jane confides to you that she feels she does not have the respect of her team members and that she feels that her opinions are not listened to or acted on. You have noticed that Jane takes a passive stance: she is overly cautious about her suggestions and speaks quietly. When she presents an idea she often puts it down first. You are reasonably certain that some of her nonassertive behavior accounts for her ideas not being picked up by the team. How would you confront her about her unproductive behavior?
4. Dr. Morton, the intern on the medical floor, has been unprofessional in his relations with you. He has teased you and made lewd jokes about you. He refuses to consult you about clients for whom you are directly responsible but goes to other nurses for this information. You want his embarrassing joking to stop and you want him to consult you about your clients. How would you confront him?

Suggested C.A.R.E. confrontations

1. "Mr. Steiger, I have observed you smoking on several occasions in the past couple of days. Smoking causes you to produce more phlegm and that makes you cough more and become short of breath. I would like to give you some information about help available to you should you choose to stop smoking. If you were able to do this your lungs would have a chance to clear and your breathing would become easier. If you don't stop smoking, then you are at risk for a serious lung infection. I know it is tough, but I think you'd be surprised to hear about the successful outcomes of people using a nicotine patch. May I tell you more about it?"
2. "Mrs. Cantor, I notice that you aren't wearing your elastic stockings and your feet are on the floor instead of being raised on the stool. Wearing your elastic stockings helps prevent blood clots from forming. I strongly recommend that you wear your stockings and raise your legs on a stool so that you prevent any more serious complications of your heart disease."

3. "Jane, I think you have some sound ideas about how we can be more efficient. I notice that when you present your ideas you seem to hesitate and speak softly and uncertainly about your views. When you start off by saying, 'This idea may not work . . .' it's almost as if you've set the team up to discount your suggestions before they have heard them. I think the value of your suggestions would be highlighted if you just gave your ideas in a more positive way. Then you and the team would both benefit."

4. "Dr. Morton, making me the brunt of your sexist jokes is distracting and demeaning, and I ask you to stop it. I'd like you to consult me about my clients when I am the primary nurse involved. If you can relate to me that way, I'm sure we'll develop a good working relationship. And I can assure you that you'll get the essential information about your clients from me in a clear and concise report."

If you require more examples, refer to Exercise 3 in Chapter 3 for situations in which clients have broken a mutually arrived-at agreement.

Exercise 2

Work in threes for this exercise. Each one of you should rotate through the roles of confronter, confrontee, and feedback giver. The confrontee will ignore the confronter as she attempts to tell you how she spent her weekend. The confrontee does not attend and does not show respect for the confronter. After several minutes the confronter will use a C.A.R.E. confrontation to get the confrontee to listen more attentively.

As the confrontee:

1. In what ways was the confrontation successful?
2. What suggestions would you make to the confronter to help her be more assertive in making a confrontation?

As the confronter:

1. Which aspects of completing a C.A.R.E. confrontation were easier for you to master?
2. Where did you run into difficulties?
3. What suggestions do you have for improving your ability to confront?

As the feedback giver:

1. Did the confronter clarify the behavior that was unpleasant?
2. Did she articulate why it was bothersome?
3. Was her request for change clear and realistic?
4. How did she encourage her confrontee to make the changes she requested?
5. Overall, how assertive was the confrontation?

Switch roles so that each of you has the opportunity to be confronter, confrontee, and feedback giver.

Exercise 3

In the next few days observe how others make confrontations to you. What do they do that makes you feel respected? Are they clear in their message to you? What do they say that leaves you feeling put down or angry? You can learn a lot about how to improve your own confrontations by observing the effect of others' confrontations on you.

Continued

Practicing Confrontation—cont'd

After you have collected your own data, compare your findings with those of your classmates. What have your observations taught you about the most effective ways to confront others?

Exercise 4

Attempt to practice confrontation in real life, whether at school, on the units, or in social situations. How effective are you at making C.A.R.E. confrontations? Have you discovered that by using this format you avoid both aggression and nonassertion? Do these guidelines for confronting provide you with more confidence?

Wit and Wisdom

You get what you tolerate.

Bumper sticker

References

Berent IM, Evans RL: *The right words: the 350 best things to say to get along with people,* New York, 1992, Warner.

Bower SA, Bower GH: *Asserting yourself: a practical guide for positive change,* Reading, Mass, 1991, Addison-Wesley Publishing.

Cox S: Nursing fix-it syndrome, *Nursing* 98 28(6):61, 1998.

Egan G: *You and me: the skills of communications and relating to others,* Monterey, Calif., 1977, Brooks/Cole Publishing (classic source).

London F: Improving compliance: what you can do, *RN* 61(1):43, 1998.

McMahon AM: Nurse-client relationship. In Haber J, Leach AM, Hoskins PP, Sideleau BF: *Comprehensive psychiatric nursing,* ed 4, St Louis, 1992, Mosby.

Murphy SZ: Don't be a doormat: personal empowerment in nursing, *Revolution* 2(2):66, 1994.

Noddings N: Learning to engage in moral dialogue, *Holistic Educ Rev* 7(2):5, 1994.

Ryan KD, Oestreich DK, Orr GA III: *The courageous messenger: how to successfully speak up at work,* San Francisco, 1996, Jossey-Bass.

Stuart GW, Laraia M: *Principles and practice of psychiatric nursing,* ed 6, St Louis, 1998, Mosby.

Tindall J: *Peer power: book one, workbook: becoming an effective peer helper and conflict mediator,* Muncie, 1994, Accelerated Development.

Suggestions for Further Reading

Alberti RE, Emmons ML: *Your perfect right: a guide to assertive living,* San Luis Obispo, Calif, 1995, Impact Publishers.

Burley-Allen M: *Managing assertively: how to improve your people skills,* New York, 1995, John Wiley & Sons.

DeMarco RF: Caring to confront in the workplace: an ethical perspective for nurses, *Nurs Outlook* 46(3):130, 1998.

Egan G: *The skilled helper: model, skills, and methods for effective helping,* ed 2, Monterey, Calif, 1982, Brooks/Cole Publishing.

In Chapter 7 of this classic text, Egan describes several methods of confrontation that can be employed in the client-counselor relationship. Many examples are given to explain the pros and cons of confrontation.

Fisher R, Ury W: *Getting to yes: negotiating agreement without giving in,* New York, 1991, Penguin.

Lerner HG: The dance of anger, New York, 1985, Harper & Row.

Long L: *Understanding/responding: a communication manual for nurses,* Boston, 1992, Jones & Bartlett.

McCallister L: *I wish I'd said that: how to talk your way out of trouble and into success,* New York, 1992, Wiley.

Orchard B: Creating constructive outcomes in conflict, AAORN 46(6):302, 1998.

Phelps S, Austin N. *The assertive woman,* 1997, San Luis Obispo, Calif, Impact Publishers.

Sundeen SJ et al: Nurse-client interaction: implementing the nursing process, St Louis, 1998, Mosby.

Taylor, PB: Setting your boundaries, *Nursing* 98 28(4):56, 1998.

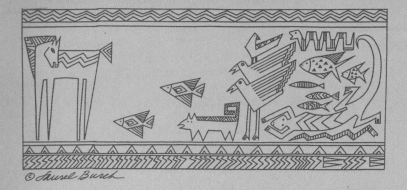

17

Refusing Unreasonable Requests

To ask well is to know much.

African proverb

OBJECTIVES

1. Discuss the importance of the right to refuse unreasonable requests from clients and colleagues.
2. Distinguish between assertive, nonassertive, and aggressive refusals.
3. Participate in exercises to build skills to refuse unreasonable requests.

WHAT ARE UNREASONABLE REQUESTS?

As nurses we receive requests from others for information, emotional support, and assistance. Week in and week out we are asked to carry out activities that will help our clients and colleagues. Each request we receive is deemed reasonable in the eyes of the person making the request. In most instances, requests from our clients and colleagues seem legitimate when we think about the request in an objective way. However, when a request is made of you, you must consider how it affects you personally because you are the one being asked to fulfill the request. It is up to you to determine whether a request is reasonable. With assertive communication skills, you learn how to refuse requests, but you choose whether to refuse depending on the situation.

Wit and Wisdom

Refusing Unreasonable Requests

You may ask of me.
I may ask of you.
We share our needs
And give our due.

I have my own needs.
My time I must measure.
I'll meet you halfway,
Each other we'll treasure.

But some things you ask
I must refuse.
Please don't your own power
With mine confuse.

Please listen to me
When I say no.
It's not an issue
of friend or foe.

Copyright 1995 Julia W. Balzer Riley.

A request may be unreasonable if it impinges on your right to provide nursing care in a way that is within your ethics, values, or beliefs. Unreasonable requests are ones that escalate your negative feelings and encroach upon your right to feel good about the work you are doing. You may be asked to perform tasks that are disrespectful of your safety or physical capabilities. It is unreasonable to respond to requests that put you in the position of hurting yourself, such as physically and emotionally stretching yourself to the point that you feel stressed, overloaded, or irritable. However, it is important to note that sometimes you choose to fulfill a request even though you would prefer to decline. You may be asked to work an extra hour because of an emergency situation. A friend may ask a favor that is inconvenient. In these cases, you make your own decision as to whether to comply. In other cases, a request may seem unreasonable to you, and yet it seems prudent to comply. You may ask yourself not whether the request is reasonable, but whether it may be reasonable to fulfill the request.

As nurses we have the right to work in a way that allows us to give our best nursing care to our clients, promotes the most congenial relationships with our colleagues, and gives us feelings of satisfaction, safety, and comfort doing our job. In Chapter One, basic assertive rights were introduced. Chenevert puts our rights as nurses in perspective: "Nurses are responsible people. We have dwelled so long and so hard on our responsibilities we are often surprised at the prospect of having rights ourselves" (1993). Review your basic assertive rights in Box 1-2.

When you consider these rights you need to use common sense. Of course, if you are a new graduate and your manager instructs you to give a pain medication at once, it would be inappropriate to say you prefer to bathe another client first. If you refuse a request, you may need to give a rationale.

Requests for our information or ideas, attention or affection, physical power or skills, all take time, energy, and commitment to fulfill. We need to check our resources before agreeing to any request. When we take on a request that overtaxes us, we lose out because we become overloaded, and others lose out because we are ineffective when we are feeling burdened. Before saying "yes" to a request, we need to check to see if it is reasonable for us to accept. If we decide it is unreasonable, then we must refuse. It is far better to refuse than to capitulate and risk a serious error. Failure to refuse can end up making you a sorry excuse for a nurse (Chenevert, 1990).

Mackay reveals that successful businesspeople tap into their own state of mind before saying "yes" to important requests for their time, money, or expertise. "In the final analysis, what your inner voice tells you is the best advice you can get" (Mackay, 1990). For making decisions in the world of business, Mackay underlines the importance of being honest enough to understand and predict our reactions if the unexpected happens. "If you know you can't handle the bad stuff, if you're not ready to make a total commitment, then you're not ready to say yes, whatever it is" (1990). We shouldn't ignore this advice.

Saying "No" Assertively

The skill in saying "no" is to refuse the request in an assertive, as opposed to an aggressive or nonassertive, style. By being assertive we protect ourselves by declining a task we cannot comfortably handle and we respect the other's rights by refusing in a polite, matter-of-fact manner. Our desire to help our clients and colleagues and our wish to be seen as helpful nurses often interfere with our ability to say "no" clearly and simply.

Ellis and Lange (1994) discuss irrational beliefs that keep us from acting in our own best interests. Review the irrational beliefs listed in Box 1-3. Let's consider one such belief, "I must be approved of at all times." "If I don't do everything people ask of me they will reject me." Such a belief escalates to "awfulizing." "It would be awful and I couldn't stand it if someone thought I considered my own needs." "They would think I am selfish" (Ellis and Lange, 1994). Get the idea? It sounds like an exaggeration, but sometimes we base our decisions on such faulty thinking. Assertive communication is based on a consideration of both parties' needs and allows that we have the right to set our own priorities on our actions and time allocation. This is difficult for some people. Jokingly, workshop participants are told that they can be taught how to say "no" but that that they will have to get counseling like everybody else to deal with the guilt (Balzer, 1992). You may at some time consider counseling if you have difficulty acting in your own best interests and find that it interferes with your ability to feel good about your work and yourself.

We sometimes fumble with wishy-washy excuses in attempts to avoid taking on a request. This nonassertive behavior makes us feel guilty and helpless and we offend the asker with our weak and irrelevant attempts to justify our refusal. A simple "no" would suffice and save both people embarrassment.

Sometimes our unnecessary or irrational guilt feelings about saying "no" make us refuse a request in a hostile, defensive manner. This aggression makes us feel ashamed that we have behaved unprofessionally, and the other person feels put down or hurt by our explosive response.

Clearly, refusing a request in a nonassertive or aggressive way does not protect our interests or those of our clients or colleagues. The assertive refusal to an unreasonable request is the only way to show respect for ourselves and others.

Saying "no" to unreasonable requests is a way of saying "yes" to yourself. Just as clients are unique individuals and you struggle to consider their individuality when providing nursing care, when you protect your rights by refusing unreasonable requests you are respecting your uniqueness. You are saying "yes" to your values, "yes" to your style of doing things, "yes" to your ways of perceiving situations, and "yes" to your ways of judging and deciding. It is freeing to remove your energy from unreasonable requests and invest it into your visions and goals.

Examples of Refusing Requests Assertively

Here are several examples of effective, assertive ways of saying "no," in contrast to ineffective, aggressive, and nonassertive ways.

Example 1

It is Tuesday. Your colleague, Elsa, asks you to be on call for her this weekend. Your in-laws are coming to visit and you have made plans to take them on a tour of the excellent countryside restaurants. Your family has been looking forward to this visit and it is unreasonable for you to work on this particular weekend. In the past, Elsa has been on call for you.

An assertive refusal:

Elsa: "Could you please be on call this weekend for me? Rob phoned long distance and he's invited me to go to New York to spend the long weekend with him. I'm so excited! Can you do it?"

Assertive you: "No, Elsa. I'm not able to switch this weekend. My in-laws are visiting from out of town and we've made reservations to do things. I hope you can find someone to switch. I can see you're really looking forward to going to New York to visit Rob."

This refusal is direct and clear. You are definite, yet you soften the refusal with the inclusion of the explanation for your refusal and your emphatic hope that she can secure a replacement.

Elsa is determined, however, and persists in her attempt to persuade you to switch.

Elsa: "I know you've got company coming, but they're just in-laws and you get to see them often. I haven't seen Rob for 3 months. I know it's last-minute, but Rob just found out he could be free and he called me as soon as he could. Oh, please, won't you be on call for me?"

Assertive you: "No, Elsa. I am not available to switch with you this weekend."

You continue to be clear and definite. Elsa is pleading and trying to make you feel guilty so that you will give in to her. Your response successfully protects your rights to have a weekend with your family and attends to her rights to be treated respectfully.

Elsa does not stop. She wants you to switch so she plies you with more guilt.

Elsa: "Remember I switched weekends with you in the spring when you wanted to go to your cousin's wedding? You agreed then that you owed me one. Well, now I'm collecting! I need you to pay me back this weekend."

Assertive you: "Elsa, I am unable to help you this weekend."

This response continues to be clear and unwavering so that Elsa is given a definite, matter-of-fact answer that is congruent with your desire to avoid becoming hostile or weakened. Although you hope Elsa will find a replacement, it is unreasonable for you to be that person this weekend.

Elsa is starting to get your assertive message.

Elsa: "Okay, okay. I see you've got plans you can't break. It's just that I'm desperate. I'll ask one of the other nurses if she can switch with me."

By being assertive you have prevented yourself from doing two things you did not want to do: be on call this weekend and come across as defensive or indecisive to your colleague Elsa.

A nonassertive refusal:

Elsa: "Could you please be on-call for me this weekend? Rob phoned long distance and he's invited me to go to New York to spend the long weekend with him. I'm so excited! Can you do it?"

Nonassertive you: "Gee, Elsa. I don't think so . . . I'm sorry."

This response does not sound convincing. Elsa would get the message that you are not really sure you can switch with her. It sounds like you are still debating with yourself, and Elsa will likely try to convince you to switch.

Elsa: "I haven't seen Rob for 3 months. I know it's last-minute, but Rob just found out he could be free and he called me as soon as he could. Oh, please, won't you work for me?"

Nonassertive you: "Gee, Elsa, I don't think I can. I'm sorry. I've got my in-laws coming and we've made plans. I don't think so, Elsa."

You still have not given a definite "no" and Elsa will likely keep asking you as long as she figures there is hope.

Elsa: "Remember I switched weekends with you in the spring when you wanted to go to your cousin's wedding? You agreed then that you owed me one. Well, now I'm collecting! I need you to pay me back this weekend."

Nonassertive you: "Yes, that's true. I guess I owe you one. Yes, I'll switch with you for this weekend."

By being nonassertive and indefinite you have agreed to a request that is unreasonable for you to take on. Giving in will most likely leave you feeling angry and your in-laws will be disappointed you have let them down. When we are nonassertive we forfeit our rights.

An aggressive refusal:

Elsa: "Could you please be on-call for me this weekend? Rob phoned long distance and he's invited me to go to New York to spend the long weekend with him. I'm so excited! Can you do it?"

Aggressive you: "Don't you know I've got my in-laws coming to visit this weekend? There's no way I can switch with you."

This abrasive, offensive reply shows no understanding of Elsa's predicament. Whereas a simple refusal would have sufficed, this response makes you appear unfriendly and inconsiderate.

Elsa is not put off and continues to try to convince you to change.

Elsa: "I haven't seen Rob for 3 months. I know it's last-minute, but Rob just found out he could be free and he called me as soon as he could. Oh, please, won't you work for me?"

Aggressive you: "I can't help it if you haven't seen Rob for 3 months. That's your problem. I've got my own problems with my in-laws coming."

Elsa: "I know you've got company coming, but they're just your in-laws and you get to see them often."

Aggressive you: "They are just as important to me as your absentee boyfriend is to you. Maybe if you got together more often you wouldn't be so desperate now."

Your insensitivity to Elsa's predicament and your judgmental, accusatory remarks will considerably damage your relationship with your co-worker. Aggressive responses are often disproportionate and fired by our irrational anger and guilt.

Elsa persists!

Elsa: "Remember I switched weekends with you in the spring when you wanted to go to your cousin's wedding? You agreed then that you owed me one. Well, now I'm collecting! I need you to pay me back this weekend."

Aggressive you: "I gave you plenty of notice—not 3 days like you're offering me. If you think I can drop my plans, you're crazy!"

Elsa: "Well, I'll never do you a favor again. Some friend you are."

You may have won the battle by refusing an unreasonable request, but you have lost the war of conducting yourself in a considerate and professional manner. If the bad feelings created by being aggressive can ever be resolved, it will take an inordinate amount of energy and time.

Example 2

You are making a home visit to a client who has right-sided weakness. You are late in visiting two clients with whom you have extensive diabetic teaching. Your child needs a ride home from school and you think you can just make it on time. Mr. Gowers, your 70-year-old client, is right-handed and has not been very successful using his left hand to write. As you are about to leave, he asks you to write a letter for him to his nephew.

An assertive refusal:

Mr. Gowers: "Could you help me write a letter to my nephew tonight? I just remembered it's his twentieth wedding anniversary and I want to let him know I'm thinking of him. He is like a son to me. I'd do it myself but I can't get the hang of using my left hand."

Assertive you: "Mr. Gowers, I will not be able to help you to write your letter today because I am running behind schedule. I can see it is important for you to get your best wishes off to this special nephew of yours in time for his anniversary. I saw your neighbor outside. How about if I ask him to come over and write the letter?"

This definite response makes it clear to Mr. Gowers that you are unable to do what he wants. Your expression of understanding about his urgency and your suggestion of an alternative solution would make him aware of your concern. You have protected your rights not to take on a task when you are already overloaded, and you have shown your client you are interested in his situation.

A nonassertive refusal:

Mr. Gowers: "Could you help me write a letter to my nephew tonight? I just remembered it's his twentieth wedding anniversary and I want to let him know I'm thinking of him. He is like a son to me. I'd do it myself but I can't."

Nonassertive you: "Uh . . . well, um, I'm not sure I can, Mr. Gowers. I'm pretty busy today, but I'll try. Maybe I can come back here on my lunch hour."

You know that you are so busy that you will be lucky to get the teaching done and pick up your son. You know you should not take on this extra task and you are already feeling more tense because it is one more thing on your long list of things to do. You have not protected your rights for a reasonable workload, and you have conveyed a lot of ambivalence to Mr. Gowers, perhaps leaving him feeling that he is imposing on you.

An aggressive refusal:

Mr. Gowers: "Could you help me write a letter to my nephew? I just remembered it's his twentieth wedding anniversary and I want to let him know I'm thinking of him. He is like a son to me. I'd do it myself but I can't write very well with my left hand."

Aggressive you: "If you think I've got time to sit down and take dictation, Mr. Gowers, you're mistaken. I'll be lucky to get my real work done today."

This hostile rejoinder protects you from doing an unreasonable assignment, but it leaves Mr. Gowers feeling devastated. He is likely feeling guilty for asking you and embarrassed at your angry refusal. Neither of you wins with an aggressive refusal.

Example 3

A physician arrives late to the afternoon prenatal clinic. Today is especially busy because more expectant mothers have kept their appointments than usual. One of your nurses is ill, leaving you short-staffed. In addition, you are responsible for all the prenatal teaching. The physician tells you he has missed his lunch and asks you to get him something to eat.

An assertive refusal:

Dr. Watts: "Will you go across to the deli and pick me up a salami on rye? I missed lunch because I was so busy this morning."

Assertive you: "No, Dr. Watts, I can't go across to get you lunch. Like you, today I am swamped with the workload."

This assertive response clearly conveys your refusal. It is polite and matter-of-fact. You have upheld your rights to do your job and treated your colleague respectfully.

A nonassertive refusal:

Dr. Watts: "Will you go across to the deli and pick me up a salami on rye? I missed lunch because I was so busy this morning."

Nonassertive you: "Um . . . uh, well, Dr. Watts, we're kind of busy here today, but, well, I suppose if I do it fast it won't take too much time. Do you want it toasted or plain? Pickles? Mustard? . . ."

Being nonassertive is probably leaving you feeling pretty angry and disappointed in yourself. It is clear to everyone that you do not wish to get your colleague's lunch. Being nonassertive this way means you lose time and lose face.

An aggressive refusal:

Dr. Watts: "Will you go across to the deli and pick me up a salami on rye? I missed lunch because I was so busy this morning."

Aggressive you: "Nurses aren't handmaidens anymore, Dr. Watts. You'd better get with the times. We're all busy, yet we managed to get our own lunches. I'm not being paid to go and fetch food for you."

Wow! You protected your rights with this response, but in the process you were rude to a colleague by the way you overreacted and attacked him. Such accusatory aggressiveness only serves to escalate bad feelings. A simple refusal would have been in order.

Saying "No" Effectively

Quite likely these examples have made you aware of some "do's" and "don'ts" when refusing unreasonable requests. Here are some suggestions to add to your observations.

Do:

- State your refusal very near the beginning of your reply so that your requester hears a clear, direct answer right away.
- Indicate concisely the reason for saying "no" if it strengthens your refusal.
- Communicate your understanding so that the requester feels you understand the predicament even if you cannot solve it.
- Suggest an alternative source of help if it seems appropriate.
- Think about your response, then speak in a forthright, calm, polite manner.
- Maintain a matter-of-fact, consistent way of refusing in the face of an aggressive requester.

Don't:

- Begin your refusal with a list of lengthy excuses against which an aggressive requester will argue so logically that you will be forced to concede.
- Stammer, pause, hem and haw, hesitate, or burst out your refusal; this will reveal that you are unsure of your response.
- Lose eye contact for lengthy periods, shift uncomfortably, or convey other nonverbal discomfort that reveals your hesitancy.
- Raise your voice or give other bodily clues of being enraged. It is your right to refuse, and you do not need to become hostile to protect this privilege.

Dare to Hold Fast to Your Principles

It is sometimes difficult to find just the right words to express your refusal even when you are convinced of your opinion. Berent and Evans (1992) offer some phrases that might be helpful.

"No!"
"No, thank you, I don't care to. I've never done that, and don't want to start."
"I can't do that."
"I make it a habit never to . . . ."
"I make it a habit always to . . . ."
"As a matter of principle, I . . ."

Moments of Connection...
Refusing to Hurry in a Managed Care World

In this day of HMOs and PPOs, insurance dictates what we as health care providers are allowed to do for our clients. I try to be a patient advocate and go beyond my nursing duties to make sure the procedures are authorized. Even though it takes up more time to teach the client and family about the financial end of health care, they are appreciative and often tell me how special they feel that I cared enough to help them answer reimbursement questions or put them in touch with someone who can. They see it as another demonstration of caring.

Think About It...
What, So What, and Now What?

Consider what you read about the right to refuse unreasonable requests and the skills to do so. Think of an unreasonable request you would like to refuse as you respond to the following questions.

What? . . . Write one thing you learned from this chapter.

So what? . . . How will this impact your nursing practice?

Now what? . . . How will you implement this new knowledge or skill?

THINK ABOUT IT

Practicing Refusing Unreasonable Requests

Exercise 1

For each of the following situations, write an assertive refusal. Compare your responses with those of your colleagues and pool your suggestions to come up with the most assertive refusal.

1. A client asks you for your home number so that he can call you "if he needs any follow-up advice." In the interests of your privacy, it is your policy not to give out your telephone number to clients.
2. A colleague with whom you are working the night shift asks you to keep an eye on the clients and an ear out for the telephone and night supervisor while she has a nap. You think this request is unreasonable because you are both being paid to do the job and if there is any trouble, two staff members will be needed.
3. A client wants you to facilitate bringing his 3-year-old son into the hospital to visit him. The rules of this unit are that no children under 12 years of age are allowed because of the high risk of infection. He says he is a single parent and really misses his son.
4. A client is being observed for withdrawal from street drugs. She asks you if she can go down to the cafeteria with her visitor to have a cup of coffee. Your preference is for her to remain on the unit where you can have frequent contact with her.
5. A client who comes once a week to receive an injection from you asks you if he could come 15 minutes later in the future. Moving back his appointment would inconvenience you, because it would mean you would be late leaving work and not make your bus connections.
6. A colleague who lives in the same area of the city asks you if he can get a ride to and from work with you. That quiet time in the car by yourself is your only peaceful time in the day. You would find it stressful to have to make conversation with another person during the commuting time.
7. The health care team has decided it will try to persuade a resistant client to receive a blood transfusion in order to save her life. As a nurse on the team, it is expected that you will participate in this coercion. Such a decision is against your beliefs about clients' rights to make independent decisions about their health.
8. A new nurse you supervise has asked you 6 months in advance if she can have Christmas off because she has small children. You know several other staff also have small children and have had to work holidays. You are reluctant to commit to an answer this soon and want to discuss with staff their ideas about how to fairly assign holiday call.

You can also use this exercise to verbally practice making refusals. One person in the vignette can role-play the manager, another the nurse, and a third can give feedback to the manager on her ability to refuse assertively.

Exercise 2

For this exercise, work in groups of three. One person will make a request, another will refuse the request, and the third will give feedback. The requester can ask for anything, and she should persist in her attempts to get what she wants. Aggressiveness in the requester is encouraged for the

Continued

Practicing Refusing Unreasonable Requests—cont'd

purposes of this exercise. The refuser will attempt to give an assertive refusal and will try to maintain that stance in the face of the requester's aggressiveness. The observer will give feedback to the refuser about her ability to refuse in an assertive way. The observer will point out where the refuser could have been more assertive or less aggressive. In debriefing, these questions can be used as a guide.

As the refuser:

1. Were you able to achieve and/or maintain an assertive refusal?
2. Where did you have difficulty being assertive?
3. What could you do to overcome these blocks and be more assertive in your refusals?

As the requester:

1. In what ways did the refuser convince you of a firm "no"?
2. Where and how could the assertion be improved?

Make sure you each get a turn in each role, and debrief after each role change.

Exercise 3

Over the next week make notes of how you make refusals to others. What do you think is effective and what could you do to improve?

Exercise 4

In the next week observe how others handle requests you make of them. Especially note how others refuse your requests. What is assertive about how they make their refusals? How do others make you feel when they refuse your requests? What is it others do to make you feel respected and understood? What is it they do to make you feel humiliated or embarrassed?

From observing others, what have you learned about effective and ineffective ways to refuse unreasonable requests?

Wit and Wisdom

An appeaser is one who feeds a crocodile—hoping it will eat him last.

Sir Winston Churchill

References

Balzer JW: Speak up and be heard—assertiveness lecture, Jacksonville, Fla, 1992, Baptist Medical Center.

Berent IM, Evans RL: *The right words: the 350 best things to say to get along with people,* New York, 1992, Warner Books.

Chenevert M: *Pro-nurse handbook: designed for the nurse who wants to thrive professionally,* ed 2, St Louis, 1993, Mosby.

Ellis A, Lange A: *How to keep people from pushing your buttons,* New York, 1994, Birch Lane Press.

Mackay H: *Beware the naked man who offers you his shirt,* New York, 1990, Ivy Books.

Suggestions for Further Reading

Alberti RE, Emmons ML: *Your perfect right: a guide to assertive living,* San Luis Obispo, Calif, 1995, Impact Publishers.

Bloom L, Coburn K, Pearlman J: *The new assertive woman,* New York, 1998, Dell.

Burley-Allen M: *Managing assertively: how to improve your people skills,* New York, 1995, John Wiley & Sons.

Davidson J: *The complete idiot's guide to assertiveness,* New York, 1997, Macmillan General Reference.

Fisher R, Ury W: *Getting to yes: negotiating agreement without giving in,* New York, 1991, Penguin Books.

Long L: *Understanding/responding: a communication manual for nurses,* Boston, 1992, Jones & Bartlett.

McCallister L: *I wish I'd said that: how to talk your way out of trouble and into success,* New York, 1992, Wiley.

Murphy SZ: Don't be a doormat: personal empowerment in nursing, *Revolution* 2(2):66, 1994.

O'Grady D: *Taking the fear out of changing,* Holbrook, Mass, 1994, Bob Adams, Inc.

Peiffer V: *The duty trap: How to say "no" when you feel you ought to say "yes,"* Rockport, Mass, 1997, Element Books.

Potash MS: *Hidden agendas: what's really going on in your relationships—in love, at work, in your family,* New York, 1990, Delacorte Press.

Stuart GW, Laraia M: *Principles and practice of psychiatric nursing,* ed 6, St Louis, 1998, Mosby.

Tindall J: *Peer power: book one, workbook: becoming an effective peer helper and conflict mediator,* Muncie, Ind, 1994, Accelerated Development, Inc.

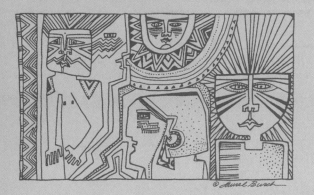

18

Communicating Assertively and Responsibly With Distressed Clients and Colleagues

My bath was too hot, I got soap in my eyes, my marble went down the drain . . . the Mickey Mouse night light burned out and I bit my tongue. The cat went to sleep with Anthony, not with me. It has been a terrible, horrible, no good, very bad day. My mom says some days are like that.

Judith Viorst,
Alexander and the Terrible,
Horrible, No Good, Very Bad Day

OBJECTIVES

1. Discuss the effect of distressed behavior of clients or colleagues on the nurse.
2. In a variety of situations, assess the situation and choose the assertive response.
3. Participate in exercises to build assertive communication strategies with distressed clients and colleagues.

WHY DISTRESSED BEHAVIOR IS A PROBLEM FOR NURSES

We are beginning to study the experience of suffering and how people find meaning in the illness experience (Pollock and Sands, 1997). Nurses witness suffering and distress. Nurses must deal with the moment-to-moment lived experience of illness. Clients convey their anguish verbally and nonverbally. Their loss of composure is a signal that they are disturbed by what is bothering them.

Changes in health status, illness, and hospitalization are just some sources of distress in clients. The work of nurses and allied health professionals is known to be stressful and ripe for causing distress. The changing health care climate causes stress for us as nurses and for our colleagues. In addition, nurses may pick up the sadness of clients, called shadow grief (Smith-Stoner and Frost, 1998), which can lead to burnout. We may find ourselves with less energy, no zest for living, and talking about our clients continuously, even on our off hours. We encounter distressed behavior frequently in our clients and occasionally in our colleagues; therefore, we need to develop ways to relate to them that soothe their distress without upsetting us. Maintaining our sensitivity to others so that we can respond in a caring way without being overcome and losing our objectivity is one of a nurse's most difficult feats.

Gerrard's (1978) review of the literature about interpersonal problems experienced by health professionals clearly reveals that our reactions to emotionally laden situations interfere with our ability to act effectively. Untoward reactions can come from within ourselves (feeling unsure or inadequate about how to act), the situation (feeling overcome or impotent), or the distressed person (distress invades the health care professional).

It has been suggested that nurses develop a protective barrier against others' pain, or become insensitive to the discomfort of others, because they encounter so much suffering in the course of their daily work. It has also been hypothesized that nurses stop responding in helpful ways because there is a dearth of positive role models (Gerrard, 1978).

If we become too involved with others' distress, we overload ourselves emotionally and become ineffective. If we avoid the distress of others by ignoring or belittling it, we are left with the feeling of not giving the attention and support that is expected. Some nurses feel helpless about how to be therapeutic with distressed persons. Others feel annoyed or irritated that clients or colleagues cannot solve their own problems. Thoughts about our own inadequacies, or judgments about the appropriateness of others' behavior, prevent us from acting in the best interests of the distressed person.

Moments of Connection...
Rx: Knowledge

We had an 11-year-old boy having a nonmalignant tumor removed from his spine. He was labeled a "brat" due to his demanding behavior. One day, I had a few extra minutes and went and sat with him. We took out his science book and talked about what was happening with his surgery and about his fears. From that time on, he was much less anxious and became one of our favorites.

Wit and Wisdom

Until You've Been There . . .

*You never can know
The suffering I bear,
But listen, just do,
My feelings I'll share.*

*I don't expect answers
Or solutions, you see.
I only want someone
To listen to me.*

*I know that you're busy
With physical things,
Tasks to accomplish,
Call bells do ring.*

*But I've never been through
This grieving, this pain.
I'm stuck in this moment,
My words, a refrain.*

*You need not come
With fancy words
Or pat, just so answers,
To calm my nerves.*

*Time is the answer
To rage and frustration
Forgive me, my dear,
Unkind aggravation.*

*I'll try to be patient
If you'll try, too.
Just give me a moment,
One moment will do.*

Copyright 1995 Julia W. Balzer Riley.

Kaufman and Wetmore (1994) suggest four common events that can cause stress: loss of control, change, sense of threat, and unrealized expectations. When nurses face distressed clients, these are the issues. Remember that it is not the situation itself that causes problems, but our reaction to it. The teaching of communication skills implies that if we say the right thing, clients or colleagues will have an "Aha!" experience; that is, they will immediately see our point of view and become both compliant and grateful. That is the paradigm, the way the game is played or the set of rules, by which we operate (Barker, 1992). Consider a new view; that is, the extraordinary set of circumstances, the distress, is not a failure or a lack of compliance, but an opportunity. This is the opportunity for nurses to learn from others' experiences and to build new skills that will increase communication effectiveness.

Ideally, we need to keep calm enough to be able to understand the reason for another person's distress, to remain nonjudgmental so that we can convey appropriate compassion for the situation at hand, and to be clearheaded enough to act responsibly on behalf of the other person. Ascher, in her memoir of grief at the death of her brother from AIDS (1994), paints a picture that demonstrates the complexity distress can present. She defines grief as a "landscape without gravity." Of her family she says:

My husband does not know I'm here, afloat. . . . They continue to communicate through normal channels as though we were all here together on the steady plane of everyday life. Grief is outside the scope of language. I can only speak in signs. The furrow of my brow, the tightness of my lips. But when they who love me entreat, 'Do you want to talk about it?' I say, 'no,' and turn away. I could say 'ouch,' I could say 'it hurts.' But language seems slight. Grief is physical and it hurts.

Ascher called it a "journey into paralysis." We must remain humble at the pain and anguish of the suffering of clients and their families, and yes, of colleagues, too, to whose stories we may have no access. What audacity to think we can so easily find just the right words!

Wit and Wisdom

Those who flow as life flows
Feel no wear, feel no tear
Need no mending, no repair.

Lao Tse

IMPROVING YOUR COMMUNICATION SKILL WITH DISTRESSED CLIENTS AND COLLEAGUES

In the rest of this chapter you will be given situations involving distressed clients and colleagues. Your task is to assess each situation, determine the request being made, and choose the most assertive and responsible communication strategy.

A critique of all the response choices for each situation is listed at the end of the chapter, beginning on p. 279. It is worthwhile reading the advantages and drawbacks of each option.

Communicating With Upset Clients

Step One: Assessment of the Data

1. Review the following situation and formulate your own assessment of the client's thoughts, feelings, and requests.

Mr. James is a 58-year-old avid outdoorsman who has been hunting in the woods near your rural hospital. While climbing steep terrain, he slipped and fell 50 feet down a ragged incline. In addition to suffering multiple bruises and scratches, he broke his glasses. Today he was admitted to your hospital for overnight observation. As you make your first round on the evening shift you go into his room to introduce yourself:

You: "Good afternoon, Mr. James. Welcome to our hospital. I'm sorry you have to be here under such unfortunate circumstances. How are you?"

Mr. James: "How long am I going to be here? Can you get me the phone? I need to reach my wife. Somebody's got to bring me my extra glasses. I can't drive. . . . I can't do anything without them. You can have your damn hospital. Just get me a phone so I can make arrangements to get out of here."

Mr. James raises his voice as he is talking and turns away from you. He squeezes the bed sheet in his hands and looks exasperated.

2. On a separate sheet of paper write down your assessment of Mr. James' thoughts and feelings. Indicate what request Mr. James is making of you, his evening nurse.

3. Compare your assessment to the assessment that follows:

Thoughts: Mr. James thinks that he cannot manage without his glasses. He is aware that he must reach his wife so that arrangements can be made to get his spare glasses.

Feelings: He is upset that he cannot read, write, or see to drive. He feels trapped in this remote rural hospital. He desperately wants to talk to his wife about arranging to get home.

Request: Mr. James wants you to understand how frustrating it is for him to be stuck in this unfamiliar hospital. He is trying to get you to comprehend how dependent and immobile he is without his glasses. He wants you to help him contact his wife. Indirectly, he may be asking to be comforted; that is, to be helped to feel more at home in this strange place.

4. Did your assessment reflect an accurate analysis of the facts as they were presented? If not, return to the original data presented in the vignette and reassess the cognitive and affective messages. If so, proceed to Step Two.

Step Two: Communication Strategies and Desired Outcomes

5. You have determined that Mr. James needs understanding, action, and comfort. On a piece of paper write which communication behaviors you would use to show Mr. James how you intend to respond to his request. Indicate the desired outcome(s) of your suggested strategy.

6. Compare your suggested strategy with this one:

It is appropriate to meet Mr. James' request for understanding and action. A warm, genuine, respectful manner will convey that you care about him. An empathic response will ensure that he knows you understand his predicament and will reduce any embarrassment he might feel for displaying his upset feelings in such a volatile way. If his upset behavior agitates you, then you can calm yourself and focus on his distress, using positive self-talk and imagery to prepare yourself to communicate assertively and responsibly.

This strategy will help Mr. James relax and feel accepted. He will likely look calmer and feel more patient with his circumstances. Your compliance with his requests contributes to the development of a trusting rapport.

Step Three: Implementing and Evaluating Your Communication Strategy

7. Now you must reply to Mr. James. Develop your own response and write it on a separate sheet of paper. Keep it handy so that you can refer to it later.

8. At this point you get the chance to compare your suggested response to the options listed below. Look over each of the response choices and turn to p. 279 at the end of the chapter to read a critique of each.

As you review the following choices, look for those that are congruent with your assessment of Mr. James' requests and your desire to communicate in an assertive and responsible way. (You will notice the choices are not listed alphabetically. This is to prevent the temptation to quickly scan all the answers without giving yourself the benefit of evaluating each response.)

Choice A: "You should be grateful to be alive. If that farmer hadn't heard you yelling and pulled you out of the ravine, you'd be out there freezing at this very minute. You don't need to snap at me. I can hear. I'll get you the phone."

Choice Z: "It's hard to be in a strange place where nothing is familiar. I know that feeling. I'll bring you the phone."

Choice J: You get red in the face, clench your fists, then turn on your heel and head down the hall to get the portable phone for Mr. James.

Choice S: "I'm sure you're eager to talk to your wife and make arrangements to get your glasses and go home. I'll get our portable phone for you right away. I can imagine it must be frustrating to be without your glasses, so please let us know how we can help you manage until you get the spare ones."

9. After you have found the most satisfactory strategy and discovered why the other options are unsuitable, go back to the suggested response you indicated earlier in this exercise. Evaluate yours in terms of how assertive and responsible it was.

Communicating With Upset Colleagues
Step One: Assessment of the Data

1. Review the following situation and formulate what you think are your colleague's thoughts and feelings. Indicate what you think your colleague is requesting from you.

Joe is the intern on the medical unit where you have been a student for the past 6 weeks. Because you are both students working on the unit at the same times, you have become good friends. This day Joe looks preoccupied and you have noticed that he is not his usual good-natured self. He snapped at you for not having your client ready for his physical examination, even though he had not warned you about his plans. Later he approaches you with:

Joe: "Shirley, I'm sorry for snapping at you earlier. I'm just not myself. Dayle just found out she's pregnant and it's all I can think about. I just can't imagine being a father. I can barely cope with being a husband and an intern. It's been the only thing on my mind since I found out 2 days ago. I can't think straight. I can't sleep. . . . I still can't believe it. I don't know what I'm going to do. We want kids, but why now?"

2. On a separate sheet of paper write down your assessment of Joe's thoughts and feelings. Indicate what you think Joe is requesting from you, his colleague.

3. Compare your assessment to the assessment that follows:

Thoughts: Joe knows his wife is pregnant and is aware that his preoccupation with this unexpected, and not yet welcome, news is causing him to be short-tempered with you. He wants to be a father but does not think the timing is good.

Feelings: He regrets that he snapped at you. Joe is shocked by the news of his wife's unexpected pregnancy and is worried about how he can cope with the added strain of being a father when he is having difficulty juggling the two roles of intern and husband. He likely is tired because he has not been sleeping, and he is upset that he cannot think straight.

Request: Joe is asking you to accept his apology for snapping at you, and he wants you to understand how the news about the pregnancy is turning his life upside down. Indirectly, he may be asking for some comfort for his predicament.

4. Did your assessment reflect an accurate analysis of the facts as they were presented? If not, return to the original data presented in the vignette and reassess the cognitive and affective messages. If so, proceed to Step Two.

Step Two: Communication Strategies and Desired Outcomes

5. You have determined that Joe wants you both to demonstrate your understanding of the shock he is experiencing and to act by accepting his apology. Identify which communication behaviors you would use to meet these two reasonable requests. Indicate the desired outcome of your suggested strategy.

6. Compare your suggested strategy to this one:

Warmth would show that you feel kindly toward Joe and you do not hold a grudge. An empathic response would convey your understanding to Joe. A self-disclosure about adjusting to the news about your own pregnancy (or another major event) would provide him with hope that getting used to the idea comes in time.

It is appropriate to meet Joe's requests. This strategy would make Joe feel relieved that you understand the reason for his outburst and that you forgive him. The hope you might give him—that he will work things out in time—would be comforting.

Step Three: Implementing and Evaluating Your Communication Strategy

7. Now you must reply to Joe. Develop your own response to Joe and write it on a separate sheet of paper. Keep it handy so that you can refer to it later.

8. At this point you get the chance to compare your response to several options listed below. Look over each of the choices and turn to p. 279 at the end of the chapter to read a critique of each option.

As you review the following response choices, be looking for those that are congruent with your assessment of Joe's requests and your desire to communicate in an assertive and responsible way.

Choice T: "It's okay, Joe. We all get upset at times."

Choice F: "Joe, I forgive you (smiling). I can see that you are preoccupied and upset with the unexpected news of Dayle's pregnancy. It seems overwhelming right now to imagine trying to squeeze in being a father when you are busy enough being a husband and getting your career launched. I, too, felt shocked when I first found out I was pregnant, but after several weeks I began to accept the idea. By the end of term I was even looking forward to Sarah's birth."

Choice V: "It's okay this time, Joe, but don't let it happen again. You really threw my whole schedule off this morning. That's great news about Dayle. So you're going to be a father, eh? I love being a parent, and I know you will too once you get used to the idea. It just takes a few weeks to get over the initial shock and then you'll be fine."

Choice O: "Apology accepted, Joe. It's easy to see that you're upset with your news. Things will turn out, Joe. You'll get used to the idea."

9. After you have found the most assertive and responsible choice and checked out why the other options are not suitable, go back to the response you wrote earlier in this exercise. Evaluate your suggestion in terms of how assertive and responsible it was.

Communicating With Clients Who Are Sad or Depressed

Step One: Assessment of the Data

1. Review the following situation and formulate what you think are your client's thoughts and feelings. Indicate what you think your client is requesting from you.

Jim is an 18-year-old client on your unit. He has just had a surgical repair after breaking his leg in a football game. Jim is an all-star athlete who knows he won't be playing any more sports this year, his senior year. He is worried about getting behind in his schoolwork because of the advanced placement classes he is taking. Every day counts if he is to keep up with the fast pace of the class. This is Jim's final year in high school and he is worrying about his grade point average slipping, because a football scholarship is now out of the question. He is tearful and seems embarrassed.

You: "Good morning, Jim. How's it going?"
Jim: "It's not . . ." (looking away from you and sighing)
You: "What's wrong?"
Jim: "Oh . . . what's the point? I've got nothing to look forward to. All my plans have gone down the tube." (Jim's voice is flat and he makes no eye contact with you.)

2. Take a piece of paper and write down your assessment of Jim's thoughts and feelings. Indicate what request Jim is making of you, his nurse for the day.
3. Compare your assessment to the one that follows:

Thoughts: Jim thinks that his academic and athletic hopes are not going to be realized. At this point in his life this injury seems like a total disaster.

Feelings: Jim probably has mixed feelings. Right now he feels discouraged and hopeless about his future. It is likely that he is frustrated that his plans have been thwarted, angry that it is his life that has been so affected, and apathetic about doing anything.

Request: Jim wants you to understand how he is feeling. He may also be wanting some help to lift himself out of his depression.

4. Did your assessment reflect an accurate analysis of the facts as they were presented? If not, return to the original data presented in the vignette and reassess the cognitive and affective messages. If so, proceed to Step Two.

Step Two: Communication Strategies and Desired Outcomes

5. You have determined that Jim needs understanding and information. On a separate sheet of paper, identify which communication behaviors you would use to respond to Jim's requests. Indicate what desired outcomes you expect by using the communication behaviors you have suggested.

6. Compare your suggested strategy to this one:

Jim's concerns are reasonable, and it is appropriate to respond to them. Warmth and genuineness would convey that you care for Jim. An empathic response would demonstrate that you really understand the unhappy situation he is in. When talking to Jim it would be important to stop whatever physical activity you are doing, face him, and give him your full attention. If his despair generates negative feelings in you (such as hopelessness or anger), relax before you respond. Visualize yourself responding to Jim in a caring and constructive way. If necessary, use your positive self-talk to remind yourself that you can be therapeutic when one of your clients is sad.

This strategy would make Jim feel cared for and give him a chance to talk. This planned intervention might lift his mood.

Step Three: Implementing and Evaluating Your Communication Strategy

7. Now you must reply to Jim. On a separate sheet of paper write down the response that you have developed. Keep it handy so that you can refer to it later.

8. At this point you get the chance to compare your suggested response with several options listed below. Look over each of the response choices and turn to p. 279 at the end of the chapter to read a critique of each option.

As you review the following response choices, look for those that are congruent with your assessment of Jim's requests and your desire to communicate in an assertive and responsible way.

Choice K: "You're young, Jim. It won't be that long until you will be up and getting back in shape again. Come on, Jim, chin up. There's no point getting depressed. You might as well make the best of it. We all have disappointments in life, I've had plenty, and you just have to make the best of things and ride through the bad times."

Choice B: "I'm worried about you, Jim. You're not thinking of doing anything like harming yourself, are you?"

Choice Q: "You're really feeling down aren't you? Breaking your leg is a big disappointment and enough to get anyone down. Maybe you're afraid you'll have trouble catching up with things in your life. You may not think so, but you'll be back to school soon. It takes time to get adjusted to the idea of something so unexpected happening to you. With all the visitors you've had, I bet it wouldn't be hard for you to find a friend to fill you in on what's happening at school. Would it help to call someone to chat?"

Choice X: "I'm sorry you feel that way, Jim."

9. After you have found the most satisfactory strategy and discovered why the other options are not suitable, go back to the response you wrote earlier in the exercise. Evaluate yours in terms of how assertive and responsible it was.

Communicating With Colleagues Who Are Sad or Depressed

Step One: Assessment of the Data

1. Read over the following situation and formulate your own assessment of your colleague's thoughts, feelings, and requests.

Petra is a fellow student whom you have come to know and like. The two of you have been in the same classes in nursing and, coincidentally, have had the same clinical rotations for the past year and a half. Now you are working on an oncology service where many of the clients are dying of cancer. Petra has been quieter and kept more to herself in the past week. She looks pale and lethargic, in sharp contrast to her usual witty and spunky self. At your coffee break one morning, you ask Petra how she is feeling and she responds with:

Petra: "I didn't think it was that noticeable. It's working with cancer patients . . . I don't think I can take much more of it. My visions of being a nurse are to cure people—to get them well again. It seems all the people we are working with now are dying and there's no way around it. It's so depressing. How can you stand it? I go home every night and all I can think is, 'Is this all there is to life?' All we do seems so pointless if this is how things end."

2. On a separate sheet of paper write down your assessment of Petra's thoughts and feelings. Indicate what request Petra is making of you, her classmate.

3. Compare your assessment to the assessment that follows:

Thoughts: Petra thinks it's pointless to prolong people's lives for a short time if they are going to feel sick from chemotherapy or radiation and die anyway. She wonders how you cope with the seeming futility of it all, and possibly she wonders if she can continue in nursing with such a hopeless attitude.

Feelings: Petra is feeling discouraged and sad about the death and dying she sees every day on the wards. She is shocked about the apparent hopelessness of nursing, since people end up suffering and dying anyway. She cannot seem to focus on those clients who do get better or those who choose to prolong their lives even for a short time. She is worried about coming to terms with her feelings so that she can continue nursing. She is frightened about the whole notion of dying. She is dispirited and wants to know how you handle similar feelings.

Request: Petra wants you to understand and accept how she is feeling. She is also asking you for information about how to handle her feelings so that they do not interfere with her ability to nurse effectively. Indirectly, she is asking to be comforted by having some of her sad feelings dissipated.

4. Does your assessment reflect an accurate analysis of the facts as they were presented by Petra? If not, return to the original vignette and reassess the cognitive and affective messages. If so, proceed to Step Two.

Step Two: Communication Strategies and Desired Outcomes

5. You have determined that Petra needs understanding and information. Identify which communication behaviors you would use to show Petra how you intend to respond to her requests. Indicate the desired outcome of your strategy. Write down your suggestions.

6. Compare your suggested strategy to this one:

It is quite a risk for Petra to reveal her feelings and questions about nursing and her fears of dying; therefore it is important to respect and accept the issues she is trying to work through. It is appropriate to respond to Petra's requests, and warmth and respect need to be conveyed to show Petra that you do not harbor negative feelings about her questions about the purpose of nursing. Accurate, genuine empathy will show her that you understand her fears about dying. To show her you are willing to share how you handle similar feelings, you might use an appropriate self-disclosure. If you wish to invite her to explore the topic of the meaning of life, you might make a gentle suggestion about how to begin.

This strategy would make Petra feel understood and possibly get her started on finding answers to some crucial questions for her personal and professional life. Her sadness is not likely to lift immediately because she is facing some major philosophical questions, but this strategy may give her some direction about how to find some answers.

Step Three: Implementing and Evaluating Your Communication Strategy

7. Now you must reply to Petra. Develop your own response to Petra and write it on a separate sheet of paper. Keep it handy so that you can refer to it later.

8. At this point you get the chance to compare your suggested response with several options listed below. Look over each of the response choices and turn to p. 279 at the end of the chapter to read a critique of each option.

As you review the following choices, look for those that are congruent with your assessment of Petra's requests and your desire to communicate in an assertive and responsible way.

Choice W: "You're wondering what's the point of nursing if clients end up dying on a unit like this one where everyone is terminally ill. When I feel discouraged, like you are now, I try to adjust my perspective. I have to remind myself that the people we see in here are a small sample of the people in our city. There are lots of older healthy people out there living active lives. Something else I try to do, even though I need to work at it more, is to strengthen my belief that dying is part of living. I think we have control over how we adjust to our dying, and I like to think I can help some of our clients live each day until they die. I think of their time with us as a very special part of their lives. They look to us to be able to listen to them without having to worry about what they say. Their family and friends can't always be helpful. These thoughts help me feel more hopeful, anyway. What do you think?"

Choice C: "Well, your sadness does show, Petra. Those clients are sad enough without having us add to their misery. Everyone has to die, Petra. You must accept that."

Choice L: "Boy, you are down about this rotation, Petra. Let's talk about something more pleasant that'll cheer you up. Are you and Gary going to the hockey game on Friday?"

Choice P: "Petra, I should have picked up that something was really getting to you on this rotation. I knew there was something, and I thought it might have to do with Gary. Gee, I don't know what to say, Petra. These are issues you have to sort out. I know it's hard to accept, but some of our clients are going to die. Yet some do get better, too. Keep that in mind. You'll feel better when we're on the next rotation in pediatrics."

9. After you have found the most satisfactory strategy and discovered why the other options are unsuitable, go back to the suggested response you wrote earlier in the exercise. Evaluate yours in terms of how assertive and responsible it was.

Communicating With Clients Who Are Crying

Step One: Assessment of the Data

1. Review the following situation and formulate your own assessment of the client's thoughts, feelings, and requests.

Mrs. Urst is a 35-year-old woman who has just given birth to her second child. Both she and her baby are healthy, and her husband and their 8-year-old son are thrilled with the new addition to their family. You have just entered her room and found her weeping. She has gone through several tissues and her eyes are red and swollen.

You: "Oh. Mrs. Urst. You are really upset. What's troubling you?"

Mrs. Urst: "Ohhhh . . . (sobs and blows nose; laughs and then starts crying again) I can't stop. It's just dawned on me that I'm now a mother of two. It's ridiculous . . . (sobs) . . . I've known for 9 months, but now I wonder how I'll cope. I've forgotten all the stuff mothers need to know and if I stay at home I'll forget all the stuff secretaries are supposed to know. Why did we get ourselves into this predicament? Oh, I'm sorry to burden you. I guess I've just got the 'baby blues' (blows nose and bites lip to keep from crying any more)."

2. On a separate sheet of paper write down your assessment of Mrs. Urst's thoughts and feelings. Indicate what request Mrs. Urst is making of you, her nurse for the day.

3. Compare your assessment to the following one:

Thoughts: Mrs. Urst thinks she is going to have difficulty being a mother of two. She wonders if she has made a mistake by having another child. She thinks she might be overburdening you with her disclosure.

Feelings: Mrs. Urst is upset and confused. She is overwhelmed by the new responsibilities she will have as the mother of a newborn, and she is worried that she will get out of practice while she is away from her job as a secretary. She is somewhat embarrassed by her outburst and tries to pass it off as "baby blues" to save face.

Request: Mrs. Urst wants you to understand her fears of being overwhelmed but she does not want to delve into her personal life in any great detail, as indicated by her referral to baby blues and her apology that she might be burdening you. She may be indirectly asking you for reassurance that she will manage.

4. Did your assessment reflect an accurate analysis of the facts as they were presented? If not, return to the original data presented in the vignette and reassess the cognitive and affective messages. If so, proceed to Step Two.

Step Two: Communication Strategies and Desired Outcomes

5. You have determined that Mrs. Urst needs understanding and comfort. Identify which communication behaviors you would use to show Mrs. Urst that you are prepared to act on her reasonable requests. Indicate the desired outcome of your suggested strategy. Write down these plans on a separate piece of paper.

6. Compare your suggested strategy to this one:

Warmth would be appropriate to show Mrs. Urst that you care that she is upset. Respect for her privacy could be demonstrated by nonjudgmental, empathic reference to her struggle between being a mother and a working person. It would be appropriate to express your agreement that some of her feelings are related to her postnatal hormonal imbalance. Your opinion that she will likely work out a satisfactory schedule would reassure her, once you have convinced her that you understand her feelings.

This strategy would make Mrs. Urst feel understood and diminish her embarrassment. In addition, your reassurance would make her feel hopeful that she can and will manage.

Step Three: Implementing and Evaluating Your Communication Strategy

7. Now you must reply to Mrs. Urst. Develop your own response to her and write it on a separate sheet of paper. Keep it handy so that you can refer to it later.

8. At this point you get the chance to compare your suggested response to several options listed below. Look over each of the response choices and turn to p. 279 at the end of the chapter to read a critique of each.

As you review the following response choices, look for those that are congruent with your assessment of Mrs. Urst's requests and your desire to communicate in an assertive and responsible way.

Choice D: "There, there, Mrs. Urst. It's natural for most women to have a crying spell after giving birth. Things will work out; they always do. Most mothers get the 'baby blues.' I see it all the time. Don't feel embarrassed."

Choice I: "It's too late to be crying over spilt milk, Mrs. Urst. You must have thought about all this when you discovered you were pregnant. You'll feel better when you are home."

Choice R: "I'm sorry you're so upset, Mrs. Urst. I'll come back later."

Choice Y: "It's likely that your tears are in part due to 'baby blues,' Mrs. Urst. But your whole world has been upset with the arrival of your new daughter; that's bound to take some adjustment. Working out a schedule between two important roles like motherhood and career is complicated. Given time to adjust to your new schedule, I'm certain you can work out something that suits you. I have some time now if you'd like to talk."

9. After you have found the most satisfactory strategy and discovered why the other options are unsuitable, go back to the response you generated earlier in the exercise. Evaluate yours in terms of how assertive and responsible it was.

Communicating With Colleagues Who Are Crying

Step One: Assessment of the Data

1. Review the following situation and formulate your own assessment of your colleague's thoughts, feelings, and requests.

Don is a nurse on the rehabilitation unit in the long-term care facility where you are working. When you go into the office to collect your purse you find him sitting in a chair with his head in his hands. When he sees you coming in he quickly rubs his eyes and turns in his chair so that you cannot see his face. He gets out a tissue and blows his nose and says:

Don: "Come on in, Kathy. Guess you caught me crying. It's the news about Mr. Kent that's got to me. (Looking at you) I really thought he would make it. I can't believe he's dead. He was making so much progress. I never thought I'd say it, but I'll even miss the way he used to act like the king of the unit."

Don is referring to Mr. Kent, an elderly resident of your rehabilitation unit, who was transferred yesterday to an acute care hospital after a cardiac arrest. Mr. Kent had been on the unit for 8 months, during which time he made himself known by his lively and sometimes overbearing involvement with all the staff. He was a well-liked, integral part of the life of your team. Your colleague Don had often been assigned as Mr. Kent's nurse because of Mr. Kent's request for a male nurse. Don and Mr. Kent had enjoyed friendly arguments about politics.

2. On a separate sheet of paper write down your assessment of Don's thoughts and feelings. Indicate what request Don is making of you, his co-worker.

3. Compare your assessment with the assessment that follows:

Thoughts: Don is having difficulty believing that Mr. Kent is dead, in view of his progress just before his transfer. It doesn't seem possible that after all that, he would die from a heart problem.

Feelings: Don is shocked and saddened by his client's death. He feels confused and amazed because Mr. Kent seemed to be improving. He misses Mr. Kent, and even longs for his more unpleasant habits.

Request: His invitation for you to enter the room, and his self-disclosure, are evidence that Don is asking you to listen to him. He is asking for understanding and some comfort.

4. Did your assessment reflect an accurate analysis of the facts as they were presented? If not, return to the original data presented in the vignette and reassess the cognitive and affective messages. If so, proceed to Step Two.

Step Two: Communicating Strategies and Desired Outcomes

5. You have determined that Don needs understanding and comfort. Identify which communication behaviors you would use to show Don how you intend to respond to his reasonable requests. Indicate the desired outcome of your suggested strategy. Write your ideas on a separate sheet of paper for future reference.

6. Compare your suggested strategy to this one:

An empathic response would show your understanding of Don's bereavement. Expressing your opinion about the comfort Don provided Mr. Kent would be respectful and give Don some comfort. Coming into the room and being with Don would be a warm gesture showing your respect for his feelings. If it felt genuinely comfortable for you, then a gentle touch would also convey your warmth and comfort to Don.

This strategy would make Don feel understood and comforted.

Step Three: Implementing and Evaluating Your Communication Strategy

7. Now you must reply to Don. Develop your own response to Don and write it on a separate sheet of paper. Keep it handy so that you can refer to it later in the chapter.

8. At this point you get the chance to compare your suggested response to several options listed below. Look over each of the response choices and turn to p. 279 at the end of the chapter to read a critique of each.

As you review the following response choices, look for those that are congruent with your assessment of Don's requests and your desire to communicate in an assertive and responsible way.

Choice G: (You sit down beside Don.) "I can't believe Mr. Kent is dead either, Don. You two had such a close relationship that I can see why you are so sad. You gave him a lot of pleasure with those heavy political discussions. It's so hard to just keep on working when you lose someone as special as Mr. Kent. Can I help you out with your assignment in any way today, Don?"

Choice N: Continuing to get your purse in the locked drawer, "I'll be out of your way just as soon as I get my purse, Don. It's awful news, isn't it?"

Choice U: "I can see that you're upset, Don, but we've got to get used to these old people dying. It's true the unit won't be the same without him, but another resident will come along and we'll all get attached to him. Do you want to come to lunch with us? We're going to try that new deli, you know the one Johnson's took over. It would do you good."

After you have found the most satisfactory strategy and discovered why the other options are not suitable, go back to the response you generated earlier in this exercise. Evaluate yours in terms of how assertive and responsible it was.

Think About It...
What, So What, and Now What?

Consider what you read about assertive communication with distressed clients and colleagues. What experience have you had? Write the answers to the following.

What? ... Write one thing you learned from this chapter.

So what? ... How will this impact your nursing practice?

Now what? ... How will you implement this new knowledge or skill?

THINK ABOUT IT

Wit and Wisdom

Rules 8 and 9 of Dale Carnegie's 12 ways to win people to your way of thinking:

8. *Try honestly to see things from the other person's point of view.*
9. *Be sympathetic with the other person's ideas and desires.*

Dale Carnegie, in *How to Win Friends and Influence People*

Practicing Communicating Assertively and Responsibly With Distressed Clients and Colleagues

Exercise 1

For this exercise work in groups of three. You will need a tape recorder. One of you will role-play a distressed client or colleague and one will be the listener; the third will give feedback to the listener on her ability to communicate in an assertive and responsible way with the distressed person. The distressed client (or colleague) will communicate to the nurse by being upset, crying, sad, or depressed. The nurse will attempt to respond in an assertive and responsible way. The feedback giver will indicate to the nurse how effective she was in employing an assertive and responsible style. Tape this interaction so that you can use the recording to complete Exercise 2.

Make sure each of you has a turn in each of the roles. Allow enough time to do this exercise, including time for feedback.

After you have each had a turn in all roles, join the rest of your classmates. Together as a group discuss what you have learned about helpful and nonhelpful ways to communicate with distressed clients and colleagues.

Exercise 2

Transcribe into writing 10 paired interactions (what the distressed person said and what you said is one paired interaction) from the tape recorded interview you did in Exercise 1. For each statement that the distressed person made, write down your assessment of the thoughts, feelings expressed, and whether it is appropriate to meet the request being made. Examine the strategy you used to respond to your "client" or "colleague" and evaluate whether it met the request. If not, come up with an alternative response that would be assertive and responsible. This review of your communication will help you develop more effective communication skills with distressed clients

Critique: Choices of Responses to Distressed Clients and Colleagues

Choice A: You are defensive and hostile in this response. You have taken Mr. James' remarks as a personal insult, when they were only a release of his intense frustration and worry. By responding so aggressively you have escalated bad feelings between you and your client and not respected your right to communicate in a caring way. You have not shown Mr. James that you understand his feelings and that you care about his predicament. Although you did not meet his request for understanding, you did meet his request for the action of getting the telephone. This response is not assertive; it is aggressive. Mr. James would likely feel angry and embarrassed by your outburst, not understood or comforted. The only responsible part of this retort is your offer to get the telephone.

Choice B: Your opening words show that you are concerned about the changes you have observed in Jim over the past week; however, by beginning this way you have put the emphasis on yourself instead of on Jim. It is an aggressive approach because it puts your feelings first, at the expense of your client's. Your reflection that Jim is not like his old self is aggressive in its undertone of disappointment and scolding. By asking Jim if he is contemplating harming himself you are reading more into his symptoms than he presented. Jim might suspect that you are more worried about yourself (should he be seriously considering harming himself) than you are about his misery. As well as being aggressive, this answer is not responsible because it does not pick up on the data Jim presented; it exaggerates and goes beyond the facts. Jim would likely not feel understood or helped by this response. He would likely be cautious about revealing any further information to you because your words suggest that you do not want to get involved if there is any sign of trouble.

Choice C: Petra is likely to feel judged and reprimanded by this approach. Your confrontation would likely sting. It is judgmental and puts down your colleague. You proceed to lay on a lot of guilt about how she should hide her feelings to protect her clients, without giving her the right to have the feelings that she does. This approach is aggressive and uncaring. By not picking up on both her requests, you have used an irresponsible strategy.

Choice D: This strategy is not responsible because it tunes in neither to the information Mrs. Urst gave about her conflict between career and motherhood, nor her stark realization that she is now the mother of two. Your patronizing choice of words is aggressive and demeaning. Mrs. Urst would not likely feel understood or comforted by this response. She might feel that you are insensitive to her concerns. She might feel like a child that has just been dismissed.

Choice F: This response is assertive and responsible. Your warmth and slight teasing shows Joe that you forgive him for his lack of consideration. By quickly focusing on his reason for being upset, you show him that you understand his situation. Your empathic remarks about his feelings are accurate and specific, leaving Joe no doubt that you understand him. Your self-disclosure is appropriate because Joe wants to be a parent, and your own experience will likely give him hope that he will adjust. Joe would probably feel accepted and reassured by these words.

Choice G: By sitting down you showed respect for the importance of Don's feelings. Your self-disclosure let Don know that you understood his feelings of shock at the news of this resident's death. Your acknowledgment of the joy that Don brought to Mr. Kent would be pleasing to Don. Your offer to help him with his work for today was respectfully offered because of the gentle phrasing. Your response is assertive because it offers Don helpful communication while respecting your right to be helpful, and it is responsible because it tunes in to all the data Don presented.

Choice I: This choice is aggressive because it judges and punishes Mrs. Urst for having normal doubts and fears. It is not a responsible strategy because it misses out on the data about her conflict of roles and her shock about being the mother of two. Mrs. Urst would likely feel insulted that you question her decision making and angry that you did not give her a chance to respond. Your insensitive suggestion that she will see things differently when she gets home is arrogant and would likely frustrate Mrs. Urst. You have not respected your right to communicate in a caring way.

Choice J: By not saying anything you have lost the opportunity to show Mr. James that you understand how he feels about his situation. Your nonassertive actions of blushing and looking flustered make you feel disappointed that you concentrated on your feelings without conveying any compassion to your client. Although you missed out meeting his request for understanding, you did offer him the telephone. Mr. James would likely be more discomfited, and possibly embarrassed, that he upset you. This response is not assertive and is only minimally responsible.

Choice K: This choice is irresponsible because it does not acknowledge Jim's feelings of lethargy and disappointment in a therapeutic way. This response is judgmental and demanding. Jim is not accepted for feeling the way he does. This aggressive approach bulldozes over Jim's sadness. It protects neither his right to feel the way he does nor your right to relate to your client in a sensitive and caring way. Jim would not feel understood by this strategy, and it is unlikely he would look to you for advice on how to get himself out of his unhappy state. He has received the facile message from you that it is easy to stay happy: just keep your chin up in the face of any troubles.

Choice L: Petra would likely feel ignored by this strategy. By diverting the conversation from your classmate's important self-disclosure you have minimized the importance of what she is saying, and you have overruled her right to be understood and respected. By avoiding the sensitive area of her feelings you have been nonassertive; neither her rights nor yours have been attended to with this reply. This retort is irresponsible because it does not pick up on the information embodied in Petra's plea.

Choice N: This is a nonassertive and irresponsible response. By not pausing to show consideration for Don's reaction you evaded giving him the support he could have appreciated. Your opening remarks are inappropriately focused on you, and they could indicate that the whole situation is embarrassing. This self-centeredness is not helpful. Your vague references to Mr. Kent's death are disrespectful in their lack of specificity. This strategy would leave Don feeling uncomfortable and hurt by your lack of respect for both him and his client.

Choice O: You have met Joe's request for forgiveness and you have made an attempt to reassure him that you think he will adjust to the situation. Your attempt is nonassertive because it does not acknowledge the specific feelings that Joe raised when he related his troubles to you. This choice is glib and is not responsible because it is not a specific reflection of the data presented. Joe would probably feel you really didn't understand the depth and turbulence of his reactions.

Choice P: Petra would likely feel understood but somewhat admonished by this strategy. At the beginning your focus is more on your guilty feelings about not picking up on Petra's changes. This self-disclosure is irrelevant. It is aggressive because it suggests that Petra's sadness is so blatant that it would be obvious to anyone. Your suggestion that she needs to work out her concerns is obvious and unhelpful. It is glib to suggest that she will feel better in the next rotation. She is likely hoping for a more personal disclosure about how you, a colleague, would handle these important issues in a similar situation. Your reply is only partially responsible.

Choice Q: This strategy is responsible because it picks up on all the data presented in Jim's opener. His feelings are acknowledged. It was assertive to ask if he wants to call a friend. This response is assertive because it meets his request for help and employs your skills in a helpful way. It is responsible because it attends to the verbal and nonverbal data about Jim's thoughts and feelings. Jim would likely feel that you understood his situation.

Choice R: This self-disclosure could have been a beautiful introduction to an empathic response; however, by itself it is inadequate. Mrs. Urst would be left to wonder why you are sorry. Is it because you do not know how to handle her crying; or because you think she should be able to snap back to her happy self; or because you care about her and are sad that she is distressed? It is nonassertive to leave Mrs. Urst without asking if you could be of some help. This response is not responsible because it does not reflect the data Mrs. Urst supplied.

Choice S: This response is the most assertive and responsible. It shows respect for Mr. James' thoughts about having to reach home and secure his glasses, and you have conveyed your understanding of his frustration at being in a strange place. Furthermore, you have offered to help him cope until his glasses arrive. Your offer is respectful because it allows him to dictate when he will need help so that he can maintain maximum independence. You offered to bring the telephone early in the response, thereby showing him you understand the importance of having contact with his wife. You can feel good about your response. You have met your client's requests and responded in keeping with your professional and caring image of yourself. It is likely that Mr. James would feel comforted by your words.

Choice T: Joe is likely to feel dismissed by this reply. You have forgiven Joe and thereby met his request for action. You have not demonstrated your understanding of his situation with your vague reference to the fact that we all get upset at times. This response would not lead Joe to feel you understand his serious and important situation. This communication strategy is nonassertive because it does not meet your colleague's right to be understood, and it does not demonstrate your ability to communicate in a caring way. Accepting his apology is responsible, but failure to act on all the data is irresponsible.

Choice U: This reply is aggressive and irresponsible. It indicates that you see Don is upset, but you neglect to show any compassion for his feelings. Your aggressive style of rushing him to consider new residents at this point is premature and disrespectful. Your invitation for lunch is intended to convey kindness, but your judgmental authoritarian approach takes the caring out of it. Your style is aggressive and would likely make Don feel angry and misunderstood. Your reply is partially responsible because you pick up that he is sad, but you have not shown understanding for the depth of Don's feelings in his bereavement.

Choice V: Although you forgive Joe for his thoughtlessness, you are somewhat stern given his special circumstances and considering that it was not his usual way of doing things. Your warning about the future is aggressive and detracts from your forgiveness. Your exuberance about the news of the pregnancy is insensitive, given Joe's reaction. Your enthusiasm is aggressive because it puts pressure on Joe to feel happy when he really feels quite desperate. This communication strategy is aggressive and irresponsible. Joe would likely feel misunderstood and judged.

Choice W: Petra would likely feel understood and accepted by your reply, and have some alternative and more hopeful ways of viewing the situation. Right at the beginning you acknowledged Petra's feelings of despair so that she would know that you understood her. This approach is assertive because it attends to her right to receive helpful communication, and it meets your expectations that you will reach out to your colleagues in a caring way. By responding to her request for respectful understanding and offering her some insights about how you sort out your feelings, you are responding to the information she gave you. In doing so you are communicating in a responsible way. You did not force your coping methods onto her; rather, you revealed how they were helpful for you and asked for her opinions. This approach is respectful of her individual style of handling events. Your self-disclosure—revealing that you have not sorted out all your thoughts on these important issues—would likely make Petra feel that she is not alone in trying to come to terms with the purpose of nursing (and life).

Choice X: This reply is nonassertive. It does not respect Jim's right to receive your helpful comments, and it deprives you of the right to communicate effectively. By not picking up on the specific information Jim gave you in his statement, and linking that to the changes you have observed in Jim in the past few weeks, you have responded without using half of the data. This reply is superficial and Jim would likely feel that the weight of his sadness had fully escaped you. He would not likely feel that he could confide any further in you after receiving this insensitive remark.

Choice Y: This response is assertive because it demonstrates your ability to communicate sensitively to Mrs. Urst. Your agreement that her tears were in part due to postnatal blues allowed her to feel less embarrassed, yet you did not ignore her real worries about juggling her roles. You did not give her advice that would have been premature, but you gave her the option of talking more about her feelings with you if she would like. This invitation allows her to choose if and when she would like to talk and is respectful of her privacy. Your accurate use of empathy would let her know you understand her confusion and ambivalence. Your style is assertive and your words are responsible. Mrs. Urst's requests would be met with this response.

Choice Z: This response is only partially assertive and responsible. It comes closer to filling his request for understanding than other options do. You have conveyed understanding of his discomfort at being in a strange place, and you have offered to get the telephone for him. Your attempt at self-disclosure is incomplete and nonspecific, and therefore would not convey the understanding you intended. What is missing is your acknowledgment of his frustration at not being able to function without his glasses, and his strong desire to contact his wife. Mr. James would probably feel somewhat comforted by your attempt to understand him, but he would be left wondering how you could possibly understand his unique predicament.

References

Ascher BL: *Landscape without gravity: a memoir of grief,* New York, 1994, Penguin Books.

Barker JA: *Paradigms: the business of discovering the future,* New York, 1992, Harper Business.

Carnegie D: *How to win friends and influence people,* New York, 1964, Simon & Schuster.

Gerrard B: Interpersonal skills for health professionals: a review of the literature, Unpublished manuscript, 1978.

Kaufman P, Wetmore C: *The brass tacks manager: getting down to what really counts in the workplace,* New York, 1994, Bantam Doubleday.

Pollock SE, Sands D: Adaptation to suffering, *Clin Nurs Res* 6(1):171, May 1997.

Smith-Stoner M, Frost AL: Coping with grief and loss: bringing your shadow self into the light, *Nursing* 98 28(2):49, 1998.

Viorst J: *Alexander and the terrible, horrible, no good very bad day,* Hartford, Conn, 1972, Connecticut Printers.

 Suggestions for Further Reading

Dickerson SS: Cardiac spouses' help-seeking experiences, *Clin Nurs Res* 7(1):6, Feb 1998.

Faulkner A: Communication with patients, families, and other professionals, *Br Med J* 316(7125):130, Jan 1998.

Johnson JL, Morse JM: Regaining control: the process of adjustment after myocardial infarction, *Imprint* 19(2):126, 1990.

Nuland SB: *How we die: reflections on life's final chapter,* New York, 1994, Alfred A Knopf.
  An intimate account of how various diseases take away life, a portrait of the experience of dying.

Purdy AM: The disabled patient: the grief that never ends, *Imprint* 37(1):68, 1990.

Rosen SL: Stillbirth: what the nurse should and should not do, *Imprint* 37(1):65, 1990.

Schubert J: Comparing the grief reactions of a rehabilitation and a psychiatric patient, *Imprint* 37(1):59, 1990.

Slyk MP: Managing difficult behaviors in head trauma patients, *Nurs Homes Long Term Care Manag* 47(5):26, 1998.

Straka DA: Are you listening? Have you heard? *Adv Pract Nurs Q* 3(2):80, 1997.

Thompson DR, Webster RA, Meddis R: In-hospital counseling for first-time myocardial infarction patients and spouses: effects on satisfaction, *J Adv Nurs* 15(9):1064, 1990.

Ward-Collins D: Noncompliant: isn't there a better way to say it? *Am J Nurs* 98(5):27, 1998.

Wells N et al: Work transitions, *J Nurs Admin* 28(2):50, 1998.

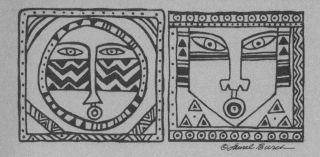

19

Communicating Assertively and Responsibly With Aggressive Clients and Colleagues

An appeaser is one who feeds a crocodile—hoping it will eat him last.

Sir Winston Churchill

OBJECTIVES

1. Describe the problems presented by aggressive behavior.
2. Identify strategies to communicate effectively with aggressive clients and colleagues.
3. Given situations involving aggressive behavior, formulate an assessment and intervention.
4. Participate in exercises to build skills to communicate with aggressive clients and colleagues.

WHY AGGRESSIVE BEHAVIOR IS PROBLEMATIC FOR NURSES

Aggressiveness refers to rejecting, hostile, abusive, and manipulative behaviors. Aggressive behavior may be a result of anger, an emotion in response to feeling powerless or out of control. Aggressiveness may also indicate another person's lack of respect for our feelings or a violation of our right to be treated with courtesy and consideration. In any case, aggressiveness is unpleasant.

Most of us would like to stand up for our right to be treated with respect in a way that is firm, effective (puts a stop to the aggressive behavior), and embarrasses neither us nor the other person;

284

Moments of Connection...
When Pain Changes Behavior

In our cancer pain center we had an elderly woman with "failed back syndrome," severe scoliosis, and degenerative disc disease. On my first encounter with her, she backed up to the wall and said, "You're not going to stick me with a needle are you?" I assured her I was just doing an assessment. Knowing that the doctor wanted to do 3 epidural blocks, I spent a lot of time explaining the procedure as she paced back and forth in the examination room. She rubbed her hands and was very anxious. On the surface she seemed uncooperative and not very nice. Her daughter confirmed that her behavior had changed with the increasing pain. The whole team spent time to explain the benefits of the procedures. I accompanied her for these procedures and later for an intrathecal pump. Today she has excellent pain relief and visits our office on holidays to bring treats. She always gives me a hug and thanks me for "giving me back my life." We really made a difference.

in other words we want to handle the aggression assertively and at the same time consider the other person's point of view. Our fears are that we will become enraged and lash out at the other person, fueling the fires of escalating aggression, or that we will remain tightlipped and slink away, carrying around the smoldering wish to more effectively deal with an attacker. Our fears of losing control or embarrassing ourselves, or our insecurity in our ability to communicate assertively and deal with the oppression, keep us from acting effectively.

When we encounter aggressive behavior, our self-esteem and physical safety are threatened. This chapter will help you deal with aggression so that you feel confident and comfortable.

Communicating Effectively With Aggressive Clients and Colleagues

Jakubowski and Lange (1978) outline the following ways of dealing with aggression from others.

Get to the Source of the Problem

Asking for more information—so that you are clear about the reason for your aggressor's discontent—will demonstrate your interest and open up a dialogue that can lead to resolution of the problem. Finding out what is causing the aggressor to attack you is a logical place to begin.

For example, you might ask your supervisor, who has just reprimanded you for telephoning the intern on call about one of your seriously ill clients, this question:

Assertive you: "I see that you are angry that I phoned Dr. Jones about our client's unstable vital signs. Could you tell me what upsets you about my calling her?"

This respectful acknowledgment of your aggressor's message allows him to clarify the problem. Using an empathic response demonstrates your understanding of the other's feelings and can disarm him enough to minimize the aggression. The open-ended phrasing of your questions is less threatening than an aggressive approach like: "Why are you trying to stop me?"

Wit and Wisdom

It's Not Just Nice People Who Get Sick . . .

Some people are nice
And they get sick.
Make them well
And they're nice, real quick.

Some people are mean
And they get sick.
We might make them well,
But nice? There's a trick!

We think with just
The right magic words
We can fix everything.
Oh! How absurd!

Some people's problems
Are bigger than me.
Maybe they'll get well
But nice, they won't be.

Some people's problems
Run deep and wide.
We care for them,
But take it in stride.

Copyright 1995 Julia W. Balzer Riley.

Increase Your Aggressor's Awareness of Abusive Behavior and Its Negative Effects

Asking questions to determine whether your aggressor is aware of the insulting impact that aggression can have, pointing out the effect of the behavior, is a technique to heighten the awareness of an aggressor. Be aware that some people are beyond caring about the effects of their behavior when they are losing control; therefore it is a judgment call as to when to use this strategy.

For example, after repeated abuse and criticism from the resident-on-call, you inform him:

Assertive you: "Dr. Smith, you may not realize that you are raising your voice and swearing at me. This approach makes working with you unpleasant. I would be glad to talk with you when you can lower your voice and not swear at me." (When someone is repeatedly aggressive, using the "I feel . . ." portion of the assertive statement may give the person more ammunition. Comment, instead, on the results of the behavior and then your request for a behavior change.)

Remaining calm and controlled in the face of an aggressor provides a contrast that may help that person realize that aggressive behavior is out of line.

Limit the Aggressive Behavior

Employing a C.A.R.E. confrontation (Chapter 16) lets your aggressor know, in no uncertain terms, what bothers you about his behavior and what changes you would like to see. Sometimes, ignoring or dismissing the aggression and continuing with your own agenda takes the wind out of an aggressor's sails and puts the emphasis on more pressing items.

For example, you are giving the end-of-shift report to the evening staff and one evening nurse repeatedly interrupts, quizzing you on an irrelevant matter. You curtail her aggression with:

Assertive you: "Sharon, I'd like to finish the report, so please hold your questions and talk to me about it later."

For each aggressor and situation you will have different expected outcomes and want to use different assertive strategies. The important point is that you develop skills for dealing assertively with aggression so that you can maintain your self-respect while being courteous, and that you have "a constructive impact on the other person" (Jakubowski and Lange, 1978). As a nurse, you must not tolerate continued aggression against yourself if you intend to preserve your self-esteem and credibility with clients and colleagues.

Improving Your Communication Skill With Aggressive Clients and Colleagues

The work you will do in this chapter will give you practice in dealing assertively with aggression so that in real-life situations you will feel and act more confidently. The forthcoming examples will help you overcome some of the barriers to relating with aggressive clients and colleagues and generate more effective responses to aggression. You will be given situations involving aggressive clients and colleagues. Your task is to assess each situation, determine the request being made, and choose the most assertive and responsible communication strategy.

A critique of all the response choices for each situation is at the end of the chapter, beginning on p. 303. It is a good idea to review all of them to learn about the strengths and limitations of each.

Communicating With Rejecting Clients

Step One: Assessment of the Data

1. Review the following situation and formulate your own assessment of the client's thoughts, feelings, and requests.

Mr. Hunter has been a client on your medical-burn unit for 6 weeks. He has extensive burns to his arms, upper body, and face as a result of trying to rescue his daughter from a house fire. He has been in isolation for the duration of his hospitalization. Chris, your colleague who has been his primary nurse since his admission, has left for a vacation. As the student having your clinical experience on this unit, you have been assigned to care for Mr. Hunter in Chris's absence. His wounds require extensive debridement and frequent dressing changes.

You are changing a dressing on Mr. Hunter's shoulder when this conversation takes place:

You: "I'm going to let that soak for 5 minutes, Mr. Hunter. Then I'll remove it and do your other shoulder. Your burns are healing nicely."

Mr. Hunter: "That's thanks to Chris. She's a wonderful nurse. You've replaced her on her days off before and you don't do things like she does. I want you to be careful and do things like they are supposed to be done. You're just a student and I'm going to watch you carefully; if you do anything out of line I'm going to report you to your instructor."

2. On a separate piece of paper write down your assessment of Mr. Hunter's thoughts and feelings. Indicate what request Mr. Hunter is making of you, his "replacement" nurse.

3. Compare your assessment to the one below:

Thoughts: Mr. Hunter is afraid you might do something to undermine Chris's effective nursing care of his burns. He thinks that because you are a student you might not care for his wounds with the same safety and skill that "his" nurse did.

Feelings: He misses the consistent care he had from daily interaction with his primary nurse, Chris. He feels threatened and at the mercy of your care, in which he does not have confidence. He is afraid that you might do something to set back the progress of his healing.

Request: The aggressiveness of his threat tells you how much Mr. Hunter wants you to take precautions to ensure continued healing of his burns. He wants to be reassured by your actions and words that you will give safe nursing care. His requests are for understanding, comfort, and safe burn treatment.

4. Did your assessment reflect an accurate analysis of the facts as they were presented? If not, return to the original vignette and reassess the cognitive and affective messages. If so, proceed to Step Two.

Step Two: Communication Strategies and Desired Outcomes

5. You have determined that Mr. Hunter needs to be understood and comforted by your actions and your words. Identify which communication behaviors you would use to respond to Mr. Hunter's requests. Indicate the desired outcome of your strategy. Write your suggestions down on a separate sheet of paper for future reference.

6. Compare your suggested strategy to this one:

Remaining calm would be important to avoid escalating his aggression. Relaxation will help you focus and avoid hostility yourself. Visualize responding in a compassionate way and use positive self-talk to remember not to explode at his aggressiveness. Empathic acknowledgment of his respect for Chris's care would reassure him that you understand the importance of safe care to ensure continued healing. Informing him that you will give your best care, and explaining what you are doing would dispel his apprehensions about your abilities. Ignoring his threat to report you would likely diminish his hostility.

These interventions would likely let Mr. Hunter know that you understand both his vulnerability as a client and his longing for the consistent care from his primary nurse. Your directness, confidence, and calmness would likely make him optimistic and hopeful about the quality of care he will receive from you.

Step Three: Implementing and Evaluating Your Communication Strategy

7. Now you must reply to Mr. Hunter. Develop your own response to Mr. Hunter and write it on a separate sheet of paper. Keep it handy so that you can refer to it later.

8. At this point you get the chance to compare your suggested response with several options listed below. Look over each of the response choices and turn to p. 303 at the end of the chapter to read a critique of each.

As you review the following response choices, look for those that are congruent with your assessment of Mr. Hunter's requests, and your desire to communicate in an assertive and responsible way.

Choice E: "Report me if you want to Mr. Hunter. You don't honestly think my clinical instructor would give me the responsibility of caring for you if she didn't think that I could do it, do you? If you'd just give me a chance, you'd see what a good nurse I can be."

Choice A: "If you want a graduate nurse I can arrange to transfer so you can feel safer, Mr. Hunter. It sounds like you want a fully qualified graduate assigned to you."

Choice M: "You're welcome to watch what I do and ask any questions. I'm sure my way of doing things is a little different from Chris's, but I do guarantee that what I'm doing is safe and in keeping with your physician's orders. It is hard when things are done differently by each nurse, and you are likely missing Chris's style since you worked closely together for the 6 weeks you have been here. Do you want to ask me anything about what I've done so far in changing your dressing?"

Choice Z: "You're just missing Chris, Mr. Hunter, and taking it out on me. I don't want to be compared to another nurse, and I won't have you making threats to report me to my instructor. I am one of the top nurses in my class, and I don't want you to question my care any more in the future. You had better get used to the idea that I am going to be your nurse."

9. After you have found the most satisfactory strategy and discovered why the other options are not suitable, go back to the suggested response you generated earlier in this exercise. Evaluate yours in terms of how assertive and responsible it was.

Communicating With Rejecting Colleagues
Step One: Assessment of the Data

1. Review the following situation and formulate your own assessment of your colleague's thoughts, feelings, and requests.

You are a student nurse who has just spent the past 6 weeks' clinical experience in obstetrical services of the hospital. During that time your clinical instructor has been meticulously thorough in her supervision and teaching of the skills needed for obstetrical nursing. This area of nursing is one you love and you think you might pursue a career in this field. You feel you are adept at the physical care of both mother and baby, and you have been influential in helping mothers and fathers adjust to caring for their newborns. Your teaching sessions to mothers have been rated as outstanding, and the head nurse in postpartum has indicated that she is pleased with your work.

Despite your certainty that you are doing a good job and the positive feedback from clients and staff, you have never received a word of praise from your clinical instructor. In fact, she takes every opportunity to tell you where you could improve and is petty in her reprimands about your small errors. You are disappointed that your instructor is not more encouraging and enthusiastic about your successes. Today she is meeting with you to give you feedback on the bath class you gave to the fathers. You have had a chance to look over the fathers' evaluation forms and they clearly state that your manner and content were reassuring in their first experience of bathing their newborns. Your instructor has just listed everything you did wrong and made suggestions about how you could improve such a class in the future.

Instructor: "Overall, you need to polish your professionalism. You are much too casual; you always are, for that matter. How do you expect anyone to treat you like a professional if you are lax and don't have a tight rein on things? You need to shape up in that regard so you'll command a lot more respect."

2. On a separate sheet of paper write down your assessment of your instructor's thoughts and feelings. Indicate what request she is making of you, her nursing student.

3. Compare your assessment to the one below:

Thoughts: Your instructor thinks you need to be more professional, and that if you could cultivate this demeanor you would gain more respect.

Feelings: She is disappointed in your overall consistent lack of professionalism. It is highly likely that she feels a great responsibility to shape you into her image of a perfectly functioning nurse.

Request: She wants you to change your behavior on a consistent basis to a style of operating that matches her image of professionalism. She expects you to put up with negative feedback in this evaluation, as she has during your complete rotation.

4. Did your assessment reflect an accurate analysis of the facts as they were presented? If not, return to the original data presented in the vignette and reassess the cognitive and affective messages. If so, proceed to Step Two.

Step Two: Communication Strategies and Desired Outcomes

5. You have determined that your instructor is making an unreasonable request of you. You are disappointed and angry that she continues her unwillingness to give you legitimate praise for the good work you have done. Identify which communication strategies you would use to handle her request. Indicate the desired outcomes of your suggested strategy. Write this information on a separate piece of paper for future reference.

6. Compare your suggested strategy to this one:

It would be important to relax and visualize yourself responding assertively in the wave of such rejecting aggression. A request for more specific comments would be in order because the instructor has not really explained what she means by being more "professional." It would be appropriate to express your opinion that the evidence you have received from the two classes indicates that you are performing well as a maternity nurse. A C.A.R.E. confrontation would be acceptable to let her know that you are disappointed in the absence of positive feedback and that you would like to receive some from her in your final evaluation as a student on the unit.

Strategies like these would let her clearly know—in a way that respects her as your instructor—that you want to be treated with respect.

Step Three: Implementing and Evaluating Your Communication Strategy

7. Now you must reply to your instructor. Develop your own response to her and write it down on a separate sheet of paper. Keep it handy so that you can refer to it later.

8. At this point you get the chance to compare your suggested response to several options listed below. Look over each of the response choices and turn to p. 303 at the end of the chapter to read a critique of each.

As you review the following response choices, look for those that are congruent with your assessment of your instructor's requests and your desire to communicate in an assertive and responsible way.

Choice H: "I can see you are giving me some advice that you believe is very important, but it's not clear to me. What exactly do you mean by 'professional'? If you explain what you mean it'll be clearer to me so that I will be more likely to improve."

Choice B: "I'm tired of your suggestions for my improvement. You have never once said anything positive in the 6 weeks I have been here. The staff and clients give me more strokes than you do. I need some positive feedback from you, too."

Choice Y: "Well, I'll try to do my best to be more professional in the future."

Choice J: "I know that when you give me all those suggestions about improving you are trying to help me be the best obstetrical nurse I can be. It's disappointing that you haven't also noted some of the good things I've done and some of the ways in which I've acted professionally. I have received enough super evaluations from the clients and encouraging comments from the staff to support my belief that I am doing some things well. Before I leave this rotation I would like you to give me some positive feedback in addition to your suggestions for improvement. Will you do that for me?"

9. After you have found the most satisfactory strategy and discovered why the other options are not suitable, go back to the response you generated earlier in this exercise. Evaluate yours in terms of how assertive and responsible it was.

Communicating With Hostile Clients

Step One: Assessment of the Data

1. Review the following situation and formulate your own assessment of the client's thoughts, feelings, and requests.

Debbie is an 18-year-old client on the medical unit where you work. She is a recently diagnosed diabetic and is terrified of receiving her insulin injection. When you try to administer it, she screams and kicks. It requires two staff members to hold her down securely in order to give the insulin safely. You know that this situation is unsatisfactory because Debbie will soon be discharged and will have to give herself her own insulin. She will have to overcome her fear and gradually take on more responsibility for her self-care.

You decide to talk with Debbie about your desire for her to be more involved in her diabetic care. You have started the conversation by explaining that you have some ideas about how she can overcome her fear and learn to be more confident in giving her insulin. Debbie interrupts you with:

Debbie: "Hold it! (Raising her voice) I'm not, repeat, NOT EVER going to give myself insulin. Get out, you bloodsucking vampire! You enjoy torturing me every morning. Well, FORGET IT! GET LOST! Go find someone else to bug. Just get off my back about this insulin junk." (Debbie comes face to face with you, and looks you right in the eye. She is red in the face and has her fists clenched and raised.)

2. On a separate sheet of paper write down your assessment of Debbie's thoughts and feelings. Indicate what request she is making of you, her nurse.

3. Compare your analysis to the assessment written below:

Thoughts: Debbie thinks you are cruel to "force" her to get more involved in taking her insulin.

Feelings: Debbie is terrified of giving herself insulin and is probably having trouble accepting that she is diabetic. She is enraged and fiercely trying to keep you at bay to protect her denial and fear. Her attack on you comes from her insecurity.

Request: Her obvious request is for you to leave her alone. The rational part of her (which is overshadowed by her fear) knows that you are right and that she will have to learn to be calmer about her insulin. Directly, Debbie is requesting to be understood and she wants you to act by leaving. Indirectly she is requesting to be comforted.

4. Did your assessment reflect an accurate analysis of the facts as they were presented? If not, return to the original data presented in the vignette and reassess the cognitive and affective messages. If so, proceed to Step Two.

Step Two: Communication Strategies and Desired Outcomes

5. You have determined that Debbie is requesting understanding, action, and comfort. Identify the communication behaviors you would use to show Debbie how you intend to respond to her requests. Indicate the desired outcomes of your suggested strategy. Write down your ideas on a separate sheet of paper.

6. Compare your suggested strategy to this one:

It is reasonable to meet Debbie's request for understanding and her implied request for comfort. She has a great adjustment to make as a diabetic and you can help her by showing you understand. It is unreasonable to meet Debbie's request for action by leaving. She is frightened and needs someone to be in control. If you leave by walking away, or become aggressive, her fear and anger will escalate out of control.

Remaining calm will help you think more clearly and might help calm Debbie. Being calm indicates that you are in control. If it is difficult for you to remain calm in the face of such enraged hostility, you could focus and visualize yourself reacting in a collected way. An empathic response to Debbie's fear and anger about having to take insulin would let her know that you do understand. A firm expression of your opinion—that she needs to learn how to be calmer about receiving her insulin—would indicate that you are in control, want to help her, and will not be put off or reject her because of her angry outburst. A gentle suggestion about how you would like to proceed to help her might make her reconsider your plan and decide that it might not be so terrifying.

This approach would show Debbie that you understand her and that you will stick with her to help her through her fear and anger; it will also give her hope of regaining self-control. She will not likely feel happy for some time, but this response will help diminish her terror.

Step Three: Implementing and Evaluating Your Communication Strategy

7. Now you must reply to Debbie. Develop your own response to Debbie and write it down on a separate sheet of paper. Keep it handy so that you can refer to it later.

8. Here is where you get the chance to compare your suggested response to several options listed below. Look over each of the response choices and turn to p. 303 at the end of the chapter to read a critique of each.

As you review the following response choices, look for those that are congruent with your assessment of Debbie's requests and your desire to communicate in an assertive and responsible way.

Choice C: (Reaching out and putting your arm around Debbie's shoulders) "There, there, Debbie. Don't be so angry. It's just a matter of time before you'll feel okay about taking your insulin. I'm just here to help you. You'll see that you'll be feeling calm about the whole thing in a few weeks."

Choice K: "Don't you talk to me like that, young lady. You'd better show a little more respect for me or you'll be in trouble. I know what's best for you. I've had lots of experience, so if you're smart you'll cooperate."

Choice Q: "I know it is scary to receive a needle every morning, Debbie. It's a big thing to adjust to, especially for someone as active and as healthy as you. I can help you to feel quite confident, and eventually even comfortable, about taking your insulin. What I'd like you to do is to sit down with me right now and listen to my plan. I want you to hear me out, and then you can ask any questions and consider whether you'd like to try it."

Choice X: "Debbie, I was only trying to help you" (you say before you leave Debbie's room).

9. After you have found the most satisfactory strategy and discovered why the others are not suitable options, go back to the original strategy you generated earlier in this exercise. Evaluate yours in terms of how assertive and responsible it was.

Communicating With Hostile Colleagues

Step One: Assessment of the Data

1. Review the following situation and formulate your own assessment of your colleague's thoughts, feelings, and requests.

You are a nurse working in an outpatient mental health center. There are small interviewing rooms that can be booked for private interviews with clients and their families. As usual, space is an issue and scheduling of rooms is essential. In the past 3 days your interviews have been 5 minutes longer than the half hour that you had booked. By going overtime you have delayed the interviews of others. Your colleague Karen has been annoyed but understanding because you are not usually so inconsiderate.

Today you booked the room for 45 minutes so that you could complete your interview without holding up others. However, your client has just revealed some serious information about her marriage and is upset and crying in the interview room. You know you need about 5 minutes over your time to help your client calm down before vacating the interview room. Karen has booked the room after you. She has knocked on the door twice already to remind you that your time is up. When you come out with your client she blasts you with:

Karen: "It's about time. This is the fourth time this week that I've had to wait for you to leave the room when I've booked it. This has got to stop. My client's family is here on their lunch hour. You aren't the only one with important things to do, you know" (Karen's voice is raised and her hands are on her hips).

2. On a separate sheet of paper write down your assessment of Karen's thoughts and feelings. Indicate what request Karen is making of you, her nurse colleague.

3. Compare your analysis to this assessment:

Thoughts: Karen thinks you are rude and inconsiderate to go beyond your allotted time in the shared interview room.

Feelings: Karen is annoyed because you have gone over into the time she had planned to be in the room. She is feeling pressured because the family she wants to interview only has a limited period of time. She is worried about seeming to be rude to them by not being able to get into the only private room available. Karen is frustrated and disappointed that you have behaved in such an inconsiderate way.

Request: Karen wants you to understand how inconvenienced she and her clients were by your thoughtlessness. She wants you to act more responsibly in the future by vacating the room after your time is up.

4. Did your assessment reflect an accurate analysis of the facts as they were presented? If not, return to the original data presented in the vignette and reassess the cognitive and affective messages. If so, proceed to Step Two.

Step Two: Communication Strategies and Desired Outcomes

5. You have determined that Karen wants understanding and action. Identify which communication behaviors you would use to respond to Karen. Indicate the desired outcomes of your strategy. Write your ideas down on a separate sheet of paper so that you can refer to them later.

6. Compare your suggested strategy to this one:

Karen's requests for understanding and future consideration are legitimate. It is reasonable to respond to them with an empathic reply and a promise to be more careful in the future. It is unreasonable to accept Karen's hostile aggressiveness, especially since she embarrassed you in front of all three clients and any other staff members in the vicinity. It would be important to stay calm and make a C.A.R.E. confrontation to Karen, asking her to speak more courteously to you about issues that bother her. It would be better to wait until later in the day to speak with Karen, at a time when you both have an opportunity to complete your discussion.

This strategy would make Karen feel assured that you respect her rights and would make her aware of your rights, too.

Step Three: Implementing and Evaluating Your Communication Strategy

7. Now you must reply to Karen. On a separate sheet of paper develop your own response to Karen and keep it handy.

8. At this point you get the opportunity to compare your suggested response to several options listed below. Look over each of the response choices and turn to p. 303 at the end of the chapter to read a critique of each.

As you review the following response choices, look for those that are congruent with your assessment of Karen's requests and your desire to communicate in an assertive and responsible way.

Choice D: "I apologize to all of you (looking at Karen and her clients) for this inconvenience." (Later, at a mutually convenient time when you and Karen are alone) "Karen, I'd like to talk with you about how you handled my overstaying my booking time this morning. Is this a good time or would a little later be better?" (Proceeding after Karen agrees to do so) "I will really try not to inconvenience you by going over my booked time in the future. I know I put you in a tough spot, and I was very embarrassed that you 'scolded' me in front of our clients in the middle of the hall where everyone could hear. In the future, I would appreciate it if you would ask to talk about any complaints you have in private. Then no one would be embarrassed and we can keep our staff quarrels separate from the clients. Could you do this, Karen?"

Choice L: (At the time) "Just a minute, Karen. What do you mean? I wouldn't deliberately try to annoy you by overstaying my time. You should know there's a very good reason for my delay. I'm not deliberately trying to inconvenience you. The room is yours now."

Choice P: (At the time) Getting red in the face and avoiding eye contact with Karen and her clients, you walk right past them. Later, when you have an opportunity to have contact with Karen you avoid her. You refuse to make eye contact and you do not initiate conversation with her even though you do with the rest of the staff.

Choice W: (At the time) "I'm sorry, Karen."

9. After you have found the most satisfactory strategy and discovered why the other options are not satisfactory, go back to the suggested response you generated earlier in this exercise. Evaluate yours in terms of how assertive and responsible it was.

Communicating With Abusive Clients
Step One: Assessment of the Data

1. Review the following situation and formulate your own assessment of your client's thoughts, feelings, and requests.

Mrs. Suit is a 60-year-old client who has been admitted to the coronary care unit with chest pain. She has diabetes, which is poorly managed, and arthritis. She has been very demanding, especially on the days when her husband is unable to get up to visit her. Today she has put her call light on repeatedly and this time she has asked you to bring her fresh water in a glass with a straw. You start out for the kitchen but are waylaid by the distraught son of another client. He is almost in tears and wants to discuss with you the news of his father's forthcoming surgery. You pause to talk with him before you get Mrs. Suit's drink. When you get back to Mrs. Suit's room she lambastes you with:

Mrs. Suit: "Damnation. You could die here before you get a simple glass of water. You're such a smartass; you probably think I'm just a sick old lady, but I've got just as much right to service as anybody in this hospital. What in the hell were you doing, melting some ice? Damn it! Just give me the straw; you're slower than molasses in January. I'll open it myself. If I let you do it you could take all night. You can go now. You smartassed nurses think you're so damn important but you can't even get an old lady a drink of water without messing things up."

2. On a separate sheet of paper write down your assessment of Mrs. Suit's thoughts and feelings. Indicate what request Mrs. Suit is making of you, her nurse.

3. Compare your assessment to the one below:

Thoughts: Mrs. Suit thinks you took your time bringing her the water because you don't think either she or her request is important.

Feelings: Mrs. Suit's feelings are hurt because of her assumption that your tardiness is associated with lack of respect for her. Her abusiveness is her defense against her hurt feelings of being rejected. It is likely that she is frightened of the monitor and lonely today because she did not receive a visit from her husband. These factors may be compounding her attack on you.

Request: Mrs. Suit is asking you to treat her with more respect by following through on her reasonable requests (like getting a glass of water). Indirectly, she is asking you to understand that she feels insecure and frightened. Obliquely, she is requesting comfort from you and reassurance that you care about her. This request for comfort is for present and future interactions.

4. Did your assessment reflect an accurate analysis of the facts as they were presented? If not, return to the original data presented in the vignette and reassess the cognitive and affective messages. If so, proceed to Step Two.

Step Two: Communication Strategies and Desired Outcomes

5. You have determined that Mrs. Suit needs understanding and comfort. Identify which communication strategy you would use to respond to her requests. Indicate the desired outcomes of your strategy. Write your ideas down so that you can refer to them later.

6. Compare your suggested strategy to this one:

Mrs. Suit's requests are all legitimate. Her way of expressing them is aggressive and irritating, and it would be easy for you to become offended. The best approach is to stay calm and extend warmth to this upset woman. It might be appropriate to explain your delay to prove that you were not delaying disrespectfully. Some reassurance of your interest in her would be supportive for her. In the future you could make efforts to ensure that she is made to feel important and cared for by coming in when she has not called and by asking her if there is anything else you could do to make her feel more comfortable before you leave the room.

This strategy would make her feel cared for and respected.

Step Three: Implementing and Evaluating Your Communication Strategy

7. Now you must reply to Mrs. Suit. On a separate sheet of paper develop your own response to Mrs. Suit and keep it for future reference.

8. At this point you get the chance to compare your suggested strategy to several options listed below. Look over each of the response choices and turn to p. 303 at the end of the chapter to read a critique of each.

As you review the following choices, look for those that are congruent with your assessment of Mrs. Suit's requests and your desire to communicate in an assertive and responsible way.

Choice AA: "Mrs. Suit, I'm sorry I was so long in coming with your water. It's not that I don't care about you. I was delayed by an upset family member who needed to talk about his seriously ill father. I'm sure you can now understand why I was delayed. I am free for a few minutes now, though, if there's anything you'd like to talk about."

Choice I: "Mrs. Suit, I went out of my way to get you your water. The least you could do is say 'thank you'" (you turn and leave).

Choice R: "Sorry, Mrs. Suit." (Facial expression is flat and you leave after giving her the straw.)

9. After you have found the most satisfactory strategy and discovered why the other options are not suitable, go back to the original response you generated in this exercise. Evaluate yours in terms of how assertive and responsible it was.

Communicating With Abusive Colleagues

Step One: Assessment of the Data

1. Review the following situation and formulate your own assessment of your colleague's thoughts, feelings, and requests.

You have been a student nurse on a surgical unit for 3 weeks. For the past 3 days you have been the medication nurse. On this unit the job of giving out medications is particularly difficult and time consuming. Clients are often downstairs having diagnostic tests, having their dressings changed, or working at physical therapy; all of these make it difficult to give out the medications smoothly. In addition, there are many intravenous drips to be regulated. You find it confusing to keep track of the IVs, the regular medications, and clients' requests for postoperative analgesics.

Your clinical instructor has encouraged you by assuring you that you are doing a fine job. She has remarked that you are safe and careful with distributing the medications and has informed you that speed will come with practice. The team leader on the floor has not been so supportive. From the first day you took over as medication nurse she has been hostile and insulting. She has said such destructive things as: "I know you students have to learn but we've got sick people here who can't wait all day for their medications. You're going to have to speed things up." and "Look out. Here comes speedy!" (to another nurse at the nursing station). She has undermined you by coming to get the medication keys from you and giving some clients narcotic pain relievers, saying: "If she has to wait for you to get there her pain will have her on the ceiling."

You are just returning to the nursing station after distributing your morning medications. Your hostile team leader is at the station and confronts you with:

Team Leader: "Well, what do you know? You're finally here. While you've been poking along out on the floor I've given three clients their pain killers. I bet you haven't remembered your IVs, have you? Well, speedy, I've been keeping my eye on them and you'd better change the bag in room 25. I don't know how you're going to function as a graduate when you don't have someone like me looking over your shoulder."

2. On a separate sheet of paper write down your assessment of your team leader's thoughts and feelings. Indicate what request she is making of you, the student nurse giving medications on this surgical unit.

3. Compare your analysis to that below:

Thoughts: Your team leader thinks you are far too slow as a medication nurse. She has the notion that you are incapable of taking charge of all the medication nurse's responsibilities at this point.

Feelings: She is concerned about those clients who need their postoperative medications, and she is worried that the IVs will run dry. She is irritated by your slowness and is unwilling to remember that it takes practice to become faster at this complicated task. Her annoyance makes her take out her frustration on you.

Request: Your team leader wants you to be faster as a medication nurse. She wants you to simultaneously keep track of IVs, regular medications, and PRN orders for analgesics. She also wants you to develop accurate speed immediately. She is requesting that you understand what she wants and that you comply with it immediately.

4. Did your assessment reflect an accurate analysis of the facts as they were presented? If not, return to the original data presented in the vignette and reassess the cognitive and affective messages. If so, proceed to Step Two.

Step Two: Communication Strategies and Desired Outcomes

5. You have determined that the team leader wants understanding and action. Identify which communication behaviors you would use to respond to her requests. Indicate the desired outcome of your strategy. Write down your ideas so that you can refer to them later.

6. Compare your suggested strategy to this one:

Your team leader's request for understanding is legitimate, but her request for immediate increased speed as medication nurse is unreasonable, given your lack of experience. It would be important to keep calm and remain calm so as to respond to her in a clear, direct way. If you get out of control, you may be upset for the rest of the day and increase your chances of making an error.

Remain calm, using imagery and positive self-talk to help you stay focused on responding assertively and responsibly to your team leader. It would be appropriate that you thank her for the help she has given you. However, it is also necessary that you ask her to consult you before giving out medications to anybody, to ensure that you as the person in charge of medications are kept informed and that no duplications are made. A C.A.R.E. confrontation to request that she have more patience with your beginning skill would let her know how it would be more helpful for her to relate to you.

This approach will let your team leader know that you do understand the need for speed and accuracy in a medication nurse, but that her request for immediate action is unreasonable. She may not like your assertive response because it will point out to her that she has been aggressive and that you do not intend to tolerate being treated in such a destructive manner. Your strategy may change her behavior in a positive way; however, if she escalates her abusiveness to you, you can confront her again and indicate a more serious consequence (such as reporting her aggressiveness to your clinical instructor).

Step Three: Implementing and Evaluating Your Communication Strategy

7. Now you must reply to your team leader. On a separate sheet of paper develop your own response to her. Keep it for future reference.

8. At this point you get the chance to compare your suggested response to several options listed below. Look over each of the response choices and turn to p. 303 at the end of the chapter to read a critique of each.

As you review the following response choices look for those that are congruent with your assessment of your team leader's requests and your desire to communicate in an assertive and responsible way.

Choice F: "I hope when I am a graduate I am more considerate of students than you are. Don't you remember what it was like when you were learning? Your insults aren't helpful at all."

Choice N: "I guess it's hard for you to sit back and have someone less experienced give out the medications. I understand the concerns you have about the clients receiving their medication on time; however, I have to learn, and it will take a few more days before I am faster at this new job. It would be helpful if you would let me know when clients are asking for, or have received, their analgesics so that I can keep track of who's had what. I appreciate your giving the clients their medications these past days but I would like to try to do the whole job of being a medication nurse now that I'm getting the hang of it. Will you let me do that?"

Choice S: "Oh. I'll go and attend to those IVs right away. Sorry I'm so slow; it must drive you crazy."

After you have found the most satisfactory strategy and discovered why the other options are not suitable, go back to the suggested response you generated in this exercise. Evaluate yours in terms of how assertive and responsible it was.

Moments of Connection...
Taking Our Work Professionally Rather Than Personally

I was busy on my 3-11 shift on a medical surgical unit. One woman was constantly on the call bell and yelling out her needs when we didn't respond as quickly as she expected. By 10 PM, things were calmer and her roommate was finally able to get to sleep. We went to the room to do brief HS care. We fluffed her pillow, talked several minutes, and brushed her hair. She looked up at me, patted my hand, touched my cheek, and said, "You are all my heroes." Somehow we had given her something . . . you never know what touches a client or what means a lot; sometimes it's the small things.

Communicating With Manipulative Clients

Step One: Assessment of the Data

1. Review the following situation and formulate your own assessment of your client's thoughts, feelings, and requests.

Mr. Gilmour is a 58-year-old gentleman on your rehabilitative stroke unit. He is a heavy smoker and because he burns holes in his clothing it is the policy to keep his cigarettes at the nursing station, ensure that he wears a nonflammable smoking jacket, and supervise him when he smokes. Since this is a nonsmoking facility, it is necessary for a staff member to take him outside for a cigarette. Mr. Gilmour has a knack of asking for cigarettes at the most inconvenient times. He knows he is supposed to wait until report is over before he asks for a smoke, but he invariably bugs the nursing staff at report time. You are the nurse in charge of the day shift and you want to complete the report to the evening staff so that you can go home. Mr. Gilmour has already interrupted your report three times to ask for a smoke. You gave him a cigarette 30 minutes ago. His fourth manipulative attempt goes like this:

Mr. Gilmour: "Aw, come on. I'll smoke it right here where you can see me. I promise I won't start a fire. (He moves his wheelchair closer and closer to the small area where you are having report.) It won't hurt you to give me one little smoke. Come on. No one else cares about these stupid hospital rules. I haven't had one all afternoon. Give a guy a break. I had to go for that stupid x-ray so I missed my after-lunch smoke. Just one and then I won't bother you again."

2. On a separate sheet of paper write down your assessment of Mr. Gilmour's thoughts and feelings. Indicate what request Mr. Gilmour is making of you, the nurse in charge on days.

3. Compare your analysis to the one below:

Thoughts: Mr. Gilmour thinks he deserves a cigarette and believes that if he bugs you enough he will get what he wants. He knows it is inconvenient for you to take him outside and hopes he can get you to break the rule.

Feelings: He is annoyed that you are not giving into his requests. He feels especially justified in persisting because he has not had a cigarette for what he thinks is a few hours.

Requests: Mr. Gilmour's request is for understanding (about his craving to have a smoke) and action (you giving him a cigarette).

4. Did your assessment reflect an accurate analysis of the facts as they were presented? If not, return to the original data presented in the vignette and reassess the cognitive and affective messages. If so, proceed to Step Two.

Step Two: Communication Strategies and Desired Outcomes

5. You have determined that Mr. Gilmour wants understanding and action. Identify which communication behaviors you would use to respond to his requests. Indicate the desired outcomes for your suggested strategy. Write your ideas down for future reference.

6. Compare your suggested strategy to this one:

It would be tempting to lash out aggressively at Mr. Gilmour, but this attack would only hurt his feelings, make you feel bad, and embarrass everyone. Even though you are frustrated by Mr. Gilmour's manipulative persistence, it is important to stay calm and handle the situation assertively and responsibly. It would be wise to be consistent with the rule the unit has made of refusing cigarettes during report. You know that report will be finished in 5 minutes and that it is not unreasonable for Mr. Gilmour to wait that long. A firm refusal to comply and a request that Mr. Gilmour wait until you complete your nursing report would both be appropriate. It would be important to ensure that he does get to smoke a cigarette right after report.

This strategy would demonstrate to Mr. Gilmour that he cannot break reasonable rules that have been established for good purposes. Your firmness would respect your own right to finish report without being interrupted and would treat Mr. Gilmour with respect.

Step Three: Implementing and Evaluating Your Communication Strategy

7. Now you must reply to Mr. Gilmour. On a separate sheet of paper develop your own response to Mr. Gilmour and keep it handy for future reference.

8. At this point you get the chance to compare your suggested response to several options listed below. Look over each of the response choices and turn to p. 303 at the end of the chapter to read a critique of each.

As you review the following response choices look for those that are congruent with your assessment of Mr. Gilmour's requests and your desire to communicate in an assertive and responsible way.

Choice G: "Get out of here and leave us alone so that we can finish our report. As soon as we are finished we will take you out for a cigarette."

Choice U: "Mr. Gilmour, please do not interrupt us while we are having report. We will finish in 5 minutes if you stop interrupting us. It's only been 30 minutes since your last cigarette, and when our report is finished one of the evening nurses will take you outside. If you do not leave us alone now, then we will delay giving you a cigarette for another hour."

Choice BB: "Ohhhh! (exasperated). At this point I'd do anything to get this report over so I can leave. Here's a cigarette. Put it out if you see someone coming."

9. After you have found the most satisfactory strategy and discovered why the other options are unsuitable, go back to the suggested response you generated earlier in this exercise. Evaluate your response in terms of how assertive and responsible it was.

It is important to note that manipulation is a method of attempting to get one's needs met and is a behavior that can be seen on a continuum from positive and resourceful to negative and destructive. Whenever a nurse feels annoyed with a client, it is useful to examine the interaction and consider if there is another issue besides the one at hand that is contributing to the annoyance. These issues are explored more thoroughly in psychiatric nursing.

Communicating With Manipulative Colleagues

Step One: Assessment of the Data

1. Review the following situation and formulate your own assessment of your colleague's thoughts, feelings, and requests.

You are a nurse in an outpatient clinic that keeps sample medications on hand to give to clients. It is midway through the day. Your colleague, Noreen, has suffered a splitting headache all night, and she is concerned that it will develop into one of her immobilizing migraine headaches. You are the only one with the keys to the medication cabinet. She approaches you with this request:

Noreen: "Leslie, I can't take this headache of mine any longer. I feel like my brain has dried up into a hard ball and it's knocking against my skull. On the outside it feels like a vise locking in on it. I've already tossed up what little supper I could eat. Leslie, could you give me some of that new analgesic for my head? I've used it in the past and it stops me from vomiting and somehow eases my head, too. My doctor would agree to it, I swear; so won't you please help me out of my misery? It's not like it's a narcotic I'm asking for. What do you say? I might be of some help to you for the rest of the day if you give me the analgesic."

2. On a separate sheet of paper write down your assessment of Noreen's thoughts and feelings. Indicate what request Noreen is making of you, her colleague on the evening shift.

3. Compare your analysis to the assessment below:

Thoughts: Noreen thinks that the analgesic will help her to feel better. She thinks it is reasonable for you to give her the analgesic without an order from her physician.

Feelings: Noreen is feeling pretty sick with her impending migraine headache and feels hopeful that you will help her by giving the analgesic.

Request: Noreen is asking you to understand that her head is making her feel violently ill. She is requesting action in the form of your giving her the analgesic.

4. Did your assessment reflect an accurate analysis of the facts as they were presented? If not, return to the original data presented in the vignette and reassess the cognitive and affective message. If so, proceed to Step Two.

Step Two: Communication Strategies and Desired Outcomes

5. You have determined that Noreen wants understanding and action. Identify which communication strategies you would use to respond to her request. Indicate the desired outcomes of your suggested strategy. Write your ideas down so that you can refer to them later.

6. Compare your suggested strategy to this one:

Warmth and an empathic reply would convey your compassion for Noreen. Her request for you to give her prescription medication without a physician's order is unreasonable because it puts you in jeopardy of disciplinary action from your professional nursing association. Furthermore, you would be unwise to administer anything that might be damaging to your colleague since she has not been examined by a physician. A firm refusal to comply with her request would be appropriate, as would be a suggestion that she leave work to attend to her health.

This strategy would show Noreen you understand and care about how she is feeling, and make it clear that you want her to handle her health problems through the correct channels.

Step Three: Implementing and Evaluating Your Communication Strategy

7. Now you must reply to Noreen. On a separate sheet of paper develop your own response to Noreen and keep it handy for future reference.

8. At this point you get to compare your suggested response to several options listed below. Look over each of the response choices and turn to p. 303 at the end of the chapter to read a critique of each.

As you review the following response choices look for those that are congruent with your assessment of Noreen's requests and your desire to communicate in an assertive and responsible way.

Choice O: "Are you serious, Noreen? I can't give you anything. If you're that sick you'd better go home."

Choice T: "Well, I guess that would be okay, Noreen. Do you really think so? You're right, it's a drug you have used before. OK, I'll do it. Do you really think we're doing the right thing?"

Choice V: "Noreen, you sound terrible. I think if you're that uncomfortable you'd better go home. I will not give you any medications, and I don't think you should take anything until you've checked with your doctor. It's been a slow day and I know I can manage. Who could we call to come and get you?"

9. After you have found the most satisfactory strategy and discovered why the other options were unsuitable, go back to the suggested response you generated earlier in this example. Evaluate yours in terms of how assertive and responsible it was.

A Final Note

The situations described above and others you will face are not so easily handled on the spot. These techniques give you a framework from which to work. You have studied techniques in this book that help you promote your own calm, confident approach to difficult situations. You are equipped to start your own journey to understand the human condition. Perhaps you are reading this book because you've already learned you need to know more. Do not be fooled; your education just begins when you leave school, but practice helps, so more exercises are included!

Think About It...
What, So What, and Now What?

Consider what you read about communicating assertively with aggressive clients and colleagues. Have you already begun to deal with these challenges? Write the answers to the following questions.

What? . . .   Write one thing you learned from this chapter.

So what? . . .   How will this impact your nursing practice?

Now what? . . .   How will you implement this new knowledge or skill?

THINK ABOUT IT

Practicing Communicating With Aggressive Clients and Colleagues

Exercise 1

(You will need an audio tape recorder.) For this exercise work in groups of three. One of you will role-play an aggressive client or colleague, another will be the nurse, and the third will give feedback to the nurse. The aggressive client (or colleague) will communicate to the nurse in a rejecting, hostile, abusive, or manipulative way. The nurse will attempt to respond in an assertive and responsible way. The feedback giver will indicate to the nurse how effective she was in employing an assertive and responsible style. Tape the dialogue between client (or colleague) and nurse so that you can use the recording to complete Exercise 2.

Make sure each of you has the chance to role-play all three roles. After you have done this exercise in your small groups, rejoin your colleagues in the rest of the class. Pool together what you have learned about communicating effectively with aggressive clients and colleagues.

Exercise 2

Transcribe into writing 10 paired interactions (what the aggressive person said and what you said is one paired interaction) from the tape-recorded interview you did in Exercise 1. For each statement that the aggressive person made, write down your assessment of his thoughts and feelings, and whether it is appropriate to meet the request he is making. Examine the strategy you used to respond to your "client" or "colleague" and evaluate whether it met his request. If not, generate an alternative response that is assertive and responsible. This review will help you develop more effective communication skills with aggressive clients and colleagues.

Critique: Choices of Responses to Aggressive Clients and Colleagues

Choice A: This is a nonassertive reply. You have acknowledged Mr. Hunter's need for secure, safe, nursing care, but you have not given any credit to your ability to provide this care. You have not respected your own skill and abilities. Mr. Hunter may feel reassured that he can get a registered nurse instead of you, a student nurse, but he would not be impressed with your lack of confidence in your own abilities. This response is not responsible because you missed data about his difficulty adjusting to his primary nurse's absence. This strategy might make Mr. Hunter wonder about his safety in your hands, and it might embarrass him that you so easily crumbled under his attack.

Choice B: This response is aggressive and hostile to your instructor. You have harbored resentment about her lack of positive feedback for 5 weeks and have not appropriately brought it up at an earlier time. Today your buildup of anger and disappointment has come crashing out against her. Although this response protects your right to speak up, it overrides her right to have her feelings respected. Not only would this response make her feel threatened and angry, but it might result in a discipline case with your school of nursing. This response in no way guarantees that you will receive positive feedback from your instructor in the future.

Choice C: This approach is aggressive in style. There is arrogance in your touching Debbie and telling her not to feel the way she does. Your response is not sensitive to her right to her feelings. This response is irresponsible because it does not pick up on the obvious data that Debbie refuses to be rushed to accept her diabetes and need for insulin. It may escalate Debbie's fury to touch her at this point. Debbie would likely feel talked down to and disregarded.

Choice D: This strategy is assertive. Your apology to Karen and her clients was timely and respected their legitimate rights. Its brevity and promptness deescalated any further hostility between your two parties. This approach is responsible because it acknowledges your role in inconveniencing others. All concerned would be satisfied with this reply. Waiting until a moment when you and Karen could talk privately and freely about how she embarrassed you was considerate and respected your right to talk out this important issue. Your request to talk to Karen, and your honesty about the issue, helped to focus on the problem right away. Starting with an apology reassured her of your sincerity. Waiting for her permission to pursue your agenda was respectful. Your C.A.R.E. confrontation spelled out clearly what bothered you and how you want your colleague to behave in the future. Karen would feel that you understood her irritation with your overstaying in the room, and she would easily be able to receive your feedback about her rudeness.

Choice E: This response is aggressive and almost taunting. It would only serve to escalate the anger building between you. It attacks Mr. Hunter's vulnerability. He has no control over who nurses him, and you have threatened his security by implying that reporting you would be futile. Your sauciness about the decision of your instructor would only make Mr. Hunter feel less secure. This response is irresponsible because it does not attend to the data about Mr. Hunter's feelings of insecurity and his desire to heal without relapse. It shows no sensitivity to his feelings of missing his primary nurse. This response would likely make Mr. Hunter feel insecure and threatened himself.

Choice F: This response is aggressive. It is a direct, insulting attack on your team leader. It does nothing to respect your right to communicate in a caring way, and it ignores her concerns about your slowness. This style of responding would only make your team leader want to retaliate by being more aggressive with you in the future.

Choice G: You have responsibly acknowledged Mr. Gilmour's need for a cigarette, but your style is aggressive and rude. It does not respect your right to communicate assertively and would likely make everyone a little embarrassed.

Choice H: This response is assertive because it puts the onus on your instructor for more specificity in her suggestion about how you should change. It is her responsibility to clarify her meaning. This response is also responsible because it picks up on the data you have been given about her intention to transform you into a professional nurse. This response would likely make your instructor clarify her meaning of "professional" to your satisfaction. With this information you could then decide whether to point out any evidence you have about your professional demeanor. If she cannot be clear in her expectations, then you have the right to ask her to withdraw the accusation that you are unprofessional.

The issue of your right to receive some positive feedback from your instructor has not been dealt with in this response. Including such a request would augment the assertiveness of your response.

Choice I: This reply is irresponsible because it does not take into account Mrs. Suit's worry or anxiety. It is aggressive because it sarcastically insults her and does not respect your right to communicate in a caring way. This reply would put down Mrs. Suit and make her feel angry and embarrassed.

Choice J: This is an assertive response. You have pointed out in a C.A.R.E. confrontation exactly what bothers you and how you want her to change. Your specificity and courteous manner would protect her self-respect while you stand up for your legitimate rights. This strategy is also responsible because your instructor can pick up your hint about giving you feedback in an effort to improve your performance, and you remind her of some data she has overlooked. It is likely that this gentle confrontation will invite your instructor to look at her omissions and try to rectify the situation by being more accepting of your abilities as a maternity nurse.

Choice K: This aggressive approach would likely increase Debbie's anger. At the least, it would dissolve any rapport or trust you had developed. You have not respected her right to be treated with respect and compassion. Irresponsibly, you have not attended to the data about her fear or her need to go slowly in her acceptance. You have not respected your right to communicate in a caring way. Debbie would likely feel even more angry and helpless because you are "pulling rank" on her. It would take a long time to repair the bad feelings generated by this response.

Choice L: This choice is aggressive in style. Your opening phrase attacks Karen and escalates the hostility between the two of you. Your defensiveness embarrasses everyone—staff and clients. This response is irresponsible in its lack of attention to Karen's request for understanding and an apology.

Choice M: This reply is assertive because it confidently assures Mr. Hunter that you know what you are doing and invites him to make any inquiries about your nursing care. Your agreement about differences between nurses might reduce his anxiety over apparent variations in nursing styles. Your acknowledgment of his missing his primary nurse would show him you understand the mutuality that they had developed. Your assurance that your care is safe and congruent with doctor's orders would reassure him that you understand his urgency to be well cared for. This responsible and assertive response would make Mr. Hunter feel understood and comforted.

Choice N: This reply is assertive and responsible. It stands up for your right to be given a chance to learn, and it shows respect for your team leader. You have acknowledged her legitimate concerns about the clients and requested her help in facilitating your development as a medication nurse. This response would make it clear what behavior you expect in a way that makes it easy for her to comply.

Choice O: This response is aggressive. It blasts Noreen without showing any compassion for how she is feeling; however, it does respect your right to nurse within the limits of the law and your own convictions. Noreen would likely feel attacked, but she would definitely get the message that she should go off duty.

Choice P: This is a nonassertive approach. You have not acknowledged Karen's feelings nor have you spoken to her about your own anger at her aggressiveness. You have irresponsibly ignored Karen's legitimate requests. By sulking and avoiding her you are harboring bad feelings, instead of dealing with them in a forthright manner. You, Karen, and other staff members would all feel uptight with this strategy.

Choice Q: This response is assertive because it acknowledges both Debbie's right to be understood and your right to communicate in a caring manner and offer Debbie a way to desensitize herself to the insulin shots. It is responsible because it picks up on her need to have her fear understood. You have comforted her by taking control and offering her a plan that might help her. Leaving or getting angry would have removed your supportive backing from Debbie. This response would make Debbie feel secure that you understand her fear and you have the willingness and interest in her to help her though it.

Choice R: This is an irresponsible and nonassertive response. You have neither attended to Mrs. Suit's request to be treated with respect nor have you shown that you understand her feelings of helplessness. You have not respected your own rights as a nurse on the unit; you had another important task to accomplish that delayed you and you have the right and responsibility to communicate in a caring way to all your clients. Mrs. Suit may have felt important that you apologized, but your manner indicated only that you wanted to get out of her presence as soon as possible. Your lack of warmth and genuine respect would let Mrs. Suit know that you did not really care for her.

Choice S: This response is nonassertive. You deserve to be bullied when you encourage it with such a meek reply. You have not respected your right to be treated in a patient manner. Your passivity has invited further putdowns.

Choice T: Clearly you are doubtful about the ethics of giving Noreen the medication, but you nonassertively give in. In so doing you lose your right to act safely and you may do your colleague some unintended harm. You have not acted responsibly because you did not follow up on the data she provided about her migraines, nor did you show much compassion for her misery.

Choice U: This firm, clear reply is assertive; it respects Mr. Gilmour's dignity and your right to communicate in a respectful way. Your inclusion of a negative consequence demonstrates that you are serious about your request for him to stop bothering you during report. This reply is responsible because it takes into account that Mr. Gilmour had a smoke recently, that there is a well-established rule about the times and places for his smoking, and that you have a right to finish work on time. Although Mr. Gilmour will likely be displeased by your reply, he will know you are definite.

Choice V: This reply is assertive and responsible. You acknowledged Noreen's extreme discomfort and wisely suggested that she go home. You protected your right to avoid legal problems and your colleague's right to be properly examined before taking medication by refusing to give her anything. You did not leave her stranded but offered to call the evening supervisor and reassured her that you would manage the shift without her. Noreen might wish to try again to persuade you to give her something for her nausea but that possibility is unlikely given your firmness.

Choice W: This is a nonassertive response. You have not protected your right to relate to your colleague in a caring way. She requested understanding and a promise that you would not repeat your inconsiderate actions in the future, and you have ignored both these requests by this non-specific response. Karen would feel minimally understood. This reply ignores your responsibility to defend your right to be treated respectfully by your colleague Karen.

Choice X: This is a nonassertive response. You respected neither Debbie's right to be understood nor your own to communicate in a helpful way. Your reply focuses only on your feelings and misses the important data about Debbie's fears and need for guidance. Debbie would likely feel misunderstood and unsupported with this response.

Choice Y: This choice is nonassertive. You have buckled under to accept an unreasonable request. Not only is your instructor's request unclear, but it does not correspond with how you feel about your work and the feedback you have been getting. This response is unlikely to stop any further aggression from your instructor. It is neither assertive nor responsible.

Choice Z: This response is an aggressive overreaction to Mr. Hunter. Returning aggressiveness with aggressiveness only escalates the feud. If Mr. Hunter had been repeatedly comparing your care to Chris's and putting you down, it would then be appropriate to ask him to stop this line of attack. At this point it is irresponsible to do so, because it puts the attention on your feelings rather than his feelings of vulnerability and loss. This is not a helpful response, and it would leave Mr. Hunter embarrassed and discomforted.

Choice AA: This is an assertive response. You calmly and kindly reassured Mrs. Suit that your delay was not out of disrespect for her. The directness and conciseness of your explanation was not overly apologetic (which would have been nonassertive), nor overly defensive (which would have been aggressive). Your reply was responsible because it picked up on her need to be treated with respect. Your offer to stay with her and talk demonstrated that you truly do care about her feelings. The strategy of overlooking her coarse abusive language was probably appropriate in this situation. Her anger stems from her fear and, if you help her cope with some of her legitimate worries, her abusiveness will likely diminish. If not, you could assertively request that she refrain from using abusive language with you.

Choice BB: This is a nonassertive response. You have given in to Mr. Gilmour's unreasonable request and in the process made it difficult for other staff members to uphold the rule. You have taught Mr. Gilmour that if he persists long enough you will bend the rules. This reply would make you feel bad that you didn't stick to your decision. It irresponsibly ignores the data that he had a cigarette recently.

Reference

Jakubowski P, Lange AJ: *The assertive option: your rights and responsibilities,* Champaign, Ill, 1978, Research Press.

 ## Suggestions for Further Reading

Andrews G: Mistrust, the hidden obstacle to empowerment, *Human Resources* 39(9):66, 1994.

Bohn J: The wounded worker, *Human Resources* 39(4):74, 1994.

Buckwalter KC: Aggression management: the pivotal role of nursing, *J Gerontol Nurs* 24(5):5, 1998. Employees who have had difficult lives may see the workplace as replacement for the families in which they were raised. Strategies are offered for working with these employees.

Cullen M: *Men & anger: understanding and managing your anger for a much better life,* Brandon, Vt, 1996, The Safer Society Press.

Farrell GA: Aggression in clinical settings: nurses' views, *J Adv Nurs* 25(3):501, 1997.

Hurlebaus AE, Link S: The effects of an aggressive behavior management program on nurses' levels of knowledge, confidence, and safety, *J Nurs Staff Devel* 13(5):260, 1997.

Lipkin GB, Cohen RG: *Effective approaches to patients' behavior,* ed 3, New York, 1986, Springer.

Maier GJ: Managing threatening behavior: the role of talk down and talk up, *J Psychosoc Nurs Mental Health Serv* 34(6):25, 1996.

Medved R: Strategies for handling angry patients and their families, *Nursing* 90 21:4, 1990.

Morrison EF: The culture of caregiving and aggression in psychiatric settings, *Arch Psychiatric Nurs* 12(1):21, 1998.

Murphy TG: Improving nurse/doctor communications, *Nursing 90* 20(8):114, 1990.

Stuart GW, Sundeen SJ: Managing aggressive behavior. In Stuart GW, Laraia M: *Principles and practice of psychiatric nursing,* ed 6, St Louis, 1998, Mosby.

Smith NM, Brown L: Ask *Home Healthcare Nurse:* dealing with aggressive patients and avoiding overinvolvement, *Home Healthcare Nurse* 15(2):131, 1997.

Turnbull J et al: Turn it around: short-term management for aggression and anger, *J Psychosoc Nurs* 28(6):7, 1990.

Whittington R: Violence to nurses: prevalence and risk factors, *Emerg Nurse* 5(8):31, 1998.

Williams ML, Robertson K: Workplace violence: prevalence, prevention, and first-line interventions, *Crit Care Nurs Clin North Am* 9(2):221, 1998.

Zernike W, Sharpe P: Patient aggression in a general hospital setting: do nurses perceive it to be a problem? *Int J Nurs Practice* 4(2):126, 1998.

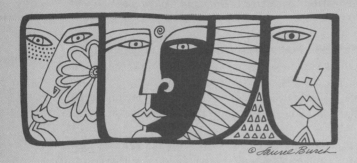

20

Communicating Assertively and Responsibly With Unpopular Clients

For the sake of the rose, the thorn is watered.

African proverb

OBJECTIVES

1. Describe characteristics of unpopular clients.
2. Identify possible reactions of nurses to unpopular clients.
3. Identify strategies to deal with negative attitudes and prevent antagonistic behavior toward unpopular clients.
4. Participate in selected exercises to build caring communication skills with unpopular clients.

WHO ARE THE UNPOPULAR CLIENTS?

It might surprise you to learn that all clients are not thought of or treated similarly. All nurses at some time have clients they do not like (Kus, 1990). Although there is nothing intrinsic that makes certain clients likable or not, there are clients whom nurses evaluate as popular or unpopular. This chapter will help you become more aware of how your prejudices about clients' behavior and personality affect how you relate to them. You will become more aware of client characteristics that trigger you to withdraw your caring. This knowledge will alert you to your negative tendencies and remind you to treat all your clients fairly, safely, and in a way that respects their dignity. Noncaring behaviors may lead to "missed diagnoses and interventions, social isolation, and minimal or negative contact with the nurse" (Maupin, 1998).

Before reading what the literature documents as the most popular and unpopular clients, take a moment to discover and examine your own attitudes toward your clients. Answer the following questions as specifically as possible:

- What are the characteristics of those clients with whom you enjoy working?
- What are the features of clients whom you find unpleasant?

Now, compare your answers to those of your colleagues in your class. Where do your views overlap? In what ways are your preferences and non-preferences for clients different? What do your collective opinions suggest to you about the client-nurse relationship?

In a classic study, Stockwell (1972) set out to determine whether there were clients whom the nursing team enjoyed caring for more than others, and whether there was any measurable difference in the nursing care afforded to the most and least popular clients. Her findings—startling at the time—still have potential impact for nurses. Stockwell reports that foreign clients, those hospitalized longer than 3 months, clients with some type of physical defect, and those with a psychiatric diagnosis figure significantly in the unpopular group. Personality factors of clients also play a significant part (sometimes the only one) in accounting for whether they are considered unpopular by the nursing team.

Stockwell's research findings reveal that unpopular clients do not generally receive individual holistic care, and that nurses withdraw their caring interpersonal communication from these clients. When clients do not fit into our molds, we become annoyed and respond to our anger by displacing it onto our clients as dislike (Gerrard, 1978).

In an investigation of the reactions of doctors and nurses to the attitudes and behaviors of surgical clients, Lorber (1975) found that medical staff label clients who interrupt well-established routines and make extra work for them as "problem" clients. Those who minimize the trouble they cause staff by being cooperative are considered "good."

Characteristics of Unpopular Clients and Their Effects on Nurses

Researchers (Kus, 1990; Lorber, 1975; Stockwell, 1972) say that unpopular clients have the following characteristics:

- Grumble or complain
- Indicate their lack of enjoyment at being in the hospital
- Imply that they are suffering more than nurses believe
- Suffer from conditions nurses feel could be better cared for in other units or in specialized hospitals
- Take up more time and attention than are deemed warranted
- Are complaining, uncooperative, or argumentative
- Have severe complications, poor prognoses, or difficult diagnoses
- Require extensive explanations, reassurance, or encouragement
- Are of low social value
- Are of low moral worth

- Have unchosen stigmata (such as sexual orientation, gender, race, or ethnicity)
- Have "own fault" diagnoses (such as alcoholism or lung cancer from heavy smoking)
- Have fear-causing conditions (such as highly contagious or incurable diseases; violent tendencies)
- Engender feelings of incompetence in nurses (have conditions about which nurses know little)

Nurses' Reactions to Unpopular Clients

Nurses feel:

- Frustrated and impatient with "grumblers and moaners"
- Afraid of being trapped or "caught" by complainers
- Irritated that unpopular clients waste their time
- Incompetent to provide the necessary care for complicated cases and psychiatric clients
- Relief when "unmanageables" are transferred
- Dissatisfaction with their jobs
- Changes in their health (such as insomnia or anorexia)

Nurses act by:

- Ignoring or avoiding demanding clients
- Indicating to demanding clients that others need their attention more
- Labeling demanding clients as nuisances or hypochondriacs
- Showing reluctance to provide necessary care if clients are thought to act inappropriately (e.g., repeated lewd behavior or aggressive language)
- Scolding and reprimanding
- Administering tranquilizers and sedatives to control their behavior
- Recommending transfer and discharge
- Requesting psychiatric consultation to manage unruly behavior
- Extending minimally adequate care
- Withdrawing from peers
- Becoming critical of the profession or the institution
- Withholding pain medication
- Ignoring clients' call lights or bells
- Being cool, detached, and insensitive
- Feeling guilty

This evidence suggests that nurses and other health professionals have definite ideas of what is acceptable client behavior and what is not. Look at the list you prepared earlier of client characteristics you dislike. How does it compare to the findings from the literature?

In contrast to unpopular clients, popular clients were found to have the following characteristics (Lorber, 1975; Stockwell, 1972):

- Were able to converse readily with nurses
- Knew the nurses' names
- Were able to joke and laugh with the nurses
- Were determined to get well again

- Were cooperative and compliant with therapeutic regimen
- Were manageable by routine methods
- Rarely complained of pain or discomfort
- Minimized the trouble they caused staff by being cooperative

Nurses demonstrated the following reactions to popular clients:

- Enjoyed interacting with clients who were "fun," had a good sense of humor, were easy to get along with, and friendly
- Gave superior care and did more for the popular client in the long run
- Treated them more leniently
- Gave them special favors and readily filled ordinary requests

Look again at your list of appealing client characteristics and compare your reactions to these findings from the literature.

We would all agree that each of our clients deserves to receive courteous care regardless of cultural background, chronicity of illness, personality, and type of illness (including the extent of complications). Is it not surprising to discover that despite the emphasis on compassion in our nursing education, we are unable to consistently extend respectful nursing care to all our clients? It is not humanly possible to like all our clients. It is, however, a professional expectation and responsibility that we treat all clients with courtesy and provide care that meets standards for nursing practice, regardless of whether or not we like our clients. Consider one nurse's admonition to

Wit and Wisdom

I'm Sick!

I'm grumpy today.
I'm sick, you see.
Please don't expect
The best of me.

The nicest of people
Can get angry and crass.
Be patient with me
And it will pass.

If I'm like this
with the flu, oh please,
Consider our clients
with major disease.

Copyright 1995 Julia W. Balzer Riley.

consider yourself lucky if the patient does complain, because this might give clues to unidentified problems and ways to improve the quality of care. A client afraid of soiling himself may express his fear as rage at the nurse who is delayed in answering the call light (Goldman, 1995).

To ignore or convey dislike to our clients is in direct contrast to the policy of nurturing a therapeutic helping relationship with them. When we show our dislike to clients, they feel unsupported. The message we convey is that they are unimportant and that we do not care about them or their problems. By extending our compassion, administering effective nursing interventions, and minimizing evidence of our dislike, we can be influential in eliminating some of the client behaviors we find problematic.

How to Overcome Negative Attitudes and Antagonistic Behavior Toward Unpopular Clients

You entered nursing so that you could be helpful to others. When you become aware of having negative feelings toward your clients, you are in a position to change such behavior. One effective approach is to try to perceive things from the clients' point of view. As trite as this sounds, it is difficult to do. Our dislikes and biases blind us from considering things from others' viewpoints. Changing your attitude will not automatically change your nursing behavior, but the effort to view your clients differently may help.

These examples will illustrate how to achieve this empathic perspective:

Situation One

Mrs. White is a 48-year-old accountant who has been diabetic since age 17. In the past 3 years she has been hospitalized for circulatory damage to her feet, resulting in amputation of two toes from both feet. She claims that she does not have time for adequate foot care as she is working long hours and is on her feet all day. On this admission she has several lesions on the remaining toes on both feet. If special skin care treatments are ineffective, Mrs. White faces the possibility of further amputations.

Your Possible Negative Attitude and Behavior

Your reaction to Mrs. White's predicament is one of disapproval. You think she is wasting valuable health care resources by occupying a hospital bed when she could have avoided the skin breakdown by a few extra minutes of attention to her feet each day. Taking better care of herself would have meant she would be out in the community leading a productive life instead of taking up expensive nursing services that others need. You resent her being on your unit and find yourself taking your time to answer her call bell, and leaving her alone for long periods. In the back of your mind you think that if she finds her hospital stay uncomfortable, she might take better precautions to avoid admission in the future.

Your awareness of how you are taking out your anger on Mrs. White by treating her disrespectfully (and possibly unsafely) is the first step in changing your behavior.

Seeing the Situation Through the Eyes of Your Client, Mrs. White

To help you change your behavior toward Mrs. White, it helps if you can see things from her point of view. Find a spot where you can think without being interrupted. Mentally put yourself in Mrs. White's position and attempt to understand how she might be thinking and feeling about being in the hospital. Your thoughts might go something like this:

"I have to wait so long for the nurse to answer the bell. It's not like I overuse the privilege. I wish they would come sooner, especially when I need the bedpan. I feel so helpless in here; I can't do a thing for myself it seems. I'm so used to being independent. I'll do anything to get healed and get out of the hospital. The pain I'm having makes me wish I'd been more stringent about my foot care. I hope they don't have to operate. I don't know if I'd be able to walk without a walker if they remove any more toes. How could I work then?"

Taking the time to imagine how you would feel in Mrs. White's position is a beginning. Instead of focusing on her neglect, this exercise may help you to pay attention to her distress here and now. Your fresh empathic viewpoint may help you treat her more respectfully.

You might now respond to her call bell more quickly and extend your warmth to her. You might seek her out when you have a few extra minutes and explore her reactions to her illness and hospitalization. Instead of aggressively taking out your anger on Mrs. White, you might be more direct and confront her about her noncompliant foot care. Your problem-solving ability and empathic listening skills will help you to assess what prevents her from performing more rigorous skin care. From there you can help her work out a plan to overcome these blocks. By making your interventions more positive, you will help her reduce her anxiety about her predicament.

It is responsible to focus your attention on becoming more empathic with this client. Empathy does not always come easily. This fuller vision provides you with more data to complete the nursing process. When you see both sides, it is more likely that you will act assertively, taking into account not only your feelings but also those of your client.

Situation Two

Mr. Evans is a 39-year-old client in the terminal stages of cancer. Although he has only been hospitalized on your unit for the past 4 weeks, he has been in and out with exacerbations for the past year. He is weak, and most caregivers are certain he will die soon. He is in isolation and requires extensive dressing changes to open areas on his legs. The ulcerated area is draining purulent matter and has a foul odor that is almost suffocating. Mr. Evans has lost 40 pounds over the last year and is emaciated. The darkened areas under his eyes, sagging skin, and low energy level create the impression that he is barely hanging on to life with each breath he takes.

Your Possible Negative Attitude and Behavior

It is painful for you to even enter his Mr. Evans' room because you are reminded of the times when he had color in his cheeks and kept you on your toes with his engaging sense of humor. You miss his former self and feel saddened about his impending death. You are distressed because you gag and feel nauseated when you change his dressings. When you go into his room to administer his care you feel trapped. You are at a loss for what to say and you just want to get your physical nursing care done so that you can leave. You work at top speed and leave as soon as his dressings are done.

Seeing the Situation Through the Eyes of Your Client, Mr. Evans

Find the time and place to quietly contemplate how Mr. Evans thinks and feels. Try to imagine things from his perspective. Your thoughts might go something like this:

"I'm ready to go. I wish I could just die soon. I'm so uncomfortable, I can't sleep, and I'm bored when I'm awake. I'd really like some company. I must be a sight to look at, though. No wonder everyone looks shocked when they see me. It's lonely waiting."

Taking the opportunity to try to imagine how Mr. Evans is reacting generates several ways you could intervene to be more helpful. This exercise in empathy helps you to focus on how he is here and now as opposed to emphasizing how he used to be.

Even though Mr. Evans does not have much energy to talk, you could arrange to spend time in his room and read to him, or arrange for some music he likes. He might be comforted by a back rub. Reading the paper to him, writing letters for him, or updating him on events are several activities that require minimal energy from him, yet allow him contact with you. Ensuring that his analgesics are administered consistently so that he is pain free, and reminding him to change his position frequently in the bed are measures that will increase his ability to relax.

Deodorizing the room frequently would make the environment more pleasant for him, his visitors, and staff. To help you manage through the dressing changes you could wear a mask and increase all the positive stimuli that you can think of (music playing, flowers within view, window open). It might help distract your attention from the unpleasant odor if you can start telling him a story when you are doing a dressing change. The activity would keep your mind focused on something more positive.

It is assertive to consider the situation from your clients' viewpoints as well as from your own. If we only concentrate on negative aspects, we are likely to act aggressively and only attempt to achieve our own goals. It is responsible to see things from other angles so that we can generate plans that consider the perspective of our clients. All our clients have the right to feel cared for.

Think About It...
What, So What, and Now What?

Consider what you read about unpopular clients. Could you identify any of your own problem areas? Write the answers to the following questions.

What? . . .   Write one thing you learned from this chapter.

So what? . . .   How will this impact your nursing practice?

Now what? . . .   How will you implement this new knowledge or skill?

THINK ABOUT IT

Practicing Communicating With Unpopular Clients

Exercise 1

Following are six situations depicting unpopular clients. Possible reactions that you might have to these "problem" clients are suggested. Your task is to put yourself in the clients' places and imagine what the situation feels like from their perspective. Then your task is to indicate how these insights would free you to interact in a more caring way with your clients. Be sure that your new approaches are assertive and responsible.

1. A 73-year-old foreign client refuses to eat his hospital food. He is on a special diet and it is important that he ingest only what the nutritionist and physician have ordered. His wife brings him food that is rich in spices and sauces. Both the client and his wife complain when the ethnic food is withdrawn and hospital food is the only choice.

You feel furious that this client is unwilling to abide by the good judgment of the physician and nutritionist. You feel disdain that he has abused his body for so many years, and are amazed that he will not take advantage of the good advice being offered by his caretakers. You avoid eye contact with this client, do not speak to his wife, and spend little time with him. You curtly order him to eat the hospital diet when you deliver his meal tray and you make a point of picking up his tray so that you can check how much he ate. When his intake has been less than adequate, you tell him you will not remove his tray until he has eaten more.

- Put yourself in this client's place and imagine what things are like from his perspective.
- With your new insight, how would you act assertively and responsibly towards your client?

2. Betty is a 16-year-old girl on your orthopedic unit. She has been in traction for 2 months after a car accident and has multiple fractures and burns. Her parents' home is over a hundred miles away, and they only visit Betty every third weekend. Betty is terribly homesick and cries for hours after her parents leave. She hates being in traction and just wants to go home. She is withdrawn and refuses to do any of the occupational therapy projects her therapist provides. She does not encourage any interaction with the other two teenagers on the unit, despite their extensive efforts to divert her attention away from her unhappy situation. She is curt and stoic with the nursing and physical therapy staff, doing the minimum of what is required of her.

You have been Betty's nurse since her admission to the unit. At first you were enthusiastic that you could cheer her up and encourage her to make the best of her situation. When she did not respond positively to your efforts and continued to be morose about being on the unit, you started to withdraw from her. Your once vivacious conversation has become almost nonexistent, and you find yourself talking to the other clients or nurses in the room instead of Betty. When you have a few spare minutes you refrain from spending them with Betty. After her parents leave one night you scold her for "acting like a baby" when you find her crying.

- Put yourself in this client's place and imagine what things are like from her perspective.
- With your new insight, how would you act assertively and responsibly towards Betty?

3. Miss Kerns is a 47-year-old school teacher who was transferred to your medical unit from the psychiatric unit upstairs. Over the past 2 years she has been admitted to psychiatry for bouts of de-

Continued

Practicing Communicating With Unpopular Clients—cont'd

pression of unknown origin. Many modalities (medication, psychotherapy, physical therapies) have been employed without success to treat her depression. She is on your unit for investigation of medical reasons for her low moods. She looks sullen and poorly groomed and mopes around in a housecoat instead of getting dressed. She rarely volunteers to speak to any of the staff, and when you initiate a conversation it is a tense situation, because she is slow to respond and often just nods or sighs.

After some time you begin to realize that you have invested little time in getting to know Miss Kerns. You have expended almost no effort finding out about her likes, dislikes, and reaction to being in the hospital. It becomes apparent that you are ignoring her because she is not easy to talk to and because you believe she does not belong on the unit. You are a bit frightened of her flattened affect, and the thought that she might be malingering bothers you.

- Put yourself in this client's place and imagine what things are like from her perspective.
- With your new insight, how would you act assertively and responsibly toward Miss Kerns?

4. Mr. Dire is a 79-year-old client who has just undergone successful cataract surgery in the outpatient surgical center where you work. Preoperatively he asked many questions and expressed fears about the surgery. You tried to reassure him, but he still kept asking for you and delayed you in your morning schedule. After a successful surgical procedure and patient teaching, he was sent home in the center's van. After he got home he began to call every 15 minutes with questions. Did he leave his raincoat there? Did you give him an appointment card for a visit to his physician? Was he eligible for a home health nurse? When he sensed impatience in your voice, he snapped at you and said, "Don't get mouthy with me, girlie! I paid good money for this surgery, and you're there to answer my questions. I'm going to report you to the doctor!"

You are angry because you have taken extra time with him and tried to be sensitive, something that is a matter of pride to you. You are embarrassed because you did tell him he should be glad he just had cataract surgery and nothing more serious.

- Put yourself in your client's place and imagine what things are like from his perspective.
- With your new insight, how would you act responsibly and assertively?

5. Mrs. Gambino delivered a healthy 6-pound boy this morning. Although she is an experienced mother (she has a 12-year-old son and an 11-year-old daughter), she acts otherwise. She asks you to supervise everything she does with her baby. She constantly asks you to repeat all your instructions. Knowing she, like many other mothers on the unit, is to be discharged within 48 hours, you feel pressured by her demands. Your attention only temporarily alleviates her anxiety, and you feel overwhelmed by her and the rest of your patient assignment. You find yourself being abrupt with her and trying to get another staff member to answer her calls.

- Put yourself in Mrs. Gambino's place and imagine what things are like from her perspective.
- With your new insight, how would you act assertively and responsibly toward her?

6. A 42-year-old man arrives at the emergency room after taking an overdose of pills. This is his third suicide attempt in 3 months. His wife moved out 6 months ago, leaving a note saying she would not return. She has had no further contact with her husband, who was left with the responsibility of raising their two teenage sons.

You are shocked that a father could be so selfish and irresponsible. You feel resentful that he is using up costly ER services when you have other clients who really need you, who couldn't help it that they are in the ER. Your first reaction is "not him again." You have an urge to tell him that he needs to stop feeling sorry for himself and get on with taking care of his boys. Your anger toward him is smoldering, yet you are uncertain about what to say or how to approach him. Deep down you are frightened by his self-destructiveness.

- Put yourself in this man's place and imagine what things are like from his perspective.
- With your new insight, how would you respond assertively and responsibly toward him?

After you have done this exercise by yourself, get together with your colleagues in your class and compare your approaches. What similarities and differences were there in your ideas about how the client in each example viewed things? Check to see when your suggestions differ and where they're alike.

Exercise 2

Think of a current client whom you consider unpopular or problematic. Make note of the specific aspects of the patient's behavior that are annoying you. Elaborate on how this client makes you feel and react. Then try to imagine how your client is viewing things. Take time to discover his or her point of view. Next, think about how your insight can help generate more positive approaches to your unpopular client. After you have done this exercise on your own, share your creative approaches with your colleagues.

Finally, carry out your more responsible and assertive plan with your client. Note how you feel and how your client reacts to your new approach. Compare experiences with your fellow students.

Moments of Connection...
A Novel Approach

A patient who had been in an automobile accident had multiple rib fractures. It was a priority for him to do his pulmonary exercises and coughing to avoid the need for mechanical ventilation. However, the patient was whiny and resistant. All of us were becoming irritated with him. Having cared for him for a while, I had the intuition to try a new approach. I walked in and said, "How is my favorite patient today?" He smiled and cooperated for the first time without whining or stalling.

Wit and Wisdom

It Has Not Happened to Me . . . Yet

I cannot see
Inside of you
To know your story
To give you your due.

When I have not walked
A mile in your shoes,
To your real pain
I have no clues.

I blame and rage at
What I cannot control.
Powerlessness and frustration
Can take their toll.

I'll suspend my judgment,
My tongue I'll hold.
I'll listen and learn
And try not to scold.

Copyright 1995 Julia W. Balzer Riley.

References

Gerrard B: Interpersonal skills for health professionals: a review of the literature, unpublished manuscript, 1978.

Goldman MC: If we're lucky the patient will complain, *Am J Nurs* 9(2):52, 1995.

Johnson M, Webb C: Rediscovering unpopular patients: the concept of social judgment, *J Adv Nurs* 21(3):466, 1995.

Kus RF: Nurses and unpopular clients, *Am J Nurs* 90(6):62, 1990.

Lorber J: Good patients and problem patients: conformity and deviance in a general hospital, *J Health Soc Behav* 16(2):213, 1975.

Maupin CR: The potential for noncaring when dealing with difficult patients: strategies for moral decision-making, *J Cardiovasc Nurs* 9(3):11, 1995.

Stockwell F: *The unpopular patient,* London, 1972, Royal College of Nursing, White Friars Press, Ltd. (Republished in 1984 by Groom Helm Limited, London.)

Suggestions for Further Reading

Barnes KE: An examination of nurses' feelings about patients with specific feeding needs, *J Adv Nurs* 15(6):703, 1990.

Beebe LH: Reframe your outlook on recidivism, *J Psychosoc Nurs* 28(9):31, 1990.

Boland BK: Fear of AIDS in nursing staff, *Nurs Manage* 21(6):40, 1990.

Carey N, Jones SL, O'Tolle AW: Do you feel powerless when a patient refuses medication? *J Psychosoc Nurs* 28(10):19, 1990.

    Clients have the right to refuse medications, and this study reports nursing responses to this behavior. This article expands nurses' understanding of common nursing reactions to medication refusal. The first step in acting differently to unpopular client behavior is to know our own reactions.

Korniewicz DM, O'Brien ME, Larson E: Coping with AIDS and HIV, *J Psychosoc Nurs* 28(3):14, 1990.

Lowenhaupt MT, Tselikis P: Consider the underlying motives of difficult patients, *Ophthalmol Times* 23(17):36, Sept 1998.

    Detailed information for an office setting.

Myers IB: *Gifts differing,* Palo Alto, Calif, 1980, Consulting Psychologists Press.

    This readable, comprehensive book on personality type describes how our differences in preferences for perceiving and thinking can lead to lack of appreciation and discrimination of others with unfamiliar and different preferences. Guidelines for communicating effectively with different types are outlined.

Sharp D: Difficult patients, *Hippocrates* 12(3):50, 1998.

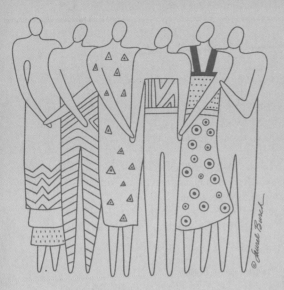

21

Managing Team Conflict Assertively and Responsibly

Work hard, keep the ceremonies, live peaceably, and unite your hearts.

Hopi Indian proverb

OBJECTIVES

1. Define conflict.
2. Identify four categories of conflict.
3. Describe behaviors in the four stages of team development.
4. Identify the steps of win-win conflict resolution.
5. Contrast win-win, lose-win, and win-lose methods of handling team conflict.
6. Participate in selected exercises to build assertive conflict-resolution skills.

WHAT IS CONFLICT?

"Conflict arises when individuals hold incompatible or seemingly incompatible ideas, interests, or values, but conflict can only occur where interdependency exists. For this reason conflict resolution is necessary to preserve and improve relationships with others as well as meet one's own needs" (Cushnie, 1988). Whenever two people come together, there is potential for conflict. Although conflict is sometimes inevitable, it can result in advantageous outcomes when handled in assertive and responsible ways.

Wit and Wisdom

The soul would have no rainbow if the eyes had no tears.

Minquass Indian proverb

Cushnie (1988) identifies the following four categories of conflicts intensifying in degree of difficulty from top to bottom:

Facts

Differences about data. These disagreements can be resolved by terminating debate and seeking information from reliable sources.

Methods

Differences about how something is done. Conflict about methods occurs when there is no absolute standard shared by all parties affected by the issue. Resolving conflicts of this kind includes acknowledging that there is more than one way to accomplish the same goal or task. A way to minimize this type of conflict is to establish criteria for method selection.

Goals

Differences about desired outcomes. Discussion often reveals that parties share a common concern. If they are able to identify a common goal, this redefinition opens up new opportunities for problem solving.

Values

Differences in belief systems are the most complex type of conflict, requiring a high level of motivation from involved parties to understand each other's beliefs. If parties can avoid the divisiveness of allocating others' viewpoints to rigid categories of "right" or "wrong," and find compatible goals, they are on their way to conflict management (Cushnie, 1988).

There are several forms of conflict (Kinder, 1981):

- Intrapersonal conflict occurs within an individual.
- Interpersonal conflict occurs between two individuals or among members of a group.
- Intragroup conflict occurs within an established group.
- Intergroup conflict is the struggle between groups.

The focus of this chapter is on interpersonal conflict in the context of a workplace or school setting.

Health care teams are composed of people with many different backgrounds. A variety of professional outlooks are found in a team of nurses, physicians, clergy, nutritionists, occupational

---

Box 21-1   **Team Members: the 4 Cs**

1. The *Contributor* provides good information, is dependable, does detail work, but may need assistance to see the big picture and understand the background for the project at hand.
2. The *Collaborator* is open, flexible, imaginative, and willing to implement projects, but may need to be focused on steps to be taken.
3. The *Communicator* helps facilitate the team, builds consensus and enthusiasm, and resolves conflict, but may need to be refocused from the process to team results.
4. The *Challenger* helps the team take risks, is adventuresome, and has principles, but may need to be diverted from more risky ideas and focus on realistic steps to get team results.

From Pillemer K, Johnson PT, 1998.

Box 21-2   **Stages of Team Development**

Conflict is a normal, healthy part of team development. Without healthy disagreement, quality problem solving is compromised. Four stages are forming, storming, norming, and performing. Think about individual development, and consider how the stages compare. Forming is like childhood. Storming is like adolescence. Norming is like young adulthood. Performing is like adulthood.

In *forming,* people are polite yet impersonal, testing the water, unsure about their commitment. The team is figuring out team goals, testing out group relationships, and beginning to get a clear idea about the work to be done.

In *storming,** overt or covert conflict may be evident; people may be hostile, engage in power struggles, be apathetic, and not do great work. People are resisting the process of teamwork. People resist cohesion and collaboration and do not have a commitment to the team.

In *norming,* the group is getting organized, figuring out necessary rules and norms to get the work done, confronting problems and issues in a constructive way, and giving feedback. People clarify the goals of the team and define the tasks and procedures for the work to be done. People move into cohesion and collaboration, and they demonstrate commitment.

In *performing,* the work is getting done. People are open, can collaborate, and are flexible and productive. People begin to do quality work, respect and support one another, motivate others by group achievement, and become flexible in their roles.

Modified from Balzer Riley J, 1997.
*This is a vulnerable time for teams if members do not understand that conflict is normal and necessary at this point for team development.

and physical therapists, social workers, and others. In addition to the differences in socialization that these professionals bring, they carry personal views based on sex, age, cultural origins, socioeconomic situations, and life experience. This potpourri is a potential source of conflict on any health care team (Box 21-1).

This variety gives birth to different perceptions about an issue, and the role and obligations each should fulfill. When team members do not see eye-to-eye about the situation or their respective roles, then the potential for conflict is great.

Many times team members have different (or opposing) ideological views on a situation. Their views may come from having different objectives or from endorsing different priorities among the objectives. Conflict results when team members do not agree on what to do, how to do it, and when to do it (Box 21-2).

Occasionally conflict will resurface between team members who have had a long history of disagreement. The degree of trust and collaboration has been worn down between these people, and their competitiveness is sharpened. Such a situation fuels conflict.

CONFLICT RESOLUTION

You know you cannot avoid conflict. What you can avoid is feeling impotent or uncomfortable when you encounter conflict situations. By now you are familiar with assertive and responsible communication. These approaches will help you resolve conflicts in constructive ways.

Resolving a conflict means acting in such a way that an agreement is reached that is acceptable, and even pleasing, to both parties. If both parties cannot agree on a resolution, the conflict will continue. When conflict drags out and team members do not see a hopeful resolution on the horizon, then helplessness prevails. Any health care team that is stuck in this hopeless situation is not working at its full capacity. Harrington-Mackin (1994) advises dealing with conflicts in a timely way and suggests that most people find it difficult to openly discuss and work through conflicts. Instead, they collect grudges and use techniques such as procrastination and sniping to "get even." Client care and morale suffer when conflicts are unresolved.

You can approach conflict resolution in three ways: win-win; lose-win; or win-lose. Although win-win is preferable, there may be times when a workable compromise is the best solution possible to avoid having both parties lose. Throughout this book the point has been made that assertiveness is a matter of choice. There may be times when you feel obligated to insist on your solution to a problem, in parenting a small child, for example. There may be times when you choose to allow the other person to win, such as when you recognize that a colleague has been pushed to the limit and your position seems less important than the peace of mind of your colleague.

The win-win approach to conflict resolution requires you to be assertive and responsible. This approach results in a solution with which you and your colleagues are happy. Not only is the outcome satisfactory, but using a win-win approach uses your full creativity and often results in a unique and innovative resolution.

The lose-win approach is one where you allow your colleagues to resolve the conflict at your expense. Either you are not happy with the outcome or you permit your colleagues to walk all over you. This approach is nonassertive and irresponsible.

The win-lose approach is the opposite of the lose-win approach. You may resolve the conflict in a way satisfying to you, but in the process you bulldoze right over the rights of your colleagues. This approach is aggressive and irresponsible.

Any win-lose/lose-win approach creates forces that aggravate the struggle and do little to discover constructive solutions acceptable to all involved (Likert, Likert, 1976). A conflict is more constructive when the outcome is satisfying to all the participants than if it is satisfying to only some. Conflict at some point is inevitable, so it helps to know how to use it as an opportunity to be constructive—because the alternatives have unpleasant consequences.

A win-win conflict management strategy involves covering each of these steps:

1. See the problem in terms of needs (what is required) instead of solutions (what should be done) in order to facilitate a mutual problem-solving approach; detach yourself from biases and stay focused on the actual data.
2. Consider the problem as a mutual one to be solved, requiring the active involvement of all affected.
3. Describe the conflict as specifically as possible, using undistorted data.
4. Identify the differences between concerned parties before attempting to resolve the conflict.
5. See the conflict from another point of view.
6. Use brainstorming to arrive at possible solutions instead of using the first or most convenient idea.
7. Select the solution that best meets both parties' needs and all possible consequences.
8. Reach an agreement about how the conflict is to end and not recur.
9. Plan who will do what and where and when it will be done.
10. After the plan has been implemented, evaluate the problem-solving process and review how well the solution turned out (ANA, 1990).

Table 21-1 summarizes three different approaches to conflict. The assertive/responsible attitude toward conflict and approach to conflict resolution are contrasted with the nonassertive/irresponsible approaches.

Assertive and Responsible Ways to Overcome Conflict

On health care teams, conflict can involve all members or only a few. How to manage conflict using a win-win approach in both these instances is explored.

A Conflict Situation Involving the Whole Health Care Team

1. Before you can do anything to resolve a conflict, you need to fully understand the conflict, including your thoughts and feelings about the situation, as well as the thoughts of your colleagues. If you try to resolve a conflict without completing an assessment, you will probably overlook an important factor that could result in an unsatisfactory resolution.

Example: You believe that clients have the right to be informed about any untoward side effects they might experience when taking a prescribed medication. On your unit, few clients are told in advance of the potential side effects. This omission is incompatible with your beliefs about good nursing care and client rights. You discover that many of your colleagues, the other nurses and physicians on your team, prefer to keep knowledge of side effects from clients so that they will be more likely to take the medication. Here the conflict is incompatible activities (informing/not informing) and beliefs (autonomy/dependency) about clients' rights.

2. To fully understand your side of the conflict, you need to examine your own thoughts and feelings. You cannot complete this step in a hurry. You need to sit down (with paper and pencil if necessary) and discover your answers to the following questions:

What is it about this conflict that bothers me?

In thinking about the conflict you might have some of the following thoughts:

- "It bothers me that clients are not warned about side effects they might get from the medications."
- "It's not right that they don't have full knowledge of the treatment, and that they are choosing to take the pills without fully understanding the implications."

- "I feel that it is dishonest to withhold information about side effects from clients."
- "I believe that people have the responsibility to decide what they should do about their health. By withholding information, we are keeping the control of clients' health in our hands."

Answering this question makes it clearer what the conflict means to you. You have a strong value that clients should be given the information they need to make the best decision about what health behavior to adopt.

Our initial reaction to a conflict situation is often influenced more by emotion than intellect. The tension or anxiety creates a "fight or flight" stress response, and the intensity of the stress response varies in relation to the degree of threat perceived (Cushnie, 1988). Taking time to sort out your emotional reactions as you just did helps to control your emotions and facilitate your effectiveness in conflict management.

What resolution to this conflict would be satisfactory for me?

In thinking about how you would like to have the conflict resolved, you come up with the following idea:

"The most satisfactory resolution for me would be to institute a policy that all clients will be informed in advance about any possible side effects of any medication prescribed for them."

It is important to answer this question. Often we know there is a conflict but we are uncertain about how we want it resolved. The clearer you can be in answering these questions, the more articulate you will be to others about your stand on the issue.

3. Discover what your colleagues' responses are to the same two questions you just answered yourself. This step requires you to invest time and energy, but you need this information to have a complete understanding of the conflict. The best approach is to arrange a time to sit down with your colleagues and find out:

What is it about the conflict that bothers them?

Your colleagues may come up with some of the following ideas:

- "If we told every client about possible side effects, it would take too much time."
- "If clients knew all the possible side effects, they might not take the medications and then they'd never benefit from them."
- "I believe that we should not scare clients by telling them everything that can go wrong. After all, they're already sick. Why add to their worries?"

You are learning that your colleagues have their clients' interests at heart when they avoid telling them about the side effects. They have raised a significant point about the time factor as well. Discovering alternative viewpoints will expand your awareness of conflict you encounter.

What is a satisfactory resolution to the conflict for your colleagues?

These are some examples of what your colleagues might tell you:

- "The only solution I can see is to tell only those clients who ask about the side effects."
- "I think we should only give out information about the most common and significant side effects so that clients will be inclined to take their medication."
- "I think we should continue as usual. I've never known any client who was upset about not knowing the side effects of the medications. They need the medications to get well again."

TABLE 21-1	Assertive/Responsible Versus Nonassertive/ Irresponsible Ways of Handling Team Conflict		
Characteristics	**Win-win**	**Lose-win**	**Win-lose**
Attitude toward conflict	Assumes conflict is inevitable and occurs whenever people work together	Assumes conflicts are sent to try us	Sees conflict as a challenge to be won
	Assumes conflict can be managed so that creative solutions are achieved	Assumes in a conflict the other person always wins	Considers manipulation needed to win conflicts is never ceasing and thinks fighting is required to get what you want
	Assumes controversy involves everyone in the issue and increases members' commitment	Assumes it is a foregone conclusion that the plan to resolve the conflict will satisfy only others	Feels the other person is trying hard to win
	Assumes conflict can be resolved in ways that are satisfying to all team members	Wonders why there must be conflict in the workplace	
Approach to conflict resolution	Employs a systematic problem-solving approach	Decides in advance that the other person will win and gives up	Keeps fighting with biased information that supports own viewpoint
Data collection	Examines own thoughts and feelings objectively	Prematurely closes data collection	Only seeks, examines, and submits data that support own desired resolution
	Listens empathically to colleagues' points of view	Assumes it is hopeless to collect data because of irrational belief that others will win regardless	
	Seeks relevant information from appropriate resources (literature, consultants)	Dwells on how bad things will be when the conflict is resolved in "opponent's" favor	

TABLE 21-1	Assertive/Responsible Versus Nonassertive/ Irresponsible Ways of Handling Team Conflict—cont'd		
Characteristics	**Win-win**	**Lose-win**	**Win-lose**
	Shares knowledge of conflict with all others involved	Passively participates in information sharing	
	Does not make inferences in data collection phase		
	Remains objective		
Assessment	Formulates an accurate definition of the conflict	Defines conflict in terms of how it affects colleagues	Does not seek out colleagues' assessment of the conflict
	Shares assessment with colleagues	Gives up defining conflict from own point of view	Overwhelmingly argues own assessment of the conflict
	Acknowledges colleagues' perceptions of the conflict		
Resolution generating	Considers resolutions that satisfy all involved	Contributes little to this planning because of assumption that winner will tell loser what to do	Only considers or supports plans that agree with own interpretation of the conflict
	Chooses resolutions that maximize the benefits and minimize the drawbacks		Sabotages plans that oppose own view
Evaluation	Maintains vigilance to ensure that resolution continues to satisfy self and colleagues on the team	Complains that resolution could never be successful; is disgruntled	Ignores the fact that others are not satisfied with the resolution

These suggestions from your colleagues tell you that they value something more than client autonomy: they value compliance and recovery from illness. You have learned that some of your colleagues are agreeable to informing clients about side effects under certain circumstances.

Finding the answers to these questions will take your best interpersonal communication skills. When you are invested in an issue, it becomes harder to see other points of view. In a conflict situation it is important to listen actively to what your colleagues have to say and check out that you have understood their side of the issue.

4. In addition to information obtained from the thoughts and feelings of the people involved in the conflict, you may need information from other sources. In this example you could seek the counsel of the hospital's legal advisor about the rights of your clients. There may be a Clients' Rights Committee that could advise you.

For example, your legal counsel may advise you that "Clients have the right by law to be informed of any likely untoward effects of any treatment regimen, unless such information would be considered by the caregivers to be threatening to the client's well-being."

A guideline like this is sufficiently nonspecific so that your health care team would have to make its own interpretation of its application.

5. Once you have fully explored how you and your colleagues feel about the conflict and you have acquired any other relevant information, the next step is to search for a resolution that will be satisfactory to all of you. This is no easy feat; the win-win approach takes time and effort.

One creative approach at this stage is to brainstorm. Out of brainstorming is likely to come a creative and original resolution to your conflict (D'Zurilla, Goldfried, 1971). It is important that everyone involved in the conflict has an opportunity to contribute ideas about how to resolve it. In this example, there should be representation from nurses, physicians, and clients.

In the brainstorming process it is important that every idea be considered and that no ideas are ridiculed or deleted. Using this rule means that team members must acknowledge and respect each other's ideas. This action of listening to one other will help to diffuse any hostility that may have arisen as the conflict grew. In a conflict, competition often reigns, with individuals wanting to get their own way; brainstorming ensures that team members communicate in a cooperative way.

In this situation the following suggestions for resolution of the conflict were put forward:

- Give information about side effects only to clients who ask for it.
- Before clients start on a medication they must be able to recite its benefits and side effects.
- Leave a copy of the drug description manual in the clients' common room so that any clients who wish to check on the side effects can do so.
- Give clients copies of the telephone numbers of the pharmaceutical companies so that they can call a representative and find out any information about drugs that are prescribed for them.
- Have the pharmacist prepare information sheets about the side effects of clients' drugs that would be available for them to keep and review.
- Give a card to every client admitted to the unit that defines the "right to know" policy concerning side effects of treatments and medications, and indicates that clients need only ask the staff to receive this information.
- Wait until clients experience side effects and then clearly explain them.
- Initiate a policy of inviting questions from clients about the side effects of a medication.

You can see that the suggestions represent a variety of points of view.

6. The next step is to choose an acceptable resolution from the many suggestions put forth. The most expedient action to take on this unit is to form a committee composed of staff members representing both sides of the conflict, as well as clients and administrators of the unit.

You are selected as a member who favors informed consent. Another nurse—with the point of view that informing clients can cause unnecessary problems—is also selected. The head nurse, one physician, and a representative from the Clients' Rights Committee, complete the membership.

This committee has the responsibility to develop a policy about what information to give clients concerning side effects of their medications. The decision it makes must meet certain criteria in a win-win approach to conflict resolution. It must satisfy both points of view, be feasible to carry out on the unit (in terms of cost, staffing abilities), and be legally sound.

7. The next step is to systematically review the pros and cons of the eligible resolutions remaining. At this stage, team members must remain open to others' points of view and give all members a chance to defend or refute points. When a group is trying to reach the best decision, it must create a climate that allows members to speak freely.

Consider the effect that the possibility of territoriality or competition among members might have on communication. Members sabotage each other by providing misleading or biased information that leads to mistrust. When the communication breaks down this way, it is unlikely that the best decision will be chosen because the database will be incomplete and inaccurate. It takes a concerted effort by the members and the leader to ensure that all points of view are encouraged and respected.

8. After considerable discussion, the group narrows down the choices for resolution to the following:

- Give a card to clients when they are admitted to the unit that advises them that they have the right to know the side effects of any medications, and that they need only ask the staff to receive this information.
- Nurses and physicians should initiate a policy of inviting questions from clients about the side effects of their medications at the time clients are started on a new medication.
- Before clients start a medication, they must be able to recite its benefits and side effects.

After much deliberation, the committee decides that distributing cards for clients would be too expensive. The members come up with the idea of adding the following paragraph to the "Permission For Treatment" sheet that all clients must sign on admission:

I am aware that all treatments, including medications, have benefits as well as potential untoward effects. I am aware that I have the right to ask my caregivers about these possible negative effects, and that I can expect to have any information explained to me in language that I am able to understand. I am aware that, if after careful consideration I refuse to comply fully with the suggested regimen (treatments and medications), this action will in no way jeopardize the care I receive by the health care team in this hospital.

Signature _____ Date_____
Witness _____

This action appeals to all members of the committee. They feel it would inform clients of their rights at the beginning of their hospital stay and instill the idea that their questions would be welcomed and answered in a clear way.

The second decision made by the committee is to endorse as unit policy the following suggestion:

Each time clients start on a new medication they will be informed of the benefits and untoward effects in a simple, clear way. At this time they will be invited and encouraged to ask any questions.

It takes the committee a lot of time to arrive at this decision. None of the committee members has difficulty with the suggestion of telling clients about the benefits of medications, but they are reluctant to explain the potential hazards. After looking at the issue from many angles, all members agree that it is unfair to give only half of the picture to clients. A compromise is drawn whereby all concur that only the most likely side effects should be explained to clients and the probability of their occurrence would be specified. Any known corrective action would also be made known to clients (such as laxative for constipation, extra fluids and chewing gum for dryness in the mouth, avoiding abrupt movements for vertigo).

Committee members agree that the workload for launching this new policy will be shared between physicians and nurses. A physician prescribing a new medication will be responsible for explaining the rationale, benefits, and risks to clients, and will invite questions. This delegation will mean that nurses will not solely incur the extra time that implementing this policy would demand.

In addition, it has been decided that the medication nurse will follow up the physician's explanation when the first dosage of the medication is administered. At that time the nurse will find out what the clients understand about the benefits and risks, confirm the facts, correct the errors, and invite any further questions. Sharing the responsibility between physicians and nurses makes the time commitment feasible for both parties.

The committee stresses that no health professional be expected to remember the side effects of a multitude of medications. Referring to pharmaceutical references and consulting with the hospital pharmacist are encouraged.

The resolutions arrived at by the committee are satisfactory to all team members and are feasible from an administrative point of view.

9. The process does not stop at the point of agreeing on a resolution. Once the plan is implemented, a follow-up evaluation must be carried out to determine if the health care team remains satisfied with the implementation of the resolution. Questions to complete this evaluation might include:

- Do those who felt strongly that clients have a right to know about side effects feel that clients are being correctly informed?
- Do those who objected because it could be time consuming and frightening for clients feel that the new plan avoids these negative consequences?
- Are clients of the opinion that their rights are being respected?
- Is the resolution being carried out without undue drawbacks in terms of cost-effectiveness and staffing patterns?

In this example the committee decides to meet 6 weeks after the resolution has been adopted to evaluate its effectiveness.

This health care team handled its conflict using a win-win conflict resolution strategy. All sides were asked to contribute their opinions in order to resolve the conflict. This action was assertive because it prevented any one side from coloring the picture or totally biasing the issue. It was responsible because it considered all the data available in the conflict situation: thoughts and feelings of both parties and objective data from a legal perspective.

A Conflict Situation Involving Two Team Members

In contrast to the previous situation, conflict situations can be isolated to a small segment of the health care team. An example in which two team members are in conflict will be examined next.

Example: You and David are two nursing students on the same medical unit in a general hospital. You are a student in an early clinical experience and David is in his graduating year. You are studying the concept of loss and its effects on body image. You wish to have Mr. Partain as your client because he has recently had a severe myocardial infarction, and it is unlikely that he will be able to resume his former job. Since he has suffered a loss in physical function that affects other areas of his life, he would make an excellent candidate for your assignment.

David has been assigned as Mr. Partain's nurse and has been caring for him for the past 3 days. When you ask David if he would switch and let you take on Mr. Partain's care, David refuses on the grounds that he needs to learn about postcardiac care for an assignment he is doing.

At the moment, Mr. Partain is the most suitable candidate for both these students. There is a conflict over limited resources in this situation.

1. The first step to take is to uncover all the information about the conflict. Accomplishing this task involves being open and listening actively. One technique for ensuring that you really understand the conflict from the other's point of view is to reflect with empathy to each statement your colleague makes. Here is an example:

David: "I think we have a problem here because I need to continue my care of Mr. Partain to understand how postcardiac clients adjust to the limited activity level and cope with the fear of resuming normal functioning. I can't change with you."

At this point it would be tempting for you to justify that you too need to study Mr. Partain's recovery to understand his loss. Such a defensive approach would escalate your conflict. Instead, to understand the conflict from David's point of view, all you are allowed to do at this point is to reflect with empathy his thoughts and feelings. You will soon get your turn to state things from your point of view.

You: "You want to continue nursing Mr. Partain for a longer period of time so that you will really understand the reaction of postcardiac patients to changes in their activity levels."

This response allows your colleague to feel understood and encourages him to reveal more of his point of view.

David: "This is one of my last assignments before I graduate and I'm afraid if I give up Mr. Partain now I would not find another postcardiac client on whom to do my assignment."

You: "I can see why you do not wish to switch with me. You're concerned that Mr. Partain may turn out to be the last client with postcardiac regimen whom you encounter before graduation, and you need this experience."

Besides allowing David to feel understood, reflecting with empathy obliges you to fully understand the conflict from his point of view. Without this information, you could not come up with the most effective resolution.

You are entitled to describe the conflict from your point of view, and you therefore explain to David the importance of Mr. Partain to your own client assignment. You have no control over whether David will listen with empathy to your side of the conflict, but your previous active listening will increase the chances.

2. Once you understand the conflict, the next step is to work out a satisfactory resolution. The resolution most acceptable to both you and David (to have Mr. Partain as sole client) is mutually incompatible. You need to generate another suitable resolution. Unlike the first example, there is limited time in which to do so. You propose the following suggestions to David:

- When David is off duty, you will take over as the nurse in charge of Mr. Partain's care.
- You offer to share with him any information you have on loss, as it applies to the postcardiac client, in return for being able to ask him questions about Mr. Partain's adjustment.

David accepts your suggestions and offers the following ones that might be helpful to you:

- You can be present when he is talking to Mr. Partain (if he agrees) so that you can apply some of what he gleans to your study of the concepts of loss and body image.
- David informs you about Mrs. Tenn, a diabetic client on the unit, who is upset that her diabetes prevents her from becoming pregnant again. David suggests that Mrs. Tenn might make a suitable client for your study of loss.
- David offers you a copy of his paper when it is completed, since your topics overlap and you might find it helpful.

This brainstorming has generated several possible resolutions that have benefits for both of you. If you and David adopt all the suggestions, both of you will gain more than you could have if you each went your separate ways. In addition to achieving your learning goals, you both will have the opportunity to learn from each other and possibly develop a closer friendship.

3. After adopting any resolution to a conflict, it is important to check to see if the plan continues to meet your expectations. The bottom line in this situation is that both you and David complete your assignments. Any additional happenings will be bonuses.

You can see that two of the important processes in effective conflict resolution are empathy and problem solving. Ensuring that these two strategies are influential in your conflict resolution approach ensures that you will be assertive and responsible.

Wit and Wisdom

Remember: Patience gets short late in any shift.

Hammerschmidt and Meador, in *A Little Book of Nurses' Rules*

CONFLICT RESOLUTION AND THE NURSING PROFESSION

Johnson (1990) points out that conflict can be a positive force for nursing if it is used to foster growth-producing change in the profession and in the organizations where nurses work. She cautions, however, that nurses must know how to use conflict effectively if these benefits are to be realized. In addition to being knowledgeable about managing conflicts, nurses must develop a positive attitude toward conflict by recognizing the potential gains to be realized from conflict. Nurses need to become more astute at predicting potential conflicts.

Shifts in power are taking place in the health care system that will be accompanied by more options for conflict resolution. The history of a power differential between nursing and medicine has made it difficult for collaboration to be used as an effective conflict management tool because collaboration rarely works well where there is a wide difference in power between the groups involved. Johnson advises that nursing as a discipline must be concerned about empowering all nurses in the work setting in preparation for handling workplace conflicts.

Moments of Connection...
When "Just Listen to the Doctor" Won't Work

As a pain management nurse, I was concerned about a very sick client who needed a re-fill for his morphine pump. Our physician said the client had to come in to the clinic. Other staff said since I work full-time and the doctor would not get reimbursement if the client did not make a clinic visit, that I should "just listen to the doctor." I told the doctor that I could do a home visit and do the refill there. He gave his permission, and I received an orientation from the home health agency staff. I visited the home four times to refill the pump as the dosage was increased. The client and his wife were so happy. He died last month. Yes, it would have been easier to comply without question, but even though everyone anticipated there would be a problem, there really was no conflict but just a difference of opinion.

Think About It...
What, So What, and Now What?

Consider what you read about team conflict. What conflict have you observed in the clinical setting? How do you assess your own skills at managing conflict? Write the answers to the following questions.

What? . . . Write one thing you learned from this chapter.

So what? . . . How will this impact your nursing practice?

Now what? . . . How will you implement this new knowledge or skill?

THINK ABOUT IT

Practicing Managing Team Conflict

Exercise 1

Work in groups of three for this exercise. One person will act as "pro" and one "con" on the issue; the third person will act as coach. You will be presented with a conflict situation, and it is the task of "pro" and "con" to resolve the conflict in an assertive and responsible way. The coach will help "pro" and "con" to resolve the issue using the win-win approach.

Guidelines for "Pro" and "Con":

1. Use a systematic problem-solving approach to the conflict you are attempting to resolve.
2. In the data collection phase remember to delve into your own—as well as others'—thoughts and feelings about the conflict.
3. In the resolution-generating phase remember to allow as many suggestions to surface as possible before you make your final decision.
4. The resolution you choose must be one agreeable to both. "Pro" and "con" must agree that the resolution satisfies both parties.
5. For the purposes of this exercise you must follow one additional rule: whenever your colleague speaks you must reflect with empathy what she has said so that she will know you fully understand her point of view.

Guidelines for the Coach:

1. It is your job to remind "pro" and "con" to use a win-win problem-solving approach in their attempts to resolve the conflict.
2. You have the responsibility to remind "pro" and "con" to use empathic responses with each other after each speaks. Do not let them proceed with their negotiation until the listener has used empathy to show she understands the other's position. (For instance, if "con" has just argued against "pro's" point of view, before "pro" can defend her position she must acknowledge "con's" perspective.)

Here are three situations involving conflict. So that each of you has the opportunity to be "pro," "con," and the coach, each of you will take a different role in the three conflict situations.

Situation One: A Conflict of Methods

You are both nurses working on a medical unit in your hospital. Problem-oriented charting is employed on your unit, and you also use a Kardex system that contains identifying data about clients and the nursing care plan.

"Pro's" position: You think your unit should do away with the Kardex system. You claim that the nursing care plans are never kept up to date on the Kardexes and you have to refer to the chart to get the most accurate information on the client.

"Con's" position: You think it is important to keep the Kardexes. They are a handy reference for obtaining an update of the client's situation. Kardexes are especially useful for relief staff or staff returning from days off. You believe that it would be inconvenient to have to refer to the chart each time you wanted to check your clients' care plans. Furthermore, the charts are often unavailable because they are being used by other personnel.

Situation Two: A Conflict of Values Compounded by Limited Resources

You are two members of the Awards Selection Committee for your school of nursing. You have one task remaining: to select the student nurse in your class who has demonstrated the best clinical nursing practice. You have narrowed the choice down to two candidates; however, there is only one prize for this category and you must agree on one student nurse.

"Pro's" position: You believe the prize should go to Ms. James because she has consistently demonstrated excellent charting and made useful suggestions about the management of her clients' care at case conferences. She is motivated to encourage her clients and she has given them consistently courteous, caring nursing.

"Con's" position: You disagree with your colleague's choice and would like to see this prize awarded to Mr. Timms, whom you feel has gone beyond the call of duty in his nursing care. He has helped clients write letters and has spent time supporting family members of his clients. He is highly regarded by the nurses on the units for his ability to work in a cooperative manner.

Situation Three: A Conflict of Goals

You work on a surgical unit in your hospital. There is a movement to allow clients to read their own charts. All staff on your unit have been asked to put forth their views on this proposed policy. You and your colleague have opposing opinions.

"Pro's" position: You have a strong belief that clients should be permitted to see anything written on their charts. You are convinced that the charts are really the property of the clients; after all, it is their health that is being charted about. You would like to have access to your chart if you were a client.

"Con's" position: You think it is absolutely unreasonable that clients should have access to their charts. You think it would lead to all kinds of problems. For one thing, clients would not comprehend the medical jargon and might misinterpret information in their charts. Considerable time would be wasted trying to write in a way that clients would understand. In your view nurses and physicians are the experts and clients should have some faith that they will create an accurate document of their care.

Debriefing Questions

1. What was the most difficult aspect of using the win-win conflict resolution approach?
2. What benefits are there to the win-win approach to resolving conflicts?

Exercise 2

The whole class can participate in this exercise. The goal of this exercise is to resolve a conflict that involves the entire health care team.

Your psychiatric unit has been asked to participate in an investigation to study the effects of a newly developed antidepressant. This mood-elevating drug is not yet available on the market because it requires the final phase of testing with human subjects. Your unit has been asked to participate in a study in which half of the depressed clients will be given this new experimental drug and the others will receive a placebo. Researchers will document the effects (benefits and untoward reactions) of the drugs on your client population. Your health care team must decide today if it will agree to participate in this study. Six volunteers are needed to role-play the following positions on the health care team:

Continued

Practicing Managing Team Conflict—cont'd

Head Nurse: is totally against doing research on human subjects. She is adamant that the clients on her unit should not be requested to participate in this study. "We are in the business to help people, not experiment on them. Our credibility in the eyes of our consumers will be in question if we get involved in this experiment."

Physician: is all for research. "The only way to achieve new frontiers of excellence in client care is through research."

Staff Nurse 1: is dubious about asking clients to participate in research. "When people are depressed they cannot make the most informed decisions. They might think they have to volunteer in order to get good health care from us."

Staff Nurse 2: supports research in psychiatry and believes your unit should set an example by completing this study. "Wonderful cures have come from clinical research. Psychiatric research has taken a back seat too long to medical research."

Occupational Therapist: sees so many immobilized depressed clients who take so long to recover from depression that she welcomes any research that might discover a more effective treatment for depression. "We should try anything that will help our depressed clients."

Social Worker: is dubious about putting the clients and their families under one more stress at an already stressful time. "We don't know if this new drug will do any good, and it might do harm. Why should our clients and their families have that possibility to worry about?"

This team has opposing points of view about whether to engage in the drug research. This controversy represents a conflict of values.

The task of the team is to resolve the conflict using the win-win approach. As a team you must use the problem-solving approach, and each member must attempt to be assertive in her negotiations.

The rest of the class will observe the team in its deliberations and be prepared to make comments on their conflict resolution procedure.

The team will take 30 to 40 minutes to complete its resolution.

Debriefing Questions

1. What factors enhanced the team's ability to use a win-win approach to resolve this conflict?
2. What factors made it difficult for the team to use an assertive and responsible approach to resolving this conflict?
3. Was the team able to decide on a resolution that was satisfactory to all team members?
4. If the team did not get to the point of resolving the conflict in the 40 minutes of the role-play, how would you rate its progress in terms of assertiveness and responsible communication?

If you would like more practice attempting to resolve conflicts that involve the whole team, use the following situations (or develop your own) and take different roles and points of view on the issue.

Situation One

There is a 48-year-old married man on your unit who has been diagnosed with terminal cancer. There is lack of agreement on your team about whether to inform the client that he is dying. Some members take the view that he will give up hope and become depressed if he is told he is dying. Others claim that he has a right to know his prognosis because he needs the opportunity to get his life affairs in order and say his good-byes to his wife and teenagers.

Situation Two

Your team is undecided about whether to give a 38-year-old depressed woman on your psychiatric unit a weekend pass. She has made a successful recovery from a suicide attempt 1 week ago. The marital problems that were largely responsible for her suicide attempt are being worked out. Some members of the team think that she should wait a week before going home because she is still fragile. They point out that she has the energy to repeat a suicide attempt, and may be so inclined if the visit home is unsuccessful. Other team members think she should be discharged because she needs to get home to where the real problems are so that she and her husband can work on them. The added strain of her husband caring for their children and paying for baby-sitters when he comes in for conjoint appointments is causing too much unnecessary stress on their family.

Wit and Wisdom

Conflict Is Not a Dirty Word!

*It's a very clean feeling
To speak my piece,
To say where I stand
Gives life a new lease.*

*Disagree with me
That's quite all right.
Conflict resolution
Need bring no fright.*

*We both have a view.
Let's meet in the middle.
Different ideas
Need not be a riddle.*

*With positive intent
I confront confusion.
With clarity comes peace
That is not an illusion.*

Copyright 1995 Julia W. Balzer Riley.

References

American Nurses Association: *Survival skills in the workplace: what every nurse should know,* Kansas City, Mo, 1990, The Association.

Balzer Riley J: *Instant tools for healthcare teams,* St Louis, 1997, Mosby.

Cushnie P: Conflict: developing resolution skills, *AORN J* 47(3):732, 1988.

Hammerschmidt R, Meador CK: *A little book of nurses' rules,* Philadelphia, 1993, Hanley & Belfus.

Harrington-Mackin D: *The team building tool kit: tips, tactics, and rules for effective workplace teams,* New York, 1994, American Management Association.

Johnson M: Use of conflict as a positive force. In McClosky JC, Grace HK, editors: *Current issues in nursing,* St Louis, 1990, Mosby.

Kinder JS: Conflict and diploma nursing education. In *Management of conflict,* New York, 1981, National League for Nursing.

Likert R, Likert JG: *New ways of managing conflict,* New York, 1976, McGraw-Hill Book Co.

Pillemer K, Johnson PT: Learning to lead, *Contemp Longterm Care* 21(2):48, 1998.

Suggestions for Further Reading

Benton DA: *Lions don't need to roar: using the leadership power of professional presence to stand out, fit in and move ahead,* New York, 1992, Warner Books.

Fisher P, Ury W: *Getting to yes: negotiating agreement without giving in,* New York, 1992, Penguin Books.

Franko G: Upgrading staff communication, *Nurs Homes* 47(3):60, 1998.

Montebello AR, Buzzotta VR: Work teams that work, *Training and Development,* pp 59-64, March 1993. How to initiate teams and promote their smooth functioning.

Ryan K, Oestreich DK, Orr III GA: *The courageous messenger: how to successfully speak up at work,* San Francisco, 1996, Jossey-Bass.

Schwartz RM: *The skilled facilitator: practical wisdom for developing effective groups,* San Francisco, 1994, Jossey-Bass.

Solomon-Gillis C: Liberate yourself from a triangle of conflict, *Nursing* 28(4):61, 1998.

Swansburg RL: *Introductory management and leadership for clinical nurses,* Boston, 1993, Jones & Bartlett.

Part IV

Building Confidence

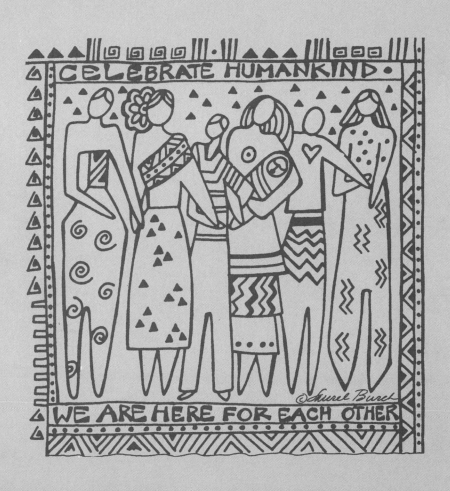

Here you will learn how to get the support you need to build your skills, how to overcome your own evaluation anxicty, and how to give and receive feedback. Information on relaxation, imagery, and self-talk provide a foundation for your continued professional and personal development. In the final chapter you will reflect on ways to respirit, reinspire, and revitalize your own practice.

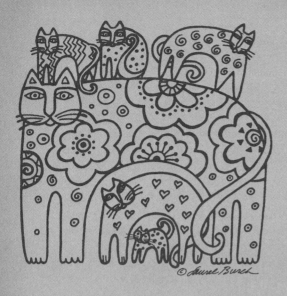
© Laurel Burch

22

Requesting Support

Kindness is like trees in a farm; they lean toward each other.

Congolese proverb

As a student nurse, and later as a registered nurse, there will be many occasions when you will need support to do your work. This chapter provides you with guidelines for making your requests for support in a way that they are most likely to be successful. You will learn how to be specific about your needs for support and how to plan an assertive strategy. The exercises will give you the opportunity to practice assertive ways to request support.

THE RELATIONSHIP BETWEEN SOCIAL SUPPORT AND HEALTH

Research on the relationship between social support and health in clients and in nurses was prolific in the 1970s and 1980s and has important implications for nursing practice today. The literature suggests that there is a positive relationship between the presence of social support and good health. Dimond and Jones (1983) summarize numerous medical studies showing that support prevents susceptibility to illness, diminishes the symptoms of illness, promotes earlier recovery from sickness, and enhances well-being. Social support is also thought to act as a buffer to maintain or regain health (Cobb, 1976; Gottlieb, 1983; Pilisuk and Froland, 1978). Social support has been linked to positive mental health. Mueller's literature review cites evidence linking inadequate social support with psychiatric illness (1980). In a sample of 170 Chinese Americans, Lin et al (1979) demonstrate that social support accounts for more variance in psychiatric symptoms than stressful life events, occupational prestige, and marital status combined.

Much of the earlier social support literature has been related to clients or potential clients. Recently more is being written about workplace support to help employees contend with occupational tensions and stresses. Some of this literature concerns support for nurses and represents a beginning acknowledgment of the necessity and benefits of support in the workplace.

The nursing literature of the 1970s and up to the mid-1980s abounded with descriptions of the stressful nature of nursing practice in a variety of clinical settings (Smith, 1986). Accompanying these portrayals was a flood of articles claiming that workplace support groups are an effective way to combat stress. The following list delineates the purported benefits of workplace support groups for nurses and other health care professionals:

- Controls or decreases staff turnover (Baider and Porath, 1981; Gray-Toft and Anderson, 1983; McDermott, 1983; Webster et al, 1982; Weiner and Caldwell, 1983)
- Reduces stress/teaches stress-reducing strategies/prevents burnout (Deming, 1984; Gray-Toft and Anderson, 1983; Scully, 1981; Webster et al, 1982)
- Increases job satisfaction/increases morale (Deming, 1984; Gray-Toft and Anderson, 1983; Hay and Oken, 1972; McDermott, 1983; Weiner and Caldwell, 1983)
- Teaches methods of conflict management (Hay and Oken, 1972; Scully, 1981)
- Assists nurses to work as a team/improves intercollegial communication/encourages working as a unit (Baider and Porath, 1981; Goetzel, Shelov, and Croen, 1983; Scully, 1981; Taerk, 1983; Webster et al, 1982; Weiner and Caldwell, 1983)
- Provides an opportunity to consult about clients/promotes nursing knowledge (Diminno and Thompson, 1980; Hay and Oken, 1972; Scully, 1981; Taerk, 1983; Webster et al, 1983)
- Provides supervision (Scully, 1981)
- Improves the quality of care provided (Jacobs, 1982; Taerk, 1983; Webster et al, 1982)
- Improves atmosphere at work (Baider and Porath, 1981; Deming, 1984; Taerk, 1983)
- Helps nurses relate to clients more positively (Baider and Porath, 1981; McDermott, 1983)
- Increases confidence in their roles/increases participation in meetings (Baider and Porath, 1981; Deming, 1984; Webster et al, 1982)
- Instills positive influence on nurses' lives away from work (Weiner and Caldwell, 1983)
- Helps nurses cope with sensory overload (Skinner, 1980)
- Allows emotional release of feelings (Diminno and Thompson, 1980; Hay and Oken, 1972; Skinner, 1980)

Although these reports on the benefits of workplace support groups for nurses are descriptive and retrospective, they attest to the enthusiasm for workplace support groups. In the current climate of change in the health care workplace support has taken on new importance. Some nurses responding to the complex demands of working with AIDS clients have established their own support groups. In lieu of support groups within the work setting, some nurses seek support and new knowledge from their involvement in specialty nursing associations. One of the recurrent demands of prospective nurse employees is for a supportive work environment (Callahan, 1990; Corcoran, Meyer, and Magliaro, 1990; Franks and Hayden, 1990; Geissler, 1990; Kinsey, 1990; Sanford, 1990; Spitzer-Lehmann, 1990; White, 1990;). What is found is that nurses tend to select—and stay with—units where they deem the work environment supportive and the professional development of the staff valued (Doering, 1990).

Wit and Wisdom

We are remembered by our good actions, not by our good intentions.

Proverb of the British Isles

DETERMINING THE SUPPORT YOU NEED AT WORK OR SCHOOL

In the broadest sense of the word, support is anything that helps you to work more effectively and feel better about how you are functioning. This general notion of support is vague and will not help you articulate specifically what you need nor guide you in getting it. If you think about support as being cognitive, affective, and physical, this conceptualization will help you assess and secure the support you need to work as a nurse.

Cognitive support helps you think intelligently about your job, decide how to approach problems, discover the how and why of doing things a certain way, and provides some criteria for doing your work. Affective support is the good feeling that accompanies open, direct communication with colleagues. The reassurance that teammates will consider your point of view and the comfort of freely expressing opinions augments your positive feelings about work. Physical support is concrete assistance given by people, computers, equipment, or spatial arrangements of the environment, all of which make your nursing more streamlined.

One method of providing nurses with cognitive support is through mentors (Kinsey, 1990). In a summary of the favorable incidents associated with mentorship, nurse leaders rank career advice, scholarly stimulation, and professional role modeling as the top three influences. Coleman describes a positive innovation for supporting and retaining nurses whereby the more experienced nurses are stimulated and challenged to advance their knowledge base and sharpen their consultative skills and then initiate changes on their units. Receiving the counsel of mentoring, as well as exploring new role options as experienced nurses, provides immense satisfaction and strengthens nurse retention. One of the strategic plans some hospitals are now implementing to attract and retain nurses is access to clinical specialists, nursing research support, staff development, staff orientation, and upward mobility (Corocoran, Meyer, and Magliaro, 1990). These reports underline how nurses today want continued stimulation and chances for professional growth.

In the realm of affective support, nurses are demanding acknowledgment for the work they do. Nurse managers need continued support and confirmation of their important role in today's world, where nursing practices are changing, client acuity is higher, and nursing shortages are real (Franks and Hayden, 1990). Respect, honor, and recognition of employees by acknowledgment of positive performance is needed frequently, not merely during an annual review (Spitzer-Lehmann, 1990). Expressing gratitude and appreciation can create feelings of goodwill and nurturance among nurses that is a form of job gratification, making them feel better about their workplaces, clients, and colleagues (Geissler, 1990; Sanford, 1990). Callahan (1990) believes that burnout occurs when nurses realize that, no matter how developed their talents are, they aren't recognized. She urges hospitals to initiate a system of Positive Incident Reports that can be posted on the unit's bulletin board and then be included in the staff nurse's personnel file. A commendation for work well done might look like this: "I'd like to commend Sheila Jersey, RN, for the empathy she showed the client in 1039 on the night of 10/12/98. Her words cut through his pain and delirium, grounding him in reality and allowing him to rest without further medication. She has a special ability to say just what the client needs to hear."

Health care employers are realizing that nurses' input is invaluable in the pursuit of continuous quality improvement. Nurses need to have a say in administrative and clinical decisions affecting client care and to be recognized for their contribution (Doering, 1990; Ligon, 1990). One hospital has fulfilled its dedication to listening to and involving nurses by incorporating their input and approval in the development and implementation of a dynamic, professional practice model (Huttner, 1990). Professional autonomy and inclusion in policy development and decision making, as well as quality assurance programs, are some of the key elements of a successful workplace for attracting and retaining nursing staff (Corcoran, Meyer, and Magliaro, 1990). Schroeder (1994) saw participation in quality improvement as an activity that will be "energizing and supportive to nurses in particular." Quality improvement involves "constant attention to better meeting the customer's needs, careful analysis of process of care and service, empowerment of front-line providers, and collaboration with others" (Schroeder, 1994). These are the issues that are important to nurses, and participation in interdisciplinary quality improvement teams is an opportunity to be heard.

The nursing literature abounds with articles related to cognitive and affective support for nurses in the workplace. Staffing requirements, an essential aspect of physical support, are discussed in the abundance of articles on retention. In this era it is believed that the provision of adequate cognitive and affective support will attract nurses. The requirements for supplies, equipment, and environmental conveniences have likely been secured in most nursing workplaces through the efforts of technology, computerization, and stringent occupational hazard and safety regulations.

As nurses, we need to be assertive about securing the support necessary to function comfortably and confidently at work. The clearer we are about what support we need to do our job, the more likely we are to secure it. We spend a lot of energy attempting to improve the health status of our clients. Getting the support we need to do our work can help us maintain our health and enhance how we feel about both our work and our co-workers.

Conceptualizing cognitive, affective, and physical components of support provides you with an

Box 22-1	**Credits and Debits in Your Support System at Work or School**

For each cognitive, affective, or physical support item ask yourself:

- Am I satisfied with the quality of support I get to do my job?
- Am I satisfied with the quantity of support I get to do my job?

	Satisfied With:			
	Quality		**Quantity**	
	Yes	**No**	**Yes**	**No**

Cognitive Support

1. *Inspiration:* You work with people whose knowledge and skill levels show how you can improve your nursing care.   — —   — —

2. *Information:* Written material (books, procedure manuals, memoranda) are available to provide clear information or instruction about relevant nursing procedures.   — —   — —

3. *Advice:* Colleagues offer expertise and willingness to help guide and/or direct you.   — —   — —

4. *Challenge:* Colleagues intellectually stimulate you by encouraging you to examine, question, and critique your nursing care.   — —   — —

5. *Direction:* Colleagues exhibit or freely share their philosophy and beliefs about nursing in a way that is helpful to you.   — —   — —

Affective Support

6. *Empathy:* Colleagues show interest in you and listen to you, and you feel respected and understood.   — —   — —

7. *Recognition:* Colleagues acknowledge the knowledge and skills you possess, and you are able to make independent decisions and use your talents properly.   — —   — —

8. *Praise:* Colleagues express admiration for your work and compliment you or show attention and genuine interest in your nursing.   — —   — —

9. *Reassurance:* Forgiveness for imperfections of omission or commission is offered with acceptance and encouragement for you to continue to do your best nursing.   — —   — —

10. *Concern:* Colleagues show warm, caring interest in you as a person, and you get a sense that they look forward to working with you; they are concerned for your welfare as a person (not just as a nurse or student).   — —   — —

Continued

organizing framework for your individual support assessment. The first step in your systematic approach is to determine whether you are satisfied with the quality and quantity of support for each facet. Quality refers to the nature or characteristics of the support; quantity refers to the amount of support.

Look at the checklist in Box 22-1, grab a pencil, and check off the pluses and minuses in your support system.

Box 22-1	**Credits and Debits in Your Support System at Work or School—cont'd**

	Satisfied With:			
	Quality		**Quantity**	
	Yes	No	Yes	No
Affective Support—cont'd	—	—	—	—
11. *Feedback:* Honest, forthright evaluation of your work is offered or is available to you when you ask for it; constructive criticism is given in a straightforward, clear manner and is worded in such a way that you can accept it.	—	—	—	—
12. *Cooperation:* Colleagues share ideas with you; there is little greedy competitiveness, and nurses enjoy working together to improve client care.	—	—	—	—
13. *Enthusiasm:* Nurses and others are keen about what they are doing and the atmosphere is lively; creative ideas to improve nursing care are encouraged.				
Physical Support	—	—	—	—
14. *Adequate personnel:* Staff with essential knowledge and skills are available to carry out the necessary nursing functions.	—	—	—	—
15. *Sharing:* When circumstances dictate, colleagues share the workload and help each other; rarely do colleagues avoid helping or refuse to pitch in and lend a hand.	—	—	—	—
16. *Supplies:* Sufficient nursing or administrative supplies are consistently available to allow you to smoothly carry out your work.	—	—	—	—
17. *Equipment:* Equipment on your unit is efficient, in working order, and easily accessible.	—	—	—	—
18. *Environment:* The physical layout and decoration of your working environment allows you to work without inconvenience, hassles, or unpleasant distractions.				

From Smith, 1984.

After you have completed this checklist, take note of those areas where you do have the support you need at work or school. It is easy enough to take for granted the support we do have, and noticing the benefits makes us more appreciative.

Next, have a look at those areas where the support you would like is not available. Answer the following questions about those instances in which you are not satisfied with the quantity or quality of the support you receive:

- What exactly dissatisfies me about the quantity or quality of support?
- If I had a choice, how would I change things to ensure that I receive the support I need?

Be as specific as possible when answering these questions. The clearer and more detailed you can be about the gaps in your support system at work or school, the greater your chances of rectifying the situation. By answering these questions you indicate your desired outcome.

MAKING REQUESTS FOR THE SUPPORT YOU NEED AT WORK OR SCHOOL

The first step is to identify your needs for support. The next step is to decide if you wish to pursue acquiring this support. Can you manage without it, or would the presence of that support really enhance your working situation? Once you have decided to go after the support, your next step is to design your strategy. You need to answer the following questions:

- Who is the best person to ask for this support?
- What is the best way to seek this support?
- How can I present my case in a way to increase the probability of securing the support I want at work or school?

Let us take an example from each of the cognitive, affective, and physical domains, and demonstrate effective and ineffective methods of seeking support.

Making a Request for Cognitive Support

You are a student nurse in a small college. Although the school has several computers with access to databases, you and most of your classmates have your own computers and would prefer to work in your dormitory rooms. You could work more efficiently if there were telephones in each room for the use of modems. In the area of cognitive support, you need better access to information. Knowing that several other colleges have recently decided to equip rooms with telephone jacks, you decide to approach the dean of your school of nursing with your request.

After making an appointment with the dean, you begin to prepare your strategy. In the 20 minutes you have been allotted, you must make the dean aware of the problem and how it is affecting the students' ability to access recent information. You want to urge the dean to explore your recommendation so that you and your colleagues will have the support you need.

You obtain information on comparably-sized schools in your region and learn that these schools have completed or begun the process of providing in-room telephone access. Next, you survey your classmates to see how many have computers or would get them if they had the facilities to use modems, and how many have used modems in the past. You also get specific information from your colleagues about how often they have been delayed in their work by having to wait for computer access in the library.

Armed with this information, you next prepare yourself for the interview with the dean. You envision yourself looking relaxed and calm. In your mind's eye you see yourself presenting your arguments in a clear, straightforward, assertive manner. You notice how the dean is paying attention to what you are saying and taking notes. You visualize the dean agreeing with your concerns and promising to explore the feasibility of installing the necessary equipment.

Here is an example of how your interview with the dean might go if you were assertive:

An Assertive Approach

Assertive you: "Thank you for seeing me, Dr. Thomas. I want to talk to you about the library resources and the students' concerns about their ability to do timely literature reviews by computer."

Dr. Thomas: "Oh? Is that the case? Can you tell me any more about the situation?"

Assertive you: "Yes, I can. Although our library has excellent computer access to information, there are too few terminals to allow us to get our work done in a timely way. Most of us have our own computers or would bring computers if we had phone access in our dorm rooms. I have checked with other schools of comparable size in this region and can show you their progress on this issue. I have surveyed the student body and have responses that indicate how many students are affected by the problem. I have made a copy of the information I have compiled that you may keep [hands dean a well-organized information packet]. We are excited about the quality of education we are getting here, and the complexity of the assignments makes them challenging. We believe we could work more efficiently if we could use modems in our rooms, especially since, as you can see by the survey, most of us have been accustomed to doing our research in this manner."

Dr. Thomas: "I can't argue with your facts. You have certainly done your homework. Your suggestion sounds like a good solution to the situation. I certainly want our students to have access to the most current information. I assure you that I will bring the matter up at the next faculty meeting. We have been talking about this, and your concern and initiative on behalf of the students to get the support you need is impressive. We have a faculty meeting this week. I'll share your data and get back with you in one week. Thank you for bringing this important matter to my attention."

Your assertive approach has brought the students' concerns to the dean's attention. By thanking Dr. Thomas for seeing you, you showed your respect for her busy timetable. You reinforced your awareness by getting right to the point of your visit. Your acknowledgment of the assets of your school library told the dean that you were appreciative of the positive resources available and were not just complaining. You clearly outlined the situation, indicating why it is a problem, and respectfully offered a possible solution. Your research and approach to the dean helped you present your needs and provided data to increase the possibility that the cognitive support requested could be provided.

In contrast to this assertive approach, you could have used a nonassertive or aggressive approach with the dean. Let us examine the consequences of both these less effective approaches.

A Nonassertive Approach

When we act nonassertively in any situation we come across as being unsure, undecided, and without confidence. These nonassertive qualities give others the message that we do not expect to receive what we are asking for. Messages of uncertainty work against us by putting doubts about our requests in the minds of potential providers. Here is an example of a nonassertive approach:

Nonassertive you: "I appreciate you seeing me, Dr. Thomas. It's about the computer problem. Uh, . . . did you know that we have trouble getting the information we need?"

Dr. Thomas: "What's this about a computer problem? What problem?"

Nonassertive you: "Well, I'm not the only one who has had to wait to use the computer to get the information I need for my assignments. It's quite a problem you see . . . I mean, it takes a lot of time to get this information."

Dr. Thomas: "Yes, I know. Library research is very time consuming. Is there a problem with the computers?"

Nonassertive you: "Well, no. You see, that's just the problem. There aren't enough computers. We have some in our rooms. What I mean to say is, I think we need to be able to use modems in our rooms."

Dr. Thomas: "Well how big a problem is this?"

Nonassertive you: "Well, last week I had to wait a long time for access to a computer in the library. Others are complaining, too."

Dr. Thomas: "If you want my assistance, I need to know more about how many students are affected by this problem, to see if any action is necessary. I'll be happy to look into this matter when you provide me with the information to do so."

When we are nonassertive we are asking to have our requests for support ignored. In this example you were not armed with the information you needed to convince Dr. Thomas of the importance of the problem. Your content was not delivered in an objective, forthright manner. On counts of style, delivery, and preparation, being nonassertive lost your case.

Let's look at an aggressive approach.

An Aggressive Approach

When we are aggressive we go after what we want in a way that is upsetting, disrespectful, or threatening to others. When we attack other people in our endeavors to get what we want, we create bad feelings that take considerable energy and time to overcome.

Here is an example of what an aggressive approach might be like:

Aggressive you: "Thanks for seeing me, Dr. Thomas. You've just got to do something about this computer situation. I'm fed up having to go to the university library to get the stuff I need to complete the assignments required for this program when I could use my modem if I had a telephone in my room. It's got to change. It's unfair to students when we can't get the latest information. How would you like to hand in assignments based on half-baked ideas?"

Dr. Thomas: "I can see you are upset about this, and it sounds quite important. When you have calmed down and can talk to me rationally about the problem, I'll be glad to meet with you."

Being aggressive did not get you what you were seeking. But it did create an unpleasant relationship between you and your dean. Now there are two problems. When we are aggressive, we are often out of control and do not present our arguments in a logical, clear way. A rational, well-planned, assertive approach is more likely to secure the needed support and maintain a good relationship.

Making a Request for Affective Support

You are a third-year nursing student in a four-year baccalaureate nursing program. You have noticed that as each academic semester begins your colleagues are becoming more and more competitive about grades. When grades are posted, students converge on the posting and hover around checking out how each student did. Some students are very upset or depressed for days if they receive anything less than a B+.

There is less sharing of articles, ideas, and material that would help colleagues do well on assignments. Students are starting to hoard materials, as if hoping that another person will not do well if the material is not easily accessible. Trying to get the academic edge is the name of the game, and it has resulted in bickering, unfriendliness, and backbiting. You are aware of the loss of cooperation among your colleagues. This situation leaves you feeling isolated and bereft, and you sense it makes others feel that way too.

You decide to try to rectify or reverse the situation. After giving the matter some thought, you decide that the best strategy is to get your closest colleagues together and raise your concerns. Having the whole group present would provide more influence than trying to reach each person individually. You decide to invite your group over for coffee, with the plan to bring up your agenda.

In preparation, you think through how you will approach the topic. You decide to allow some time for chitchat and for everyone to get reacquainted. You plan to have coffee and snacks to break the ice and get everyone mixing. You decide that the best way to broach the subject is to begin with your feelings of loss. You don't want the discussion to disintegrate into a gripe session, so you come up with several suggestions that the group could consider.

In addition to planning the content, you spend time preparing yourself emotionally for the meeting with your fellow students. You envision yourself and your colleagues looking relaxed. You imagine that when you raise the issue of lack of cooperative support your classmates look interested and agree with your assessment of the situation. In your mind's eye, others look eager to return to your more cooperative ways of relating to each other, and there are even suggestions from the group members.

When you are prepared, you carry out your plan. Following is what an assertive approach to your request for support might be like.

An Assertive Approach

After your colleagues have enjoyed getting reacquainted, you bring up your issue in the following way:

Assertive you: "I'm really enjoying seeing all of you again. It's like old times. Something I've noticed as we get further along in the program is that we are becoming more obsessed with grades. It's really bothering me that we don't share ideas and material the way we used to. It's like we are all operating in isolation—each student for herself. It's too cutthroat for me. I'd like to propose that we restart our weekly study group so that we can share our ideas and knowledge, and our books and articles too. I think we could really help each other, and it would make us feel more like we were in this thing together instead of in competition. What do you think?"

Colleague: "I think it's a great idea. I've been feeling lonely for our shared times, but I guess I just assumed you guys were so 'nose to the grindstone' that you didn't need our group support. I'd love to start meeting again."

Another colleague: "I think it would be a good idea to make a list of what projects we are working on and circulate it. Then when we find articles on someone's topic we could let them know. It wouldn't take any more time, and it would really help us all out."

Another colleague: "I'm housesitting for my brother and he has a huge dining room table that we could use for our meetings."

Your assertive strategy worked. By putting effort into setting the scene and allowing the opportunity for people to realize how much they had missed each other, you furthered your cause immensely. By expressing your feelings, you avoided blaming anyone. Including a suggestion got the ball rolling and gave others a chance to put forth their ideas. It is likely that your strategy has set things in motion for securing the cooperative support you were after.

Consider how things might have gone if you had chosen a nonassertive approach.

A Nonassertive Approach

When we are nonassertive, at some level we are conveying that we do not have much faith in ourselves or our ideas. If we are not able to convey that we believe strongly in what we are saying, then it is highly unlikely that we will convince anyone else. Being nonassertive involves little advance preparation and little visualization of positive outcomes. When we are nonassertive, we look unsure and sound hesitant. Here is what your strategy might have been like if you had taken a nonassertive approach:

You invite your colleagues over for coffee and sooner or later the conversation rolls around to school and grades. Soon every one is comparing how they are doing on their assignments and an uncomfortable atmosphere of competition surfaces. You attempt to intervene with:

Nonassertive you: "Uh, . . . this is the kind of thing I find so disappointing. . . . I mean, all we ever talk about any more is grades and who's got an A . . . ."

Colleague: "Well, it's only natural. That's what we are here for. Grades are the most important things in our lives as students."

Nonassertive you: "Well, they are important, I agree. But so is feeling good and sharing things with friends."

Colleague: "Yes, but when we get good grades that's the thing that makes us feel good these days."

Nonassertive you: "Well, I was wondering if we could help each other out more, like we used to do. Don't you ever long to get our study group together?"

Colleague: "Those days were fun. Now, though, we hardly take any of the same subjects. I'm afraid it would take more time and energy than I've got to get us together and make it time well spent."

Nonassertion got you nowhere except feeling more discouraged about the situation. By not presenting a positive, concrete solution to your complaints, you missed an opportunity to influence your colleagues' outlook on the situation. You avoided emphasizing the benefits of sharing, and consequently, your colleagues swayed the argument to the negative aspects of meeting. Not only did you fail to get cooperation, but you are likely feeling disappointed in your lack of assertiveness.

Consider how the scene might change if you were aggressive.

An Aggressive Approach

Although we may get what we want when we are aggressive, we lose out on the good feelings between ourselves and the other person. Sometimes the bad feelings generated by aggressiveness take extensive time to repair.

Here is one possible scenario if you were to use an aggressive approach:

Aggressive you: "Come on you guys, stop talking about school and grades. I've had enough of it. You've got your heads buried so deeply in the books that you can't even take time to have fun. I remember when you used to be a fun group to be with. Now I get the feeling that if anyone does well it's like stealing points from each other. When are you going to wake up and realize that those little numbers on your papers aren't nearly as important as having some contact as people?"

Colleague: "Well, you may not care about grades, but I do. I might want to go to graduate school some day, and my grades have to be good. You don't even take that into consideration."

Another colleague: "If you can't even see how important school is to some of us, then there's no point in getting together. I think we're on different wavelengths."

By being aggressive you have further ostracized yourself from your colleagues. Your demonstration of insensitivity about the value your friends put on school has cost you their cooperation. By not seeing things through their eyes, you have lost your connection to a valuable source of support.

Making a Request for Physical Support

You are a nurse working on a surgical unit in a general hospital. About 6 months ago the head nurse asked all nursing personnel to complete a health history on newly admitted clients. Part of this history involves asking personal questions about, for example, drug use, religious beliefs, and sleeping habits. Any information that might be important for the nursing staff to know about clients who will be undergoing an anesthetic is included. There is no place to interview clients in private on your unit, and you have felt uncomfortable asking clients some of these questions within the hearing range of other clients and staff on the unit. To complete these initial histories you need the physical support of adequate private space.

You have identified what dissatisfies you about the lack of private space; now you need to decide how you would like to see things changed. You know there is absolutely no possibility of getting a room designated for interviewing alone because of budget cutbacks. What would be satisfactory is a room that could be booked in advance for a private interview with clients and used for other purposes as well. There is a room on the unit, which is designated for Dr. Gait, the physician in charge of the unit. She makes rounds each morning and occasionally uses her room then, but at other times it is not used by anyone. You decide to attempt to secure access to Dr. Gait's office for the purpose of completing the initial histories on clients. It is important to have the privacy, and you feel certain that you can complete the histories more accurately if you had it.

Having decided to seek support, the next step is to determine how to go about acquiring it. The interpersonal style you use to make your request will greatly influence the outcome. A meek or indirect approach leaves you open to being misunderstood or ignored. An aggressive or overly confrontational presentation will put others on the defensive and likely result in rejection. A balance of speaking up for your rights for support without hurting others is what the situation requires.

You already know that the other nurses on the unit agree that a private room is necessary. The lines of communication on the unit dictate that you should make your request to the head nurse. You decide that she needs some advance notice about the issue, and you approach her with a request for a meeting time to discuss the issue. Your request for a meeting is simple, straightforward, and clear:

Assertive you: "Ms. Peters, I would like to make an appointment with you to discuss the need for some private space in which to conduct our initial histories. I'm on duty for the next 3 days. Do you have about 15 or 20 minutes during that time when I can discuss this matter with you?"

Once the meeting has been arranged, you need to plan your strategy for the meeting. You have asked for about 15 minutes during which time you must convince Ms. Peters of the importance of having a private place to interview clients. You prepare for the meeting by itemizing all the reasons you and your colleagues have come up with for needing privacy. You are well aware that you will have more success at having your request granted if you can present a reasonable solution, so you itemize the reasons for using Dr. Gait's office.

Having secured your facts, you now ready yourself for your encounter with Ms. Peters. You prepare by visualizing yourself talking to her in a relaxed, confident manner. In your mind's eye, you envision her listening to you intently, nodding her head in agreement with the points you are making. You imagine yourself successfully counteracting any arguments she has against the use of Dr. Gait's office. All in all, your mental rehearsal of the meeting is successful, increasing your confidence.

Here is an example of how your meeting with your head nurse, Ms. Peters, might go if you were assertive.

An Assertive Approach

Assertive you: "Thank you for setting aside the time to meet with me, Ms. Peters. As you know, I wish to discuss the need for some private space to complete the initial health histories on our clients. I've talked to the other nurses and we all agree that the histories provide some important information about our clients that increases their safety in undergoing anesthesia. Also it gives us a chance to relax the clients and put them at ease. However, there is one major problem we have encountered. There is no designated space for us to talk to our clients, so we end up interviewing them in the corridor, or their rooms, or in the sunroom; in all these locations what they say can be overheard by other clients and staff. We are concerned that some clients may hold back information about themselves that might be important because of the lack of confidentiality. We would like to have a room where we could take newly admitted clients and interview them in private. A little checking shows that Dr. Gait rarely uses her office in the afternoons. The other nurses and I suggest that Dr. Gait's office might be a place we could use. What do you think of this idea?"

Ms. Peters: "I can see your point about the privacy. As you know I'm interested in having the histories completed, so I would like to push for a room if the privacy will mean the histories will be more accurate. In the past Dr. Gait has wanted her office off limits to nurses because she has done her dictating and teaching to her residents in there. But from what you are saying, she doesn't use the office for those purposes any more. I will talk to her about making her office available to our nursing staff in the afternoons. Thank you for your interest and your suggestions."

Your assertive strategy worked. By stating that you and your colleagues supported the histories, you avoided putting your head nurse on the defensive and you invited her to listen. Your reasons for needing a private room were sound on two counts: client safety and client respect. Your astute inclusion of the data about the vacancy of Dr. Gait's office added credibility to your suggestion. You ended your suggestion by respectfully inviting the head nurse's opinion. Your delivery was forthright. Never once did you beat around the bush or sound hesitant. You did not even have to rush since you had already made an appointment with your head nurse.

Here are some examples of ineffective ways to make the same request for a private room.

A Nonassertive Approach

When we are nonassertive, we do not give full credit to our needs. We act shy or make light of factors that are really important to us. When we avoid expressing ourselves clearly and forthrightly, we waive control over our legitimate rights. Being nonassertive invites others to walk all over us.

In this situation a nonassertive nurse would not likely book time with her manager, but probably would take the chance that she could catch the head nurse's attention without advance notice. Nonassertive nurses would not likely plan an effective strategy in advance and would not envision themselves being successful. Verbally nonassertive approaches are limp, unclear, and do not convey confidence or conviction. Here is an example of nonassertion.

Nonassertive you: "Uh, Ms. Peters, do you have a few minutes?"

Ms. Peters has no idea what you want to talk to her about, nor how long it will take. If she is a typically busy head nurse, she will probably have other things planned for that moment.

Ms. Peters: "I can see you briefly. What is it about?"

Nonassertive you: "Well, it's about those histories you want us to do on the new clients. I think it's rather hard . . . . I mean, sometimes there are so many people around. It's hard to talk to the clients when there's no privacy, do you know what I mean? Something's really got to be done, I think."

It is possible that this approach may put Ms. Peters on the defensive. You have given the impression that completing the histories is difficult by not finishing your sentence. You have provided no rationale for the idea that privacy is essential. By not clearly explaining your points you are ensuring that Ms. Peters will not understand, and then she will not be sympathetic to your cause.

Ms. Peters: "Well, I realize that it might be difficult to do the histories, but it's essential that the information be collected. Client safety in the OR depends on this information."

Nonassertive you: "Uh, yes . . . it is important. It's just that, you know, it's hard to talk to the clients when there are other people around. Isn't there a quiet place we could go to? How about Dr. Gait's office?"

Ms. Peters: "Well, you know that she needs her office to be available to her. You can always use a quiet corner of the sunroom, or even ask the other clients to leave the room if you want to have a private interview."

Nonassertive you: "Yeah . . . I guess so. I haven't tried that yet. Maybe that'll work . . . . I hate to ask a client to leave, . . . but I'll give it a try."

You have lost your case. By not being clear about what you wanted, and not defending your suggestion, you have permitted your manager to overlook your suggestion and to force you to continue the way you have been. Had you better prepared your defense and your speech you may have secured the support you were requesting.

An Aggressive Approach

When we behave aggressively we forget to give due respect to the other person's rights. We become so intent on getting what we want that we tend to bulldoze the other person. Here is an example of an aggressive approach to trying to secure a private place for interviewing.

Aggressive you: "Ms. Peters, I need to see you as soon as possible about the initial histories. When can you see me? Today?"

This rush on Ms. Peters does not give her much breathing space. You have indicated there is an urgency about your need to see her that is out of proportion to the truth. In no way have you respected her own timetable or any agenda she may wish to complete. Already she is probably on the defensive.

When you get to see Ms. Peters, you begin with:

Aggressive you: "You've got to do something about getting us a quiet place to do these initial histories you want done on all the clients. It's impossible to do them when everyone can hear what you are saying. How would you like to spill your guts about your sex life or pills you take when every client and staff member around can hear? If you don't get us a quiet place then they just won't be done right. Why can't we use Dr. Gait's office? We nurses don't have any private space and this one doctor has a whole office to herself, even when she's not around."

Ms. Peters: "It's not up to you to dictate how the office space will be assigned on the unit. When you've learned proper etiquette and protocol, I'd be glad to discuss this issue with you. In the meantime, do the best you can. That'll be all for today."

You have made your dissatisfaction very clear. However, in the process of doing so you have put your manager on the defensive and created a rift between you. There are now two problems to be solved: the lack of privacy and the discord between the two of you. When we attack other people, they are likely to divert energy to their injured feelings instead of the issue for which you are fighting. Using an aggressive approach like this diminishes the chances that you will secure the physical support you were hoping to get.

The Importance of Planning an Assertive Strategy for Making Requests

The preceding examples illustrate the importance of planning and implementing an assertive strategy for seeking cognitive, affective, or physical support. If it is important for you to have the support you have identified, then it is important to invest the time and energy in securing it. As a nurse, you spend considerable energy trying to meet your clients' needs for support. If you can secure the support you need at work or school, then it is more likely that you will have the energy to extend support to your clients and colleagues. Nurses who keep on giving without adequate cognitive, affective, or physical support are draining their own reserves. We spend a lot of time trying to get our clients to take care of their health; securing the support we need as nurses provides them with an example to follow.

Just because you use an assertive approach does not mean that you will get the support you are after. Sometimes support is not forthcoming, no matter what strategy is used. On occasion your colleagues may not have the interest or skills to support you. Other times there may not be the money or time to provide you with the support you are seeking. At those times you must decide whether you can continue to work in the system without the support. If you cannot secure the support you need from others at work or school, you may be able to get some support from friends or family to see you through. Only you can decide whether the support is adequate. Since you are the seeker and receiver, it is your perception of the support that is important.

Providing Support at Work and School

The CAPS (Cognitive, Affective, Physical Support) framework is helpful for articulating exactly what support you need at work and school. It can also be a guideline to help you determine your colleagues' need for support. Support is a nebulous concept; breaking it down into cognitive, affective, and physical components helps you to decipher your colleagues' needs for support. One way to get support is to offer it to others. In so doing a bond is built between you that encourages both parties to give and take.

Whether in the classroom or in the workplace, the work of nursing can be stressful. The literature indicates that efforts to counteract this stress have been effective. Several authors describe how structured group support meetings may relieve the negative impact on nurses working in intensive care areas (Scully, 1981; Skinner, 1980). The absence of pathological symptoms in palliative care nurses has been attributed to the availability of a support group (Quenneville, Falardeau, and Rochette, 1981-1982). Another study reports that it is the ongoing day-to-day support that makes hospice nurses feel energetic and cared for at work (Smith and Varoglu, 1983).

Contributing to the effort to build a solid support system at work and school will add to your feelings of confidence and competence. It is worth the effort to learn the assertive way to make requests for the support you need.

WE'RE ALL IN THIS TOGETHER

The changing health care climate makes the ability to ask for and give support an imperative. Health care and other industries are responding to economic concerns by decreasing staff, reassigning the work of staff whose positions are not filled when vacated, and by crosstraining. Charlie Brown's friend Linus clings to his tattered blanket to face change. Koerner (1994) sees Linus' strategy as similar to that of nurses who expect job security from competently performing all the tasks they have always done. She suggests that only by "rescripting our roles and relationships can true transformation occur to create a care delivery system that is relevant to the changing needs of the twenty-first century society." Like the anthropologist Bateson (1994), she sees us needing to rely on the skills of improvisation, and adds the skill of imagination. She suggests that role relationships are not predetermined but must be renegotiated. This involves the ability to be aware of the needs of others and of our own, to be able to give and seek the support necessary to cope with the ambiguity of change. Imagination helps us to see new ways of working together to respond to change. We must come to see that security lies not in the job itself but in our own demonstration of innovation and flexibility (Koener, 1994).

The ability to know what we need and how to ask for support is increasingly important to move beyond our fears to face the challenge of change. Harrington relates a moving story of a nurse who found comfort from the support of colleagues in moments of uncertainty while caring for a terminally ill pediatric patient. "Only the gang at work really understood, and since that day, I've continued to marvel at the friendship and support nurses constantly give each other" (Harrington, 1994). We truly are all in this together.

Think About It...
What, So What, and Now What?

Consider what you read about the importance of support. Can you identify your own needs for support? How can you get what you need? Answer the following questions.

What? . . . Write one thing you learned from this chapter.

So what? . . . How will this impact your nursing practice?

Now what? . . . How will you implement this new knowledge or skill?

THINK ABOUT IT

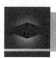 **Practicing Requesting Support**

Exercise 1

In relation to a unit where you are working, or to school, fill in the form in Box 22-1. Answer the two questions:

1. What exactly dissatisfies me about the quality or quantity of support?
2. If I had a choice, how would I change things to ensure that I would get the support I need?

Choose one area where you would like more support and plan an assertive strategy for securing it. Think about who is the best person to approach to get this support. If more than one person is involved, is it better to see them individually or in a group? What is the best approach to take? Consider whether you should provide advance notice in the form of a memo or whether your request would be better made spontaneously. Think about what data you will need to defend your request for this support. If you need information from others, make sure you give them adequate time to prepare it for you. If it would be helpful for your potential supporter to have access to any information, make sure you bring a copy with you. Consider your timing carefully. Good timing can facilitate the meeting of your request, and bad timing can ensure that your needs for support will go to the bottom of the list.

It may be helpful for you to write down your desired outcome and the strategy you intend to use. This act will formalize your intent and force you to think through your strategy. As you proceed, you will have something concrete to refer to.

Once you are satisfied with your strategy, carry it out. Attempt to be assertive in your approach, and avoid being nonassertive or aggressive.

As soon as possible after the event, review what went well and what you would like to have done differently. If you were successful in securing the support you were after, jot down what made your request so successful. Conversely, if you did not secure the support you were after, what factors contributed to this disappointment? Examine whether your success or failure was because of your strategy and approach or a result of other factors.

After you have carried out this exercise on your own, compare notes with your colleagues. In general, what factors contribute to the success of securing the support you need?

To gain competence in making requests in an assertive way, practice this exercise again for some of the other gaps in your cognitive, affective, or physical support systems.

Exercise 2

For this exercise work in groups of three. One person will request support from another in your group. The third person will give feedback on how assertively the requester sought support. When you are the requester, choose one of the cognitive, affective, or physical supports that you would like to secure. Explain to the person role-playing the provider of this support some details of her role (she is a teacher or a colleague, etc.).

When you are clear about your roles, act out a scene where you are requesting support. After you have completed your request, seek feedback from the person providing the support and the feedback giver on how assertive you were in making your request.

Continued

Practicing Requesting Support—cont'd

What have you learned about your ability to be assertive in requesting support? Where do you excel in being assertive? What suggestions do you have for improving your ability to be assertive?

Switch roles so that each of you has the opportunity to role-play the requester, the provider, and the feedback giver.

After you have done this exercise in your small groups, join your colleagues in the rest of the class and compare what you have learned about requesting support.

Wit and Wisdom

How Can I Ask?

Ask for what you really need.
I cannot read your mind.
Ask for it with confidence.
Surprised at what you find?

Ask for what you really need.
I respond to words assured.
Ask as if you mean it.
Much lost by those demurred.

Copyright 1995 Julia W. Balzer Riley.

Moments of Connection...
The Loss of a Cat, a Friend, a Companion

A nurse was finding it hard to concentrate at work and was often moved to tears. "I was just on overload. My husband had just asked for a divorce. I was worried about being a single parent and how I would survive financially. It was just so overwhelming. Then we had to have our cat put to sleep because of massive cancer. I knew only one person would really understand: the oncology supervisor. She responded right away when I told her about the cat. She's an animal lover too. I made an appointment to see her on my lunch break. She listened and really knew my grief was just compounded. It's like losing a child. She didn't make fun of me. She is so special."

References

Baider L, Porath S: Uncovering fear: group experience of nurses in a cancer ward, *Int J Nurs Stud* 18:47, 1981.

Bateson MC: *Peripheral visions,* New York, 1994, Harper Collins.

Callahan M: Applauding the artistry of nursing, *Nursing 90* 20(10):63, 1990.

Cobb S: Social support as a moderator of life stress, *Psychosom Med* 38(5):300, 1976.

Corcoran NM, Meyer LA, Magliaro BL: Retention: the key to the 21st century for health care institutions, *Nurs Admin Q* 14(4):23, 1990.

Deming AL: Personal effectiveness groups: a new approach to faculty development, *J College Student Personnel* p. 54, Jan 1984.

Diminno M, Thompson E: An interactional support group for graduate nursing students: a report, *J Nurs Educ* 19(3):16, 1980.

Dimond M, Jones SL: Social support: a review and theoretical integration. In Chinn PL, editor: *Advances in nursing theory development,* Rockville, Md, 1983, Aspen.

Doering L: Recruitment and retention: Successful strategies in critical care, *Heart Lung* 19(3):220, 1990.

Franks JC, Hayden MJ: Establishing a permanent charge nurse support group, *Nurs Manag* 21(6):46, 1990.

Geissler EM: Nurturance flows two ways, *Am J Nurs* 90(4):72, 1990.

Goetzel RZ, Shelov S, Croen LG: Evaluating medical student self-help support groups: a general systems model, *Small Group Behav* 14(3):337, 1983.

Gottlieb BH: Social support strategies: guidelines for mental health practice, vol 7, *Sage studies in community mental health,* Beverly Hills, Calif, 1983, Sage Publications.

Gray-Toft P, Anderson JG: A hospital staff support program: design and evaluation, *Int J Nurs Stud* 20(3):137, 1983.

Harrington CS: Supporting each other, *Nursing 94* 24(4):62, 1994.

Hay D, Oken D: The psychological stresses of intensive care unit nursing, *Psychosom Med* 4(2):109, 1972.

Huttner CA: Strategies for recruitment and retention of critical care nurses: a cardiovascular program experience, *Heart Lung* 19(3):230, 1990.

Jacobs R: Nurses matter too, *Nurs Mirror* p. 27, Feb 1982.

Kinsey DC: Mentorship and influence in nursing, *Nurs Manag* 21(5):45, 1990.

Koerner J: Drawing on the art of nursing practice, *J Prof Nurs* 10(2):68, 1994.

Ligon R: A blueprint for involving staff in policy development, *Nurs Manag* 21(7):30, 1990.

Lin N et al: Social support, stressful life events, and illness: a model and an empirical test, *J Health Soc Behav* 20:108, 1979.

McDermott B: A preventive approach to staff stress, *Can Nurse* 79(2):27, 1983.

Mueller DP: Social networks: a promising direction for research on the relationship of social environment to psychiatric disorder, *Soc Sci Med* 14A:147, 1980.

Pilisuk M, Froland C: Kinship, social networks, social support and health, *Soc Sci Med* 12B:273, 1978.

Quenneville Y, Falardeau M, Rochette D: Evaluation of staff support system in a palliative care unit, *OMEGA* 12(4):355, 1981-1982.

Sanford K: Nurses, let's support each other more, Nursing 20(1):109-118, 1990.

Schroeder P: *Improving quality and performance: concepts, programs, and techniques,* St Louis, 1994, Mosby.

Scully R: Staff support groups: helping nurses to help themselves, *J Nurs Admin* 11(3):48, 1981.

Skinner K: Support group for ICU nurses, *Nurs Outlook* 28(5):296, 1980.

Smith SP, Varoglu G: Support for hospice nurses. In Mitchell KA, editor: *Proceedings of the first annual Pacific Health Forum '83,* Vancouver, BC, 1983, University of British Columbia Health Care and Epidemiology Alumni Association.

Smith SP: *Support for nurses working in extended-care,* Victoria, BC, 1986, University of Victoria.

Spitzer-Lehmann R: Recruitment and retention of our greatest asset, *Nurs Admin Q* 14(4):66, 1990.

Taerk G: Psychological support of oncology nurses: a role for the liaison psychiatrist, *Can J Psychiatry* 28:532, 1983.

Webster S et al: A method of stress management: the support group, *Nurs Manag* 13(9):26, 1982.

Weiner MF, Caldwell T: The process and impact of an ICU nurse support group, *Int J Psychiatr Med* 13(1):47, 1983.

White SK: Symposium on successful recruitment and retention strategies in critical care: overview, *Heart Lung* 19(3):219-220, 1990.

Suggestions for Further Reading

American Nurses Association: *Survival skills in the workplace: what every nurse should know,* Kansas City, Mo, 1990, The Association.

This booklet helps nurses get the support they need to make the most of their skills and abilities in the workplace of the 1990s, with more complex health care services, scarcer financial resources, increasing ethical dilemmas, and personnel shortages.

Anderson G: *Healing wisdom: wit, insight, and inspiration for anyone facing illness,* New York, 1994, Dutton.

Coleman B: Advanced nursing apprenticeship program: a strategy for retention of experienced critical care nurses, *Heart Lung* 19(3):236, 1990.

Perlman D, Takas GJ: The 10 stages of change, *Nurs Manag* (21)4:33, 1990.

Smith SP: Need support at work? Think CAPs, *Can Nurse* 81(8):40, 1984.

Wilson GL, Hantz AM, Hanna MS: *Interpersonal growth through communication,* Dubuque, Ia, 1985, WC Brown.

Chapter 8, Defending and Supporting, delineates defensive and supportive communication for readers and provides ways to help nurses choose to remain supportive.

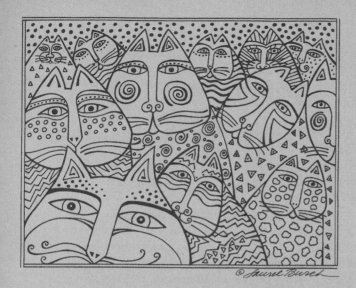

23

Overcoming Evaluation Anxiety

Not until we have fallen do we know how to rearrange our burden.

African proverb

OBJECTIVES

1. Define evaluation anxiety.
2. Describe characteristics of evaluation anxiety.
3. Identify strategies to handle job performance appraisals assertively.
4. Discuss techniques to decrease test anxiety.
5. Identify benefits of criticism.
6. Identify assertive strategies to handle difficult situations in student performance evaluations.
7. Participate in exercises to overcome evaluation anxiety.

WHAT IS EVALUATION ANXIETY?

Even though we easily toss off the old saying "to err is human," most of us prefer that someone else be the one to err! In our competitive culture we idolize excellence in personal performance, products, and services. Advertisements bombard us from billboards, radio, and TV about "better" or "improved" products. We spend years in an educational system that makes judgments about our physical and psychological abilities through a variety of examinations and elaborate grading systems.

Making mistakes is the antithesis of our cultural standard for excellence. Our preoccupation with perfection makes it difficult to accept that making mistakes is a normal part of human endeavor.

Evaluation anxiety occurs when we are upset about having our performance judged and are intimidated by the evaluation process. One form of evaluation anxiety is test anxiety, which has negative effects on academic performance. For nursing students, test anxiety can be evident in both written examinations and evaluations of clinical proficiency. Instead of focusing on relevant parts of a task, students with high test anxiety worry about their performance and how well others are doing and ruminate about alternatives (Meichenbaum, 1972). High test anxiety is associated with intrusion of such irrelevant thoughts as preoccupation with feelings of inadequacy, anticipation of punishment, and loss of status and esteem.

Accompanying these cognitive aspects of test anxiety is emotionality, the autonomic arousal aspect of anxiety, and a variety of physical symptoms including increased heart rate, muscular tension, gastrointestinal changes, changes in breathing, and dietary and sleep pattern disturbances (Meichenbaum, 1972). These physiological symptoms are distressing and need to be alleviated just as much as the negative thought processes. Learning to relax and decrease unpleasant symptoms helps diminish their negative effects.

One of the most significant and recurring problems experienced by health professionals is a fear of making a mistake and being negatively evaluated. Clinicians in practice have revealed fears about committing errors in diagnosis or treatment. In a study to identify specific clinical situations that were anxiety-producing for junior and senior nursing students, Kleehammer, Hart, and Keck (1990) found that the highest anxiety-producing situation for both groups is the fear of mak-

---

Wit and Wisdom

No Knowing, No Growing

*It's safe to perform
your tasks, do your duty.
Look inside yourself
And see only beauty.*

*Have you the courage
To ask for inspection?
Can you face hearing
You're less than perfection?*

*Have you learned yet
We're better for knowing?
To take bad with good,
A chance to keep growing.*

Copyright 1995 Julia W. Balzer Riley.

ing mistakes. Examples of other nursing situations that engender anxiety in students are the initial clinical experience on a unit, nursing procedures, hospital equipment, evaluation by faculty, observation by instructors, tardiness, and conversations with physicians.

The two major factors underlying evaluation anxiety in nurses are concern for client safety and concern for our own security.

Concern for Client Safety

Nursing involves caring for the health of fellow human beings. Health is a precious commodity, making the stakes high if a nursing error detracts from our clients' health or pushes them into illness. This responsibility underlies our anxiety about making an error in our nursing practice.

Concern for Our Own Security

Clients are becoming more knowledgeable and critical about health care and its cost. No longer content to passively submit to treatment, consumers of health care are demanding to know the rationale for regimens and to have access to a second opinion. In extreme cases clients are suing physicians and other health care professionals, including nurses, for ineffective health care. This potential threat from clients hovers as a powerful source of disapproval, with implications for career advancement and public embarrassment. The loss of one's job and financial assets could also result from unsafe care. Today, nurses are aware of accountability for the nursing care we give and of our vulnerability to investigations of these actions through the legal process.

Evaluation anxiety is an unpleasant, ever-lurking phenomenon that, as two decades of literature reports, has threatened nurses and other health professionals. As nurses, we are committed to making a positive difference for our clients, yet today's work environments are loaded with potential deterrents to this goal: inadequate staffing, higher acuity clients, technological advancements, information overload, and the uncertainty of health care reform. In its mildest form, evaluation anxiety can detract from enjoyment in the workplace and, when strong, can be overwhelming, interfering with our ability to perform competently as nurses.

As nursing students, or as practicing registered nurses, we need to develop ways to minimize evaluation anxiety so that we can confidently handle clinical or written examinations, job performance appraisals, and everyday criticisms—all naturally recurring events in the professional life of nurses.

Characteristics of Evaluation Anxiety

People who suffer from evaluation anxiety exhibit ways of thinking that make them feel uneasy and interfere with their ability to perform in adaptive ways. The following characteristics of those experiencing evaluation anxiety have been reported in the literature (Dweck and Wortman, 1982; Wine, 1982).

- *Self-focus versus task-focus.* These people spend more time thinking about their performance than they devote to the actual task. Attention to their performance detracts from the necessary attention needed to do the task adequately. Self-focused thoughts are negative and self-devaluing, and they lead to self-doubt. Not only does a focus on self versus task detract from task performance, but the focus on negative aspects of one's performance engenders feelings of anxiety.

- *Self-blame.* Some people with evaluation anxiety tend to blame themselves for their poor performance more than they do circumstances or other external factors.
- *Worry and concern about evaluation.* People with high evaluation anxiety tend to place a lot of emphasis on how they are doing in comparison to others and how the examiner is evaluating them.

Those with low evaluation anxiety react to performance evaluation with an external, situational, task-oriented focus. For those with high evaluation anxiety, failure signifies a lack of ability. Those with low evaluation anxiety generate thoughts about the task or situation that encourage solutions or completion of the task, whereas those with high anxiety give up and see themselves as the main reason for failure.

Options such as trying different strategies, or looking for an external causative factor, are not fully explored, leaving high-anxiety types with feelings of failure and uneasiness. Mistakes are interpreted as failures, not as stepping stones in the process of discovering the best solution. People with high performance anxiety tend to attribute success to factors other than their own ability, yet they readily assume failure is their doing. This view leads them to feel pressured in every new achievement situation (Dweck and Wortman, 1982; Wine, 1982). Consider, too, the effect of past negative experiences on the evaluation process. Students and nurses with previous work experience who have had a traumatic experience in performance appraisal may have so much anxiety that the process is highly emotionally charged (Marquis and Huston, 1998). It is useful to spend some time reflecting on your fears and worries to evaluate how realistic they are (Ryan, Oestreich, and Orr, 1996).

In our culture it is easy to berate ourselves when we make a mistake. In addition to our self-chastisement we sometimes invent or exaggerate disapproval from others. How we internally evaluate ourselves can be constructive or destructive.

Here is an example of constructive and destructive thoughts in relation to being evaluated.

Constructive Thoughts	**Destructive Thoughts**
"I'm doing a good job. I can't do everything I'd like to for my clients today because we're short-staffed, but I'll make sure I do the most important things."	"I've got to do everything for my clients or I'll feel like a failure." "If I don't do everything just perfectly I'll be letting down my clients and the rest of the team."
"I've done the important things I can for the clients on the unit. Now I'll prepare a concise report for the evening staff."	"How can I possibly explain to the evening staff that I didn't get everything done on the day shift? They'll think I'm incompetent and disorganized."
"One thing I didn't make arrangements for was an extra load of linen for the evening staff. Now that I know you have to put your order in before 1 PM, I won't forget in the future."	"They're going to crucify me for not arranging for an extra load of linen. They'll be mad at me for days for that mistake."
"I can go home knowing I did the best I could today. It was super busy and we were short-staffed, but we gave our clients the best care we could under the circumstances."	"What a day! All I can think about is what still needs to be done. I'll be miserable all evening mulling over how I could have done things better."

How to Gain Control Over Your Evaluation Anxiety

Since evaluation anxiety affects cognitive, affective, and psychomotor dimensions, a multifaceted approach is needed to help overcome it.

- You can use positive self-talk (see Chapter 27) to overcome your self-defeating internal dialogue. Making sure that your inner voice is reassuring will comfort you in your day-to-day activities and during these times when you are having an examination or a performance appraisal.
- Relaxation (see Chapter 25) will help you focus on the task and act more efficiently. You will feel more relaxed and overcome the negative physiological effects of evaluation anxiety when you relax.
- Imagery (see Chapter 26) will help you picture yourself performing in a way that makes you feel good about yourself. Your positive visualizations will keep you focused on performing your best and will engender positive feelings that will overpower the uneasiness generated by your anxiety.
- Learning how to make use of feedback (see Chapter 24) from others will help you prepare yourself for situations in which your performance is evaluated. Practice sessions with helpful colleagues can boost your confidence.

In addition to these four approaches, avoiding errors requires thinking before acting. Using the nursing process on a consistent basis helps to ensure that your nursing actions will be safe, ethical, and helpful.

Handling Job Performance Appraisals Assertively

At many points in our nursing careers we receive both formal and informal evaluations of our performance. For us, the purpose of these evaluations is to learn what we are doing well (so that we can continue to do it), and where we need to improve our work performance. For the employer, evaluations serve as a check on whether employees are fulfilling the expectations of the work contract.

Evaluations are helpful to both parties and should occur regularly. As the employee, you can take an assertive approach to evaluations, which will help ease your anxiety. Here are several assertive steps you can take to prepare for an evaluation. This example is for a nurse employed in service. As a student nurse, apply the same preparatory procedures for evaluations at your school of nursing.

Before Your Evaluation

1. Find out what the schedule is for evaluations in your agency. Many agencies offer an evaluation for new employees after 3 to 6 months of probationary employment and yearly thereafter.
2. Find out in advance the criteria by which your employer will be evaluating you. Having this information gives you the chance to make notes about how you think you have met the standards expected of someone in your position.
3. If your employer does not have a standard criteria for evaluation, suggest that one be instituted soon. Request that your job description or the standards of nursing care prepared by your professional nursing association be used as the reference for determining your performance level.

4. Review what you and your colleagues in similar nursing positions actually do in the work-place. Compare this time and task allotment with what your job description outlines. At your evaluation, point out any of these discrepancies to your employer. If job descriptions are not updated, you may find that a significant part of your daily work is not being acknowledged.

5. Prepare your own evaluation of your work performance before meeting with your employer. Go to your appointment armed with specific examples of how you have met the requirements of your job description. Be aware of where you need to improve and what support you will need from your head nurse to make the necessary changes.

6. Develop goals you would like to work toward. Be as clear, realistic, and specific as possible in the preparation of these work objectives so that you can articulate them clearly in your performance evaluation.

7. If the date when your evaluation should have occurred passes, request an evaluation from your employer. Evaluations protect you by providing guidelines for maintaining or changing your professional behavior. You need feedback to know if your nursing care is within the legal and qualitative expectations of your agency.

8. Prepare mentally for your evaluation interview by ensuring that your self-talk is encouraging and visualize yourself looking and feeling calm and confident during your interview.

During Your Evaluation

1. Inform your employer that you wish to discuss your goals at some time during the interview.
2. Allow your employer uninterrupted time to comment about your work.
3. Ask for clarification of any points that are not understandable. Request evidence of your employer's points so that comments are backed up with examples. These illustrations will clarify for you the kind of behavior your employer expects.
4. Your employer may have suggestions about ways in which you can improve your performance. Agree only to those changes that are realistic given your time and potential and the support available in the workplace.
5. Share your performance goals with your employer and ask for support for the achievement of your career plans. Ask your employer for a list of goals you should be working toward.
6. Do not sign your evaluation until you are fully satisfied that it records an accurate and fair assessment of how you do your job.
7. Thank your employer for the supervision and the feedback you receive.
8. Come to an agreement about the date for your next evaluation.

After Your Job Appraisal Interview

1. Take time to reflect on how you handled the evaluation. Praise yourself for the ways you handled yourself assertively. Make note of things you would like to do differently in your next evaluation interview.
2. Follow up on the goals you and your employer set. Take time to develop your strategy to achieve your objectives and set intermediate and final deadlines. Think about people and resources you can tap to help develop your talents.
3. Keep a diary of your work performance in preparation for your next performance evaluation. Mackay (1990) offers a suggestion to all job holders to ensure that they keep their jobs. His motto, "deliver more than you promise," is his sure-fire way to get you and your work noticed. Mackay urges employees: "Don't try to meet your quotas. Exceed them. Do what it

Moments of Connection...
Beyond the Call of Duty

In a chronic pain setting, a young woman with a newborn child and very poor support systems was angry at the world because of a chronic neck and back injury. She would refuse treatment and medications yet was angry that we wouldn't do anything to stop her pain. It was hard to continue to interact with her, knowing that she would be critical of everything we did. After a period of months of contact with her, just listening to her, not becoming offended by her attacks, and understanding what she was experiencing, she now relies on me as her support. In a crisis she will call. I calm her and help her think through the situation. Although this is beyond the normal attention given to a client, it is a special connection that can assist her to build her problem-solving skills, cope, and receive the care she needs, by simply offering caring and understanding.

takes to set yourself apart from the pack. Make them need you." Nurses putting this attitude into practice should not feel anxious at job appraisal time.

Assessing the Validity and Reliability of an Employer's Appraisal System

The performance appraisal process should provide nurses with an evaluative component that rates their nursing behavior against established criteria, and a career developmental component that seeks to improve their nursing performance through self-learning and growth (American Nurses Association, 1990). Many appraisal systems that fail to provide the necessary input/feedback to enhance employee performance do so for some, or all, of the following reasons:

- *The appraisal process is conducted by upper management rather than the nurse employee's immediate supervisor.* Performance appraisal is best handled at the management level closest to the nurse, by supervisors who have firsthand knowledge of the work performance.
- *A single appraisal tool is used to evaluate all employees.* A nurse's job description should form the basis of any performance evaluation, anchoring the appraisal with a pertinent and appropriate focus.
- *Evaluation and assessment focus on personal traits rather than work behavior.* Using the referent of the nurse's job description focuses on observable, measurable behaviors.
- *Behaviors that are the subject of evaluation/assessment fail to reflect the major substance of a specific job.* A job description spells out precise job content, including nursing duties, nursing activities to be performed, nursing responsibilities, and results expected by the nurse's employer.
- *The weighting of traits and behaviors does not reflect their significance in the performance of a specific job.* Ideally a nurse and a supervisor develop the job description in concert so that both parties have a clear understanding of the job expectations at the outset.
- *Criteria for identifying an acceptable level of performance are vague, leaving it open to varying interpretations.* Tasks included in a nurse's job description should be specific, comprehensive, and stated in action verbs, minimizing the likelihood that the nurse will be eval-

uated on insignificant job behavior or personal traits. Acceptable levels of nurse performance must be clearly defined. If rating scales are used, the meaning of each rating should be open to a single interpretation.

- *There is little or no informal feedback on job performance and formal evaluation occurs infrequently.* The appraisal system should allow for sufficient interaction throughout the process. Job performance appraisal should entail systematic assessment/evaluation throughout the designated period. Feedback (employment counseling or "coaching") should be ongoing, including recommendations for improvement. The more frequent the evaluation of job performance, the more likely nurses are to see the evaluation in the light of guidance and thus find the appraisal less stressful (ANA, 1990).

If you do your part to ensure that your job performance appraisals are objective, fair, and frequent, you will do much to minimize your own evaluation anxiety.

Coping With the Anxiety of Written Examinations

Taking examinations is part of student life. Even as a registered nurse you may find yourself preparing for an examination as part of a continuing education course or degree program. Your grade symbolizes the level of achievement you have secured at a given point in time. Many examinations offer only one chance to demonstrate your knowledge or skill, so you may feel anxious about performing well at the given time of the examination. Here are some assertive steps you can take to make you feel better prepared and less anxious about examinations.

Before Your Examination

1. Find out all you can about what content (or skill) will be tested on the examination. This knowledge will help you narrow down the material to study.
2. Review the objectives for the course and focus on content that directly relates to these objectives.
3. Find out the format of the examination (whether it is multiple choice or essay). This information will determine your study approach.
4. If you need guidance on how to study, go to your teachers, the counseling center, or a study guide.
5. Consider forming or joining a study group. Effective study groups can make preparation for examinations fun and fruitful.
6. Make a realistic timetable of study preparations for the examination and stick to it. Keeping pace with your schedule will help you integrate the material you are studying. If you are rushed, prioritize what is important to learn and cover it first.
7. Find out where the examination is being held and familiarize yourself with the room. Choose a seat where you will be comfortable. Be sure you know the exact hour of the exam.
8. Make sure you have all the necessary tools to help you in the exam, such as a spare calculator battery, sharpened pencils, a watch, tissues, and your good luck charm!
9. Mentally prepare before the exam by visualizing yourself in the examination room looking calm and smiling as you read the questions because you know the answers. As you study for the exam be sure that your self-talk is positive. Tell yourself that you are learning and that you are covering the material in a sensible way. Encourage yourself and do not allow self-defeating thoughts about failure or mistakes to take over your internal dialogue.

10. Put yourself through a dry run of the examination. If it is a written test, obtain exams from previous years and write them in the specified time limits. If there are no old exams, make up your own questions and answer them in a simulated exam situation. If you are being examined on your nursing technique, do the procedure in front of your colleagues. Have them evaluate you using the criteria that your instructor will use.
11. Plan a postexamination reward. This treat will give you something to look forward to and will prevent you from dwelling on the examination after it is over.

During Your Examination

1. Decide in advance what time you will be arriving at the place of the examination. If you are the type who likes to talk with colleagues before the examination, arrive early. If preexamination cramming with colleagues raises your anxiety level, time your arrival accordingly.
2. Take time to calm down before even looking at the exam. Sit calmly and do your deep breathing.
3. Maintain this focused calm throughout the exam. If you are thinking about passing or failing, instead of staying focused on the examination questions, your concentration will slip. Just as athletes don't perform their best when they are thinking about winning the gold medal or breaking a record during an event (Orlick, 1986), neither will you perform your best if you are thinking about anything other than the best response to the question in front of you. Thinking about anything else creates anxiety and interferes with your concentration on the questions.
4. If you are distracted by an external interference (like noise from other candidates or the proctors, or uncomfortable conditions in the room) that can be stopped, be assertive and ask the proctor to handle the situation. If nothing can be done about the external distractions, then tell yourself to refocus, giving all your attention to the question at hand.
5. Read over the entire exam before answering any questions. This way you will know what is expected of you and you can pace yourself throughout the allotted time.
6. Before answering any question, be sure you understand what is expected so that your answers will be at the appropriate level. If you merely describe an issue when you are expected to critique it, then you will not secure full marks.
7. Tackle questions to which you know the answers first. This strategy will boost your confidence.
8. Decide how much time to spend on any one question (usually determined by the number of points allotted) and stick to your timetable so that you are not rushed at the end.
9. If you finish before the allotted time period, read over your answers before submitting them. This review will assure you that you have answered all the questions and you may think of some points to add.

After Your Examination

1. Decide whether or not you wish to join your colleagues for a "postmortem." Sometimes going over an examination only serves to increase your anxiety.
2. Follow through with your plan for celebration after the examination. Doing something fun will help clear your mind and relax you after all the hard work you did preparing and writing the examination.
3. After you get your results, check to see where you did well and where you need to improve. Find out whether you need to study the content more or if you need experience interpreting the questions. This information will help you prepare for future examinations.

Tips for Dealing With Criticism

Many people feel anxious about receiving criticism. Here are some perceptions on criticism that shed a more positive light on the issue.

1. Think about criticism as a gift instead of bad news. Criticism offers you the chance to reevaluate your performance. People who take time to criticize you are often interested in you or the job you are doing.
2. Seek more information from the person who is criticizing you. Adler (1991) suggests asking for specific facts about the particular behavior for which you are being criticized. This information will help you determine the validity of the criticism.
3. You are not obliged to agree with all criticism sent your way. Take time to review it, extract what fits your self-assessment, and discard what does not fit.
4. If you receive criticism you have heard before, take note of it. There is likely some truth to criticism you hear repeatedly.
5. Reply to unjust or aggressive criticism; do not let it pass without speaking up. You will feel better about yourself if you confront or correct the person who is unfairly criticizing you. Some people deliver destructive criticism to make them feel more powerful or superior. You do not have to accept the criticism. You can assert yourself.
6. Realize that criticism does not mean there is something wrong with you. You may be accurately criticized for doing something ineffectively or incorrectly, but that in no way means you are a bad or stupid person.

Assertively Handling Difficult Situations Occurring in Nursing Student Performance Evaluations

Some situations increase our evaluation anxiety. We need to prepare ourselves for uncomfortable situations, such as when an evaluator is aggressive, when we are given an evaluation without time to prepare, or when serious allegations are made without evidence. Here are several examples of difficult evaluation situations with suggestions for handling them assertively.

Harshly Delivered Criticism

Your clinical instructor tells you that your charting is fine, and your treatments are carried out superbly, and she compliments you on your effective sterile technique. She also points out that your organization is poor. She notes that your rooms look disheveled and cluttered. "How can you or your clients find things you need in that confusion? Half the time your beds aren't made until after noon, and the room is a mess. This is a disgrace to the nursing profession."

You know that these comments are legitimate, even though they are delivered in an aggressive way. You tend to be disorganized and messy at home as well. Here is an assertive reply to this evaluation:

Assertive you: "Thank you for the feedback on my nursing skills. I don't know what to do about my organization. It's a bad habit I've had for years, even before I came into nursing. I always admire nurses who can do things well and keep their work space uncluttered at the same time. I don't know where to begin. Can you give me some suggestions about how I can improve?"

This reply acknowledges both the compliments and the criticisms from your instructor. Your openness to improve your organization is demonstrated by your request for help. If you really want to improve, you will follow through with some of the suggestions your instructor provides.

Unexpected Aggressive Criticism

You have been assigned to a telemetry unit in a general hospital for the past 7 weeks. It is your last week on the unit, so you decide to stop at the head nurse's office to thank her for the help she has been to you during your practicum.

Without requesting it, the head nurse gives you this piece of advice: "I'm glad you enjoyed your time with us. Here's some advice I'd like to give you before you leave us: improve your charting. It's a mess to read. I spent 10 minutes trying to decipher one of your notes the other day. You'll never make a good nurse if you can't communicate to the rest of the world what you've done."

Assertive you: "I am aware that my charting is too long and difficult to read. Miss Jameson, my clinical instructor, has also pointed out my need to improve. Do you have any suggestions to help me learn how to improve my charting?"

Wit and Wisdom

The Secret to Success

Would you like to wow them
With your high self-esteem?
Want to hear a secret,
An instructor's dream?

Be willing to listen
To others' critique.
Your strengths and weaknesses,
What make you unique.

If you knew all there was
To know when you came
Why come here at all?
Stay home, stay the same.

So be open to listen
And, yes, really hear.
Take a look at yourself
There's nothing to fear.

Don't be defensive.
Ask how you can change.
Old approaches for new
You soon can exchange.

Copyright 1995 Julia W. Balzer Riley.

This reply acknowledges the feedback from your head nurse. Although her feedback is aggressive, you maintained an assertive stance in your response. Your request for guidance invites her to contribute to your development in a more positive way.

Allegations Without Evidence

Your clinical instructor is giving you your final evaluation on your performance on the obstetrical unit where you have been working for the past 3 weeks. She has made several negative comments about your handling of the babies and your interactions with the new mothers. However, she has given no examples to support her comments and she has never observed you directly. You believe that your performance is acceptable and that it meets the standards set out in the procedure manual. You reply in the following way:

Assertive you: "My own assessment of my handling of the babies and my interactions with the mothers is that I treat them both with respect and care. I would appreciate your providing me with more concrete evidence of any rough handling, since this charge has serious implications for my career. I have worked closely with Ms. Green in the nursery and Mrs. Nuthers on the unit. Both these staff nurses could provide you with a thorough assessment of my performance. I would like to have a joint meeting with you and these nurses to discuss my performance. I will not sign this evaluation form until this meeting has taken place."

This assertive response lets your instructor know that you intend to protect your reputation. you have made a reasonable request for another evaluation. Your straightforward manner, which is neither insulting nor disrespectful to your instructor, increases the likelihood of having another evaluation.

MOVING FROM REACTIVE TO PROACTIVE BEHAVIOR

The ability to seek out opportunities for evaluation sets you apart as a person who has vision, who wants to improve rather than hide in hopes that no one will notice your mistakes. Covey (1989) suggests that "being proactive" is the first of seven habits of highly effective people. He says to be proactive means "we are responsible for our own lives. . . ." Proactive people "do not blame circumstances . . . for their behavior." The reactive person blames other people and specific situations for problems. To be evaluated can be experienced as criticism and can evoke a natural tendency to look for excuses. As your skills improve and your confidence increases, you should find yourself moving from reactive to proactive, seeking out evaluation. You give your permission for others to give you feedback. You take responsibility for corrective action without having your feelings hurt.

Wit and Wisdom

They cannot take away our self-respect if we do not give it to them.

Gandhi

Think About It...
What, So What, and Now What?

Consider what you read about evaluation anxiety. In what areas do you experience evaluation anxiety? Write the answers to the following questions.

What? . . . Write one thing you learned from this chapter.

So what? . . . How will this impact your nursing practice?

Now what? . . . How will you implement this new knowledge or skill?

THINK ABOUT IT

Practicing Overcoming Evaluation Anxiety

Exercise 1

Dr. Barbara Bunch (1994), a nurse and psychologist, recommends the following technique to minimize your state of arousal to stress, a preventive strategy that you can practice throughout the day when you feel stressed. She believes it has a cumulative effect and will decrease the effects of stress in tough situations like evaluations.

1. Smile!
2. Take two abdominal breaths.
3. Drop your jaw.
4. Drop your shoulders.

Go ahead and laugh! You may look silly, but try this for several days and share your results with another student or colleague.

Exercise 2

Your colleague in the school of nursing has an important physiology test coming up in 2 days. Over coffee in the cafeteria she says:

Nervous Nina: "I'm terrified about this exam. Everyone says Jones is such a hard grader. I did okay on the first test but the stuff we've taken since then is a lot more complicated. I can't fail because it will put my course selection out of sequence. I've put so much time into studying this stuff that I'd better pass. I'll be glad when it's over."

How would you intervene to help minimize your friend's evaluation anxiety? Prepare your suggested strategy individually, then work in groups of four to compare your suggestions.

Exercise 3

You are a staff nurse working in the operating room of a general hospital. A student doing her clinical practicum in the operating room is talking to you at coffee break. This is what she says:

Anxious Anita: "Tomorrow's going to be awful!. I've got to scrub for Dr. Shark and I've seen how he yells at students if they don't do exactly what he wants. And to top it off, my clinical instructor chooses tomorrow to evaluate me! I'll be a wreck by 4 o'clock tomorrow."

How would you help this student nurse cope with her evaluation anxiety? Prepare your own response and then work in groups of four to compare and share strategies.

Exercise 4

You are a staff nurse working in a small rural hospital. It is time for your 3-month evaluation from the Director of Nursing. In preparation for your performance evaluation interview (which you had to ask for) you search for an evaluation form. You soon discover that there is no standard evaluation form because performance evaluations are rarely done in this hospital. You also discover that your job description, which was written 4 years ago, is one that was copied from a large hospital in the city 200 miles away, and is irrelevant to your position in a rural hospital.

How would you handle this situation to reduce your evaluation anxiety? Compare your ideas with those of your colleagues.

Exercise 5

Here are several questions posed by the American Nurses Association (1990) as one means of assessing the validity and reliability of your employer's appraisal system. To how many of these questions would you answer "yes" at your place of employment (or prospective place)?

1. Are employees actively involved in determining policies and procedures for the appraisal process?
2. Is more than one type of performance appraisal tool used to evaluate an employee's performance? Are different tools used to evaluate different types of job assignments?
3. Is job performance appraisal handled at the management level closest to the employee?
4. Does the appraiser routinely collect relevant data about job performance or depend on recall to meet a deadline for completing appraisal forms?
5. Is there any type of review of a supervisor's appraisal of employees by upper management?
6. Is there a standard time frame for formal evaluation (quarterly, biannually, and so on)?
7. Does the appraisal process include setting goals? Is there sufficient opportunity to review progress in achieving these goals during the appraisal period?
8. Are the categories delineated in the evaluation tools realistic?
9. Do the categories delineated in the evaluation tools complement the job description?
10. Are the behaviors to be evaluated measurable?
11. Do the formats of the appraisal tool provide space for recording supporting evidence/concrete illustrations?
12. Are the standards/criteria for judging levels of job performance clearly defined?
13. Do the evaluation tools weigh categories of employee behavior on the basis of their importance to the job?
14. Is there a clear understanding of the impact of performance appraisal on salary increments, job status, and so on?
15. Are there clear steps available for an employee who is dissatisfied with the outcome of a job performance appraisal?

What action would you recommend if your agency does not have a fair system of job performance appraisal, making you and other employees feel more anxious about the evaluation?

Exercise 6

How can employees follow Mackay's advice to jobholders to "deliver more than you promise"? How could nurses "exceed their quotas"? Think about this question separately, then compare your views to your classmates'.

References

Adler RB: *Understanding human communication,* Fort Worth, 1991, Harcourt, Brace College Publications.

American Nurses Association: *Survival skills in the workplace: what every nurse should know,* Kansas City, Mo, 1990, The Association.

Bunch B: Handling anxiety disorders. Lecture delivered at Baptist Medical Center, Jacksonville, Florida, August 1994.

Covey SR: *The 7 habits of highly effective people,* New York, 1989, Simon & Schuster.

Dweck CS, Wortman CB: Learned helplessness, anxiety and achievement motivation. In Krohne HW, Laux L, editors: *Achievement, stress, and anxiety,* Washington, DC, 1982, Hemisphere Publishing.

Kleehammer K, Hart AL, Keck JF: Nursing students' perceptions of anxiety-producing situations in the clinical setting, *J Nurs Educ* 29(4):183, 1990.

Mackay H: *Beware the naked man who offers you his shirt,* New York, 1990, Ivy Books.

Marquis BL, Huston CJ: *Management decision making for nurses: 124 case studies,* Philadelphia, 1998, Lippincott.

Meichenbaum DH: Cognitive modification of test anxious college students, *J Consult Clin Psychol* 39(3):370, 1972.

Orlick T: Psyching for sport: mental training for athletes, Champaign, Ill, 1986, Leisure Press.

Ryan KD, Oestreich DK, Orr III GA: *The courageous messenger: how to successfully speak up at work,* San Francisco, 1996, Jossey-Bass.

Wine JD: Evaluation anxiety: a cognitive-attentional construct. In Krohne HW, Laux L, editors: *Achievement, stress, and anxiety,* Washington, DC, 1982, Hemisphere Publishing.

 ## Suggestions for Further Reading

Kabat-Zinn J: *Full catastrophe living: using the wisdom of your body and mind to face stress, pain, and illness,* New York, 1990, Dell.

See the chapter on working with fear, panic, and anxiety for techniques to decrease symptoms of evaluation anxiety.

Check the counseling or career counseling center at your college for information or classes on overcoming test anxiety and improving study habits.

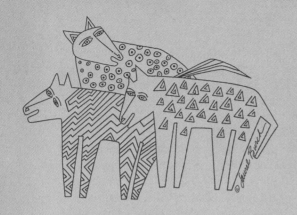

24

Feedback

One may find the faults of others in a few minutes, while it takes a lifetime to discover one's own.

Author unknown

OBJECTIVES

1. Discuss the importance of feedback in communication.
2. Identify strategies for giving feedback.
3. Discuss steps for receiving feedback to promote self-growth.
4. Practice seeking, giving, and receiving feedback in selected exercises.

THE IMPORTANCE OF FEEDBACK

Feedback is defined as a "response following an action" (Webster, 1993). Discussions about how to give feedback distinguish between positive and negative feedback, but either one can be considered a gift. Consider the two parts of the word—"feed" and "back." In one sense of the word, "feed" implies to nourish, even comfort, or to meet another's needs. "Back" in this context is to return something to another. Combining these two notions, feedback means the returning of nourishment to another person. In this sense, feedback is something positive—a gift for the other person. The gift that is given is one person's thoughts and feelings about another person's behavior.

379

Feedback helps us see our behavior from another's perspective. This reflection tells us how someone else is reacting to our communication. This picture helps us decide whether to continue acting in the same way or to change. Viewed this way, feedback is a springboard for self-growth. Feeling happy with ourselves is one of the most joyous experiences in life. This contentment is an acknowledgment of what we like about ourselves and it solidifies our self-concept. Contemplating a change in our way of behaving is really envisioning a new self-concept. Feedback has the potential for expanding our development as human beings. To be most effective, feedback on progress toward goals must be frequent and specific (Eisenberg, 1997). Consider the nursing process as an example of a feedback mechanism. Assessment, planning, and intervention can change based on feedback from the client in the evaluation phases and on additional information obtained in continuing assessment (Marquis and Huston, 1998). Improving care based on feedback has been a part of nursing since the days of Florence Nightingale (Porter-O'Grady, 1994). Continuous quality improvement (CQI), which is really just data-driven problem solving, examines processes in delivery of care to improve service and is dependent on regular feedback for excellence (Porter-O'Grady, 1994). 360 degree feedback, or multi-source performance approval data, is used as a staff development tool since it draws feedback from peers and subordinates to supplement direct observation from the manager (Coates, 1998).

There is a difference between giving feedback and giving advice. Giving feedback is merely a reflection about how another person's behavior has affected us, not advice about how a person should change. After receiving our feedback, clients or colleagues may wish to make changes in their behavior. One thing we might be asked is: "What do you think I should do to change?" Often we will have advice, but a note of caution is in order.

To avoid hurting the feelings of others, and to ensure that we are being respectful, these options should be made as suggestions for their consideration. We can never know what changes will be comfortable or suitable for another person, because each of us must decide what suits our personal style and priorities. Our suggestions will be more readily received if they are offered tentatively, such as:

"Something I've tried is this . . . ." "Perhaps adding this change will help you." Or, "When I was trying to change in the same way, my sister-in-law suggested I do this . . . . It worked for me, and maybe it will work for you."

These examples allow the receiver the final option of accepting or rejecting.

For feedback to be integrated it must be delivered in a way that is receivable, and the receiver must be open to considering the feedback. Following are some steps you can follow to increase the probability that your feedback will be accepted.

HOW TO GIVE FEEDBACK

First, check your agenda for wanting to give feedback. What is motivating you to give feedback? What do you hope to accomplish by delivering feedback? Any reasons based on the belief that your feedback will benefit the other person by increasing the opportunities for self-growth are acceptable to the intention of feedback. There are many reasons for giving feedback that are unacceptable in a caring, therapeutic relationship. Feeling irritable and wanting to lash out at another as a way of getting revenge, wanting to display our superior knowledge to "show up" another, or wanting to rigidly control the behavior of clients or colleagues because of intolerance are not good reasons for giving feedback.

Gain Permission to Give Feedback

The next step is to gain permission from your client or colleague to give feedback. Requesting permission may be done verbally by simply asking if the other person would like the feedback. Or the request can be made through a nonverbal checking out.

The following example includes verbal and nonverbal ways of getting permission to give feedback.

You have been teaching a new father to bathe his newborn, and he has given a return demonstration.

"I noticed how securely you have been holding your baby daughter—I'm sure it makes her feel safe and secure. It looks like she's enjoying the bath you are giving her and especially how you are talking to her. I'd like to point out one suggestion for improvement."

Here you pause and look at the father, who nods his approval for you to continue.

"When you allow your daughter's umbilical cord to get wet, it increases the chance that she'll get an infection. I've got some suggestions, if you'd like to hear them, for how you could keep her cord dry."

Again you make eye contact with the father and do not proceed until he conveys his interest in your information.

"Some ways to keep the cord dry are to fill the tub with less water and hold her at about a 45-degree angle. Also you can squeeze out the washcloth so that water doesn't accidentally drip on her cord. "

Be Specific

Giving feedback to clients or colleagues is not your chance to bombard them with everything about their behavior that you like or dislike. To give your feedback impact, you must focus on specific, observable behavior. The following situation between two nurses illustrates how to be specific when giving feedback.

You are on the evening shift and are still relatively new to the procedures on the unit. Before the night shift comes on you always have last minute charting and tying together of loose ends for your report. For the past 4 nights one of the night nurses has come on duty 30 minutes early and tried to engage you in a social conversation. Your hints that you don't have time to talk at that moment have been ignored, and she has persisted in bending your ear about her date or how she slept that day. You approach her with:

"Rhonda, I'd like to talk to you about how your coming on early and talking to me is affecting me."

At this point you wait until she's agreeable to discuss the issue and proceed with:

"I'd love to talk with you, but when you try to capture my attention at the end of my shift it agitates me because I'm trying to tie up so many loose ends and get things in order for the night shift. I find myself getting so tense that I can't pay enough attention to what you are trying to tell me and I don't get my work completed the way I'd like to. Do you understand what I'm saying?"

Here you must pause and give Rhonda a chance to respond. You might proceed with:

"I've got a suggestion that will allow me to get my last-minute work done and still give us a chance to visit before I leave. Want to hear it?"

Keeping your feedback to observable behavior prevents you from blurting out something cruel like: "Can't you wait till your shift starts to talk my ear off?" or, "I can't stand you bugging me like this!" Being specific helps you keep feedback realistic and acceptable.

Convey Your Perspective

When you give feedback you must remind yourself that you are reporting your view of things. Nothing is innately or objectively right or wrong about your perspective; it is simply how you see the world. Since every relationship you have with colleagues and clients, however, has importance and influence for both parties, your reactions are important to others.

When looking in the mirror after getting your hair cut in a new style, you might smile with approval, blush with embarrassment, or refuse to pay for such an outrageous coiffure! The hairdresser might glow with pleasure at your sophisticated new image and your friends may look ambivalent about the new you. Any of these reactions is legitimate, and none is better than the other. Each reaction is feedback based on the viewer's frame of reference. You need to keep in mind when you are giving feedback that, as important as your views are, the receiver may not agree with your perspective.

To ensure that you give feedback respectfully, you can couch your comments with phrases like these:

"As I see it . . . ." "I felt happy (sad) when you clapped (did not applaud)." "From my perspective . . . ." "The way I see things is . . . ."

Using the first person to convey your thoughts and feelings prevents you from accusing or labeling another person's behavior.

Being responsible for customer service training in a hospital setting, it is my responsibility to give feedback when I observe poor customer service. When I am in the role of client, I am in a good position to assess the quality of service. When I give feedback, I share my perspective of someone who has "been there." When I went to the laboratory to have my blood drawn, a woman came into the room, did not identify herself, and was wearing no name tag. When I asked her about it, I learned she was a student. A staff member came in to help and I learned that students were not routinely given name pins. I shared this information with the manager and how uncomfortable it made me as a patient not to know who was working with me. She agreed and arranged to provide the students with name tags. It is not always easy to give feedback if it requires correction, but it may help others. In this case, we were able to polish the image of the staff as professionals.

Formula for Success in Giving Assertive Feedback

In difficult situations where you need to tell others how their behavior is affecting you and request a behavior change, the following formula, used often in assertiveness training, is helpful:

1. When you . . . (describe the behavior without judging it)
2. The effects are . . . (describe concretely how it affects your life in a practical sense)
3. I feel . . . (describe your feelings without blaming. The "I" statement implies ownership of your own feelings)
4. I prefer . . . (describe what response or change you would like or if possible give the other person a chance to come up with a solution) (Carr-Ruffino, 1994).

For example:

1. When you speak in a loud voice when I am trying to listen to someone on the telephone
2. I cannot hear and I must ask the caller to repeat the message
3. I feel embarrassed that the patient might think the unit is in chaos
4. How can we handle this? Or, I would prefer you to speak more softly or finish the conversation away from the telephone.

Let's try this with the name pin issue:

When you don't wear a name pin, I can't call you by name and I don't know who to ask for if I need to talk with you later. I don't feel like I'm in a setting where people are professional and I can't even be sure you work here. Are you given name tags? No? In that case, I'd like to check into this because I think it might make other patients more comfortable, too. Would that be all right with you?

Invite Comments From the Receiver

Since the feedback you give is from your perspective, it is important to keep in mind how others might feel when receiving your comments. One way to do this is to check out their reactions with phrases like: "What do you think about my comments to you?" or, "Could you tell me your reactions to what I've just told you?" Giving feedback requires consideration. You never know how others will respond to your feedback, and you must allow them to express their reactions. People need time to grasp what you are saying, mull it over, ask for more information, and express their feelings and thoughts about what you have said.

Be Genuine

It warrants saying that those who give feedback should be honest when expressing their views. If you do not mean it, do not say it! When you are sincere in giving feedback, you build trust. If you are verbalizing something positive, but the frown on your face indicates displeasure, then the receiver of your feedback will get a mixed message. It is important to keep your verbal and nonverbal behavior congruent.

Check Out How Your Feedback Is Being Received

If you can honestly say that the feedback was given in the best interest of the receiver, if you gained permission before proceeding with your feedback, and if you were specific in your comments and gave them tentatively, then you know within yourself that you have given feedback in a caring way.

In addition to your self-assessment, you can also pick up clues from your clients or colleagues about whether your way of giving feedback is acceptable. If they indicate that they understand what you are saying, and verbally and nonverbally indicate that they would like you to continue, then you know that your manner of giving feedback is respectful. If they become embarrassed, angry, or move away from you, they may be indicating that they are not yet ready to receive any feedback from you, or at least not in the dosage you are administering. When you pick up clues that your clients or colleagues are becoming defensive about your comments, it is important that you pause and check with them on how to proceed. You might stop altogether or choose gentler and more receivable words.

HOW TO RECEIVE FEEDBACK

Feedback is an opportunity for self-growth; therefore, it is worthwhile knowing how to get the most out of the experience. Clearly, giving feedback requires risking another person's feelings and the relationship you have. Knowing about that risk has implications for how you can act when one of your clients or colleagues takes the chance to give you feedback.

Get Focused

It is important to be focused when receiving feedback. This means not thinking or worrying about some other issue but attending to the feedback and listening respectfully.

Arrange to Have Enough Time to Receive the Feedback

Being unrushed at the time feedback is being given is also important. If you know you are hurried, then say that you value learning others' ideas and you would like to schedule another time to hear them. Making another appointment is important because it indicates that you respect other people's opinions and intend to follow through. You could say:

"I am touched that you have gone to the effort of preparing some feedback for me on the inservice I gave. Could we schedule a convenient time to go over your views? I want to hear what you have to say when I'm not so pressed for time as I am today, so I can take it all in."

Make Sure You Understand the Feedback

Let feedback givers have the floor long enough to clearly state their views, and then ask questions about anything that was unclear.

After your nursing instructor has given you feedback on your sterile technique, for example, you might respond with:

"I think I understand your comments. You noticed I opened the tray before washing my hands and then I left the tray exposed to the air while I washed them. I also had the client's furniture placed in my way so I had to lean over the sterile field and I almost contaminated it. I think those were the main points where I need to improve, weren't they?"

It is not only respectful to repeat the feedback to ensure that you understood, but it is also a way of once more outlining the points as a reminder for yourself.

Request Guidance on How to Change

If you would like to make changes in your behavior because of the feedback, then ask for directions for change—if you genuinely want to hear them. Consider this example:

Your student nurse colleague has given you feedback about your leadership style during your first week as team leader. Most of her comments were positive, but she also indicated that she occasionally felt slighted or put down when you unilaterally made decisions about the nursing care for her clients.

You are surprised to hear her reaction because you had assumed that it was up to you as team leader to take charge, but you feel bad that your leadership style may cause your team members to feel unimportant or left out. You want to change to a more respectful leadership style, so you could ask your colleague:

"Thank you for your comments. I'm pleased with where I seem to be doing well, but I really want to overcome being so autocratic. What could I do differently as team leader to make you feel more included in the decision making for your clients?"

Show Appreciation for the Feedback

Thank others for their feedback. Even if you are not going to change, it has likely been of benefit to hear another person's point of view about your behavior, and for this information you can express your gratitude. Here is an example:

One of your nursing instructors tells you that she fears your habit of only taking half of the allotted time for lunch will wear you out, and she worries about your health. You respond with:

"Thanks for your concern, Mrs. Brown. I find that the physical nursing care on this medical floor demands much more of me than the ENT floor I just came from, where I had more than enough time. I'm slowly getting more accustomed to the pace in the 9 days I've been here, and I'm sure I'll soon be organized and relaxed enough to take the full break at lunch time."

Think About the Feedback You Receive

It is you who will benefit from thinking over any feedback you have been given. Take the opportunity to consider the implications of feedback given to you. Here is an example:

One of your patients, uncomfortable because of her pain, often lashes out at others. As you start her bath one morning she snarls at you:

"Oh! It's you! Miss Sugary Sweet Nancy Nurse! Your smile is sickening, and your cheeriness is just too much to take this morning! Go away and find someone else to gush over!"

Your first reaction may be one of hurt. Or you may brush off her comments and rationalize that she spoke them out of her pain and did not really mean them. As time passes you might find yourself recalling her words and wondering if perhaps you are too cheery and bubbly with your clients—to the point that you keep your distance and do not allow yourself to reach out to their sadness or fear. To be fair to yourself, you should really check out the answer to your concern about your possible insensitivity.

By reevaluating your ability to be warm and compassionate with your clients, you will learn about your strong points and areas where you could be connecting more humanly with your clients. By making use of the feedback you receive, you can grow and develop, both personally and professionally.

ABOUT SEEKING FEEDBACK

As you become comfortable with receiving feedback, you may wish to seek out feedback from others before they offer it. To seek out feedback is to publicly announce that you are ready for self-growth; it implies that you have the confidence to look at your strengths and areas where you could make improvements.

Be Sure You Are Ready to Receive Feedback

Before seeking feedback, check to see that you are really ready to receive it. When you are not fully open to receiving feedback, you will convey that message either verbally or nonverbally. Verbally, you may become angry, get defensive, or make excuses to rationalize your behavior. Nonverbally, you may physically tune out feedback by losing eye contact, turning your body away, or folding your arms to create a barrier against the penetration of the feedback. Both these verbal and nonverbal responses are disrespectful to the person from whom you are asking feedback.

There are times when we are simply not ready to hear feedback. In those cases we should protect ourselves and not seek out others' reactions until we are confident enough to examine them. Receiving feedback with implications for change when we feel shaky or unconfident may only serve to make us feel worse about ourselves. It is a risk to ask for feedback; when we are ready to receive feedback, it then has great potential for self-growth.

Be Specific in Your Request for Feedback

Clarify which aspects of your behavior you want feedback about. Delineating those areas will help your clients and colleagues focus and ensure that you receive the information you want to hear.

For example, after you complete a preoperative teaching session with your surgical client, you ask him:

"What did you think about the session?"

This request for feedback is vague and would not help your client to focus on any particular area. The following request would help your client to focus his comments:

"I included this brochure, which I will leave with you. It reviews what you can expect to happen immediately after surgery. What other questions do you have at this time?"

Feedback and Caring Communication

If you follow the guidelines for giving, receiving, and seeking feedback outlined previously, your feedback behavior will be assertive. Clearly, feedback is a responsible process because it allows participants to make use of all the information available. Behavioral science tells us that whatever behavior we reward will be strengthened or repeated. Remember to take time to comment on what your colleagues do that makes your day easier. In your interpersonal communication skills development, feedback is a crucial factor.

Moments of Connection...
Put It In Writing

One nurse manager, when asked for suggestions to build staff skills, talked about writing thank you or acknowledgment cards for staff when they were observed doing something extra for clients, family or co-workers. At Nurse Week, this manager sends each staff member a card thanking them for their contributions and mentioning at least one specific thing about each person. Staff report saving such cards and notes and reviewing them in tough times.

Think About It...
What, So What, and Now What?

Consider what you read about the importance of feedback. Can you identify your own experience with seeking, receiving, and giving feedback? How can you be open to these communication skills? Answer the following questions.

What? . . . Write one thing you learned from this chapter.

So what? . . . How will this impact your nursing practice?

Now what? . . . How will you implement this new knowledge or skill?

THINK ABOUT IT

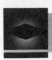

Practicing Giving and Receiving Feedback

Exercise 1

Find a partner in the class. One of you takes the role of listener, the other the role of speaker. The speaker will choose any topic and talk about it for 5 minutes. The listener will convey interest in the speaker's topic and use the communication behaviors learned in Part One.

At the end of 5 minutes the listener will make a specific request to the speaker for feedback on her listening skills. The speaker will respond by giving feedback on the specific points requested by the listener. If appropriate, the speaker will offer to give additional feedback on the abilities of the listener. The listener will respond to the feedback given by the speaker.

After you have finished this exercise, take a few minutes to answer these questions.

As the speaker:

- Was the listener's request for feedback specific?
- Did the listener look like she was open to receiving feedback from you?

As the listener:

- How specific was your request for feedback on your listening skills to your speaker?
- How openly did you respond to your colleague's feedback?
- Was the speaker's feedback to you specific, clear, and tentative?

After you have answered these questions, switch roles and repeat the exercise. This exercise provides you with the chance to seek, receive, and give feedback. What have you learned about feedback from completing this exercise? Get together with the rest of the class and compare your notes about the important and delicate communication behavior of feedback.

Exercise 2

Over the next week, pay attention to how others give you feedback. What do they do to make you feel comfortable about receiving their feedback? What could they do differently to make their feedback more receivable?

At the end of the week you may wish to meet with your colleagues and compare notes on your observations about effective and ineffective ways of giving feedback.

Exercise 3

Over the next few days, keep track of how often you seek out feedback from others. What factors make it comfortable for you to seek feedback? Observe how you receive feedback. What is your assessment of your ability to receive feedback from others?

After you have completed this exercise, in the class as a whole pool your ideas about what factors increase the possibility that people will seek out feedback and what increases the possibility that they will receive it openly.

Exercise 4

Now that you know how to seek and receive feedback, take every opportunity to get feedback on your interpersonal communication skills. Ask your classmates or instructors to observe you when you are interacting with clients, or tape record your dialogue with your clients and replay the tapes for feedback. Taking the time to get others' opinions and suggestions for improvement will enhance your ability to communicate in a caring way.

Wit and Wisdom

Feedback: A Necessity!

If I can't share
The things that I see;
How can I expect you'll
Be honest with me?

We both do want
The best patient care.
It's a responsibility
We all do share.

Some things, of course,
Are no big deal.
Others can cause
a problem for real.

Let's make a pact,
No low self-esteem.
We'll share with each other,
A norm for our team.

Copyright 1995 Julia W. Balzer Riley.

References

Carr-Ruffino N: *The promotable woman: advancing through leadership skills,* Belmont, Calif, 1994, Wadsworth.

Coates DE: Don't tie 360 feedback to pay, *Training* 35(9):68, 1998.

Eisenberg EM, Goodall Jr HL: *Organizational communication: balancing creativity and constraint,* New York, 1997, St Martin's Press.

Marquis BL, Huston CJ: *Management decision making for nurses: 124 case studies,* Philadelphia, 1998, Lippincott.

New Webster's dictionary and thesaurus, Danbury, Conn, 1993, Lexicon Publications.

Porter-O'Grady T: *The nurse manager's problem solver,* St Louis, Mosby, 1994.

Suggestions for Further Reading

Allen J: Time for a good word, *Human Resources* 37(9):136, 1992.

Brooks WD, Emmert P: *Interpersonal communication,* ed 2, Dubuque, Ia, 1980, WC Brown.
Chapter 7, Listening and Feedback, is divided into two parts. The first section discusses listening as a way of receiving feedback. The latter part of the chapter is devoted to a discussion of feedback. Definitions, types, problems, and effects of feedback are discussed.

Burley-Allen M: *Managing assertively: how to improve your people skills,* New York, 1995, John Wiley & Sons.

Ganzel R: Customer service is getting worse? *Training* 35(7):24, 1998.
Response to feedback from customers helps health care delivery systems provide quality, convenient care.

Moran RA: *Beware those who ask for feedback,* New York, 1994, Harper Business.
Humorous axioms for success in business.

Moravec M, Gyr H, Friedman L: A 21st century communication tool, *Human Resources* 38(7):77, 1993.
Discussion of the benefits of upward feedback in an organization.

Nelson B: *1001 ways to reward employees,* New York, 1994, Workman.

Weaver RL: *Understanding interpersonal communication,* ed 2, Glenview, Il, 1981, Scott, Foresman & Co.

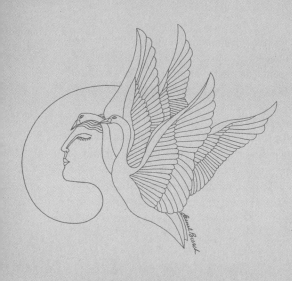

25

Relaxation

One of the greatest necessities in America is to discover creative solitude.

Carl Sandburg

OBJECTIVES

1. Discuss the importance of relaxation skills for the nurse.
2. Identify stressors in nursing.
3. Describe guidelines for beginning to practice meditation to elicit the relaxation response.
4. Identify brief, practical strategies for immediate relaxation.
5. Identify brief stretching exercises to promote relaxation.
6. Practice relaxation techniques.

THE IMPORTANCE OF RELAXING YOUR BODY

As a student in the professional program of nursing, juggling a full life in addition to your academic responsibilities, it is likely you have experienced the unwanted effects of stress. This chapter is designed to encourage you to take charge of your reactions to stressful interpersonal situations in the workplace and develop a habit of daily relaxation, a letting-go technique, to eliminate the negative buildup of stress in your body. Other chapters help you prepare your mind for communicating effectively in your interpersonal encounters with clients and colleagues. This chapter focuses on preparing your body to relax during your workplace interactions. If you are worried about something, then your mental stewing can trigger tension in your muscles, resulting in soreness, headaches, or digestive upsets. In turn, bodily tension is an aggravating signal to your mind that you are not at peace and something is "eating away at you." If you allow these physical symptoms of stress to build up, you are in danger of eventually damaging your body.

Carrying around tightened muscles, tension headaches, or digestive disturbances reflects your "dis-ease" and registers diminished well being. Built-up stress reactions steal valuable energy and put you at risk of holding back or closing off in your interpersonal relationships. In a study of high school students who received relaxation training, trait (transient) anxiety scores were reduced. This is important, too, for nursing students because high anxiety adversely affects learning (Rasid and Parrish, 1998). You can see that it is assertive to learn to minimize your tension and expand your relaxation response in the workplace. There are benefits for you, as well as for your clients and colleagues, when you are more relaxed.

Wit and Wisdom

For fast-acting relief, try slowing down.

Lily Tomlin

NURSING IS A STRESSFUL OCCUPATION

The literature abounds with documentation of the stressors nurses experience. Calhoun (1980) cites four main events responsible for workplace stress and conflict: multiple levels of authority, heterogeneity of personnel, work interdependence, and specialization. All four criteria apply to the nursing profession. As a nurse, you navigate several organizational structures to ensure client well-being: the nursing hierarchy; the medical hierarchy; and the agency's bureaucracy. To survive this organizational maze, you need effective interpersonal communication techniques and efficient management skills.

Not only do nurses require a sound knowledge in their own area of expertise but, in order to be effective in helping clients, they need to know the role and functions of other health care professionals, how to communicate clearly with other members of the health care team, and how to coordinate work efforts of all these disciplines. The changing exposure to different personnel demands that you quickly size up how to relate to colleagues effectively, adding one more stress to an already complex working environment.

One of the most frequently cited sources of stress in nursing is the excessive workload demand, giving nurses the feeling that they are always in a hurry, as if in a race with time. These factors are overlaid by nurses' day-to-day encounters with distressing and anxiety-provoking situations, as well as insufficient resources in these times of health care restraint.

Overriding all of these specific sources of stress is the well-documented strain of being a helping professional (Burke, 1985; Freudenberger, 1983). As helping professionals, each of you has a vision of what your workplace, colleagues, and clients will be like, and these images may not prepare you for the reality you encounter.

Nurses today who want to know where the health care industry is headed must read widely beyond nursing literature in such areas as business and industry. Such titles as *Upsizing the Individual in the Downsized Organization: Managing in the Wake of Reengineering, Globalization, and Overwhelming Technological Change* (Johansen and Swigart, 1994) illustrate the need for techniques of relaxation to cope with overwhelming change in health care and other industries. "Stress-related symptoms . . . account for 75% to 90% of all physician visits" (Vogler, 1998).

Whatever agencies employing nurses can do to support nurses is welcome. As individual nurses we can, and must, complement these organizational reforms with our own methods of stress reduction. This chapter invites you to empower yourself by taking charge of your individual resourcefulness for increasing your relaxation response.

Part of your health teaching with any client is reviewing the basics of health promotion such as eating nutritiously, exercising regularly, securing adequate sleep, engaging in supportive social encounters, and making time for solitude and/or spiritual contemplation. Your knowledge of the benefits of taking care of oneself physically, emotionally, socially, and spiritually is sound. With the investment you have in health, you likely try to incorporate these health behaviors in your own daily life. The return on your investment is an enhanced feeling of well-being and a readiness to handle the stress of working as a nurse. This chapter invites you to add two practices to help you relax and prepare for stress in your interpersonal relationships with clients and colleagues: daily meditation and on-the-spot relaxation exercises. Both of these techniques are designed to relax your body, putting it in a state where the fight-or-flight response or the defense-alarm syndrome of arousal is greatly diminished or eliminated, freeing your energy for communicating effectively (Pelletier, 1977).

Wit and Wisdom

Few things in life are so bad that they can't be helped by a good nap.

Sue Bale

MEDITATION AS A WAY TO AUGMENT YOUR RELAXATION RESPONSE

Meditation is an experiential exercise involving your actual attention, not your belief system or other cognitive processes. Meditation is a highly individualized and personal practice, and effective meditation does not in any way require you to adhere to rigid group norms or abdicate your life to a spiritual or secular leader. Meditation is something you do by yourself and for yourself in order to benefit from the subjective sense of deep relaxation of the body's musculature; an added benefit is that you may possibly come to know yourself more fully. Meditation is psychologically and physically refreshing and energy-restoring (Pelletier, 1977).

It has been empirically verified that the meditative process relieves nervous system stress more efficiently than either dreaming or sleeping. Marked physiological alterations have been proved to accompany meditation: reduction of the metabolic rate; reduction of the breathing rate to four to six breaths per minute; an increase in the amount of the alpha waves in the brain of eight to twelve cycles; the appearance of theta waves in the brain of five to eight cycles; and a 20% reduction in the blood pressure of hypertensive patients (Pelletier, 1977).

The regenerating effects of meditation are experienced during the meditation itself and have a carryover effect into your daily activities (Pelletier, 1977). Once you have learned the low arousal effect during the meditation practice, you can maintain this state of neurophysiological functioning in response to stressful situations. It is impossible to be relaxed and tense at the same time, and your enhanced ability to maintain relaxation during the day in the face of stressful interpersonal situations is what will help to minimize the stress effects on you. With practice you will be able to call upon your low arousal state as needed during your working day. By itself this mechanism is helpful, and your heightened feelings of being able to cope with pressures of everyday life will augment your good feelings (Pelletier, 1977). When you learn to diminish your reaction to stressors, you free yourself to deal with aspects of the interpersonal situation more worthy of your energy. Being able to shift focus from being tight or nervous to feeling calm and in charge allows you to communicate more effectively with your clients and colleagues.

Concentration is essential in all systems of meditation. Meditation will teach you to fix your attention firmly upon a given task for increasingly protracted periods of time, overcoming the habit of flitting from one subject to another. A chaplain working in a hospice setting made this remark about meditation: "When you are trying to still the mind, if a thought comes into your head, you need not invite it to tea."

When the incessant activity of your mind is stilled, you will experience that aspect of your being that is distinct from both your thoughts and attention. It is this state that has been described as transcendental awareness, cosmic consciousness, or satori (Pelletier, 1977):

This goal may seem deceptively simple. Once you have tried truly to quiet your mind, or to allow images to run through it without letting any particular one become distracting, you will understand why practice and perseverance are necessary if you are to be successful. Mental activity is a wayward and not easily controlled phenomenon. At first it seems to have a life of its own. When you exert will or volition and attempt to become quiet, it is very likely that you will be perversely and regularly disobeyed. Your mind jumps unbidden from one thought or concern to another despite your efforts to concentrate on eliminating such activity. With practice and experimentation to determine the best approach for you personally, you can gradually increase your ability to regulate your attention and reduce or rectify the mind's overwhelming tendency to generate incessant activity and distractions. At this point the subtle benefits of meditation become more pronounced (Pelletier, 1977).

GUIDELINES FOR BEGINNING TO PRACTICE MEDITATION

This chapter provides beginning guidelines for practicing meditation on your own. The meditation procedure described here is adapted from the standard clinical meditation (Cormier and Cormier, 1991). There are other forms of meditation, and you may wish to read or even take a course or individualized instruction in meditation.

Make Time to Meditate

To experience benefits from meditation you need to meditate for 15 to 30 minutes at least once a day. This commitment means setting aside that time consistently.

Many individuals say that they have an extremely busy schedule and simply do not have the opportunity to sit for such a long period of time each day. Very often a realistic examination of a person's schedule indicates that in fact there is sufficient time if the individual is conscientious and serious in his efforts. To some extent, the minor life reorientation necessitated by meditative practice may be responsible for its success. It involves a reordering of life priorities and behavioral patterns (Pelletier, 1977).

Set the Climate to Meditate

Find a quiet place where you will not be disturbed. Silence the ringer on your phone and engage your answering machine for the time you are meditating. Tell others that you do not wish to be disturbed for a specified length of time, and assure them that you will be available after your meditation. Taking these precautions frees you to relax instead of tensing at sounds in your environment. Many people find it best to meditate first thing in the morning when their home is quiet and the world has not yet started to intrude. For nurses doing shift work, other arrangements can be made. Some people choose a quiet place outside their home such as the hospital chapel.

Secure a Comfortable Position for Meditation

Find a position that is truly comfortable for you where your body is supported by minimal muscular work. Support your back and feet if necessary. Adjust the room temperature so that you are comfortable. If you are warm enough, you are more likely to stay relaxed and not be distracted.

Develop a Passive Attitude

Reassure yourself that you are not being tested on how well you meditate, and put aside worrying about your technique. Distracting thoughts are likely to occur during your meditation, especially at first when you are learning to focus. Let these thoughts pass without becoming worried about their intrusion or your ability.

Select a Mental Device

To help you shift away from logical, externally oriented thoughts, select a mental device—a phrase, a word, or a sound that you can repeat while you meditate. Repetition of this sound, called a mantra, assists in breaking the stream of distracting thoughts. Some suggestions for a mental device are single-syllable sounds of words such as "in," "out," "one," or "zum'" that can be repeated silently or in a low tone while meditating. Select a mantra that is not emotionally charged and is soothing to you. Make up a word if you prefer (Cormier and Cormier, 1991).

Relax Your Body

When you are ready to begin your meditation, start by relaxing your body. Start with the muscle groups in the head and work to the feet. Say to yourself: "Relax your face; now allow your neck muscles to thaw; let your head relax; take the tension out of your shoulders; let your chest muscles loosen; allow your abdomen to soften; let your back muscles unfreeze; take the tension out of your thigh muscles; let your calves melt; allow your feet to rest comfortably supported." As you tune into the difference between relaxation and tension in your muscles, you will be able to quickly release tightness in your body in preparation for your meditation times. Wearing comfortable, loose-fitting clothing will help you assume a posture that is relaxing.

Focus on Your Breathing

Breathe through your nose and focus on, or become aware of, your breathing. This awareness will help you relax. Breathe easily and naturally, allowing the air to come to you on each inhalation (Cormier and Cormier, 1991). Exhale slowly, allowing all the air out of the lungs. You will find this focus on your breathing very peaceful. When you are stressed, your breathing is quicker; by slowing your breathing and appreciating its rhythm, you begin to relieve tension. Remember not to control your breathing; you do not want to become lightheaded. Just breathe easily and naturally.

While you are focusing on your breathing, you can repeat your mental device silently on inhalation and exhalation. You can try saying to yourself as you inhale, "I am breathing in peace and calm." Upon exhalation, try thinking, "I am blowing out tension and negativity."

Meditate for 10 Minutes

Start off with meditating for 10 minutes, increasing the time to 15 or 20 minutes as you gain experience in being still. Close your eyes during your meditation if this helps you focus on your breathing and on your mantra. Do not think things over or try to solve problems during this quiet time. Your meditation time is time out from running your life, managing time, controlling events, and performing as an adult in your hectic world. In this quiet time, for 10 to 20 minutes, you are free to just sit and breathe. Don't expend energy judging your thoughts or criticizing any distractions; simply let them pass by and remain focused on the present, on your breathing and on your mental device.

Allow your images and thoughts to flow freely. Your mantra will come back to you. While you are meditating you do not need to expend a great effort or concentrate. Enjoy this quiet, peaceful experience. If you need to open your eyes to check the time, arrange to have a clock in view so that moving is unnecessary.

Experience Your Unique Meditation

There are no rules or "shoulds" for what you will experience in your meditations. Enjoy the peaceful hiatus in which you can unwind and experience the sensation of relaxation. You may discover sensations in your body that you were previously too busy to notice. It may happen that in addition to your peacefulness, you achieve a level of stillness in which you might be pervaded with the overwhelming and joyous knowledge that all of existence is a unity and that you are at one with it. This powerful feeling is described as dissolving all fear, including the fear of death, and an inundation of warmth, joy, and harmony (Pelletier, 1977).

Transcendental meditation, one form of meditation, has been found to be an effective tool for:

- Changing one's time orientation to the "here and now"
- Increasing one's behavioral motivation to be more inner-directed
- Developing sensitivity to personal needs and feelings

- Improving the ability to express feelings spontaneously
- Increasing self-acceptance
- Raising one's level of self-actualization (Ramaswami and Sheikh, 1989)

Such effects add to the nurse's ability to learn and maintain the perspective necessary to be able to stay connected to clients and family without becoming personally overwhelmed. Additional techniques that can be used with children are found in Rozman's work (1976).

End Your Meditation Peacefully

When it is time to end your meditation, take a pause before standing up and moving. It may be soothing to sit for a brief moment with your eyes closed before slowly opening them. Don't rush away; rather, gently leave your meditation and enter your world refreshed and relaxed.

Mindfulness Meditation

A stress-reduction clinic based on mindfulness meditation at the University of Massachusetts Medical Center was founded by Jon Kabat-Zinn in 1979. Now there are more than one hundred such clinics that offer mindfulness-based stress-reduction programs. Mindfulness involves "intentional self regulation of attention" (Roth, 1997) and is achieved by holding a focus of attention on a single object such as one's breathing, a religious figure, a sound or a single word or mantra. Through mindfulness techniques, which also include eating meditation, walking meditation, and mindful yoga, concentration is increased and this sets the stage for deeply experiencing one's life. This program has helped clients with many different disease processes to reflect on their automatic responses to suffering and modify responses.

Wit and Wisdom

Those who seek the truth by means of intellect and learning only get further and further away from it. Not til your thoughts cease all their branching here and there, not til your mind is motionless as wood or stone, will you be on the right road to the Gate.

Huang Po

ON-THE-SPOT RELAXATION EXERCISES AS A WAY TO RELIEVE YOUR BODILY TENSION IN THE FACE OF AN INTERPERSONAL STRESSOR

Meditating on a daily basis will make you more relaxed and vital at work or school. Even with this new peacefulness there will be times when a distraught client, an enraged family member, or an agitated colleague can raise your tension level. It would be ideal, but probably impractical, if you could leave the unit for some quiet time when clients and colleagues upset your peacefulness.

What can help are some on-the-spot ways to regain your relaxation response. Sweeney (1978) suggests that relaxation promotes the quality of life (Titlebaum, 1988). Techniques such as meditation or prayer will help you learn to maintain your perspective in the face of the complex demands of nursing. This chapter offers you creative techniques that you can call upon to cool down when the heat is on. So when the unit is understaffed, client census is overloaded, and you are encountering interpersonal stress, here is what you can do to relax your body.

STRATEGIES FOR RELAXING YOUR BODY WHEN YOUR STRESSOR IS IMMEDIATE

Some stressful situations provide no warning. In these instances, it helps to have in your repertoire on-the-spot methods for relaxing your body. Start by practicing a few abdominal breaths. Breathe in through your mouth, focusing on making your stomach bigger; breathe out though your nose, pushing your stomach in toward your spinal column. When working with pediatric patients, nurse researcher, Sharlene Weiss, calls these "belly" breaths and asks children to imagine blowing up a balloon in their "tummy." She explains that this simple exercise puts a brake on the sympathetic nervous system's response during stress by stimulating the parasympathetic nervous system (Weiss, 1998). Try a few abdominal breaths now and notice how you feel afterwards in contrast to before the exercise. Stop reading now and try it. Many people report feeling light-headed. Did this happen to you? We are more accustomed to shallow breathing. More oxygen to your brain can provide quicker problem-solving responses!

Each of the following brief relaxation exercises can be done on a moment's notice with no need for privacy or special equipment. Each can be done as you walk down the corridor, ride on the elevator, or stand up to face the person who is stressing you.

An Unexpected Stressful Interpersonal Encounter

Imagine it is noon on the orthopedic unit where you are in your third week of clinical work. The lunches have not arrived and the clients are hungry. You are hungry. A physician strides out of the elevator, spies you, and heads in your direction. Her forceful walk, scowl, furrowed brow, and finger pointed in your direction give you clues that she is irate about something and, since you are the only nurse in the vicinity, it is likely you will bear the brunt of her aggression.

Here are some ideas of what you can do to relax your body before tension tightens your muscles in a fight-flight response. These techniques can be done in the moment while you are awaiting the approach of the irate physician (your stressor) and even while you are communicating assertively in the face of this threat.

Sprinkling Shower

The spray from the imaginary shower nozzle is right above your head and you can feel the water trickling through your hair and warming your shoulder muscles on its way down your back. Your hunched shoulders sag with relief under the warmth. You feel the warm soapy water sluicing over your body, caressing your muscles, and heating your skin. The soapy lather massages your skin as it flows over you, warming your legs and feet before disappearing down the drain. As you lift your face up to the nozzle, you are pelted with a clear stream of fresh water. Someone has adjusted the nozzle; you sense a firm staccato pressure on your face and over your neck and shoulders.

You notice that this beating of water is simultaneously comforting and invigorating. You feel regenerated. The comforting relief you experience from the water surrounding your body makes you sigh deeply. The pressure of the water eases up to a refreshing sprinkle. As the shower turns off you are suddenly dry, and you feel warm and refreshed. As you relax, say to yourself: "This is relaxation. This is how it feels to be loose. This is what I want."

Sunbeam

Picture a radiant ball of light situated just above your head, creating a field of bright rays vibrating in a protective pyramid around your body. Feel its protective glow encircling your body to a diameter of 4 feet. Notice that the light feels warm and, as it envelops you, you are comforted by its penetrating rays. You find yourself raising your face to bask in the heat of the radiant sun. You can actually feel the light infiltrate your body, permeating your cells. This experience is comforting, and to your surprise, you can actually feel the warmth from the light circulating from your head to your toes. Now you notice that the light is twinkling and, as it touches your skin, you feel unusually invigorated. The sparkling sunbeams dance over your skin, dissipating any tension you were feeling. Your energy opens up in response to the warmth and tingling. As you relax, your muscles are overwhelmed to the core of your being with a feeling of profound comfort and safety in the rays of your own special sunbeam. As you relax, say to yourself: "This is relaxation. This is how it feels to be loose. This is what I want."

Safety Shield

Picture a clear Plexiglass shield that rises up to surround you when you sense danger. Your protective shield is about 2 feet away from your body, and it allows you to move freely while it protects you on all sides. You can see quite clearly into the outside world, just as if the shield were invisible. Inside your shield, the air is fresh and tingles your skin as it circulates around your body. This is your personal air supply and when you breathe, you notice it penetrates your lungs, invigorating your cells as it circulates throughout your body. You feel energized and nourished by this special supply of air in your protected space. You also notice that you feel calm and well defended inside your shield, because you realize that the shield deflects tension away from you. You are relaxed and free from any tensions outside your shield and you feel this assurance in your body. You notice your breathing slowing with the nourishing air, and you feel that your muscles are loose and fluidly mobile. You relax because you know you are safe. As you relax, say to yourself: "This is relaxation. This is how it feels to be loose. This is what I want."

Sweeper

A magic broom comes out of nowhere to sweep the tension from your body. It rakes through your hair, leaving your scalp tingling as the circulation is invigorated. Your head feels warm and tension-free after this stimulation. You notice your neck is mobile and relaxed instead of stiff. As it sweeps the stress from your shoulders, they relax and feel lighter. You stand less rigidly and notice your back is free from any tension. This broom is powerful and thorough in its ability to brush the stress off and away from your body. You can feel its bristles brush away the tension from your abdomen and the front and backs of your legs. When your feet are swept you feel lighter and more mobile; this sensation is energizing. You know you are tension-free and you feel safe when the stress is swept into a pan and thrown far away from your body. Without the encumbrance of stress and tension, you feel ready to handle anything. The sweeping has regenerated your batteries and renewed your energy. Your feet are moving with renewed energy and you're tempted to get up and dance on the balls of your feet. You feel alive and free! As you relax, say to yourself: "This is relaxation. This is how it feels to be loose. This is what I want."

Massage

A pair of powerful hands come out of nowhere and lay themselves across your shoulders. These large but gentle hands are unusually warm and radiate a heat to your upper back. The motion is soothing, and heat penetrates deep inside. You rotate your shoulders easily after these comforting hands have massaged away the tension. There is no effort to stand or move. You are relaxed. The hands move up to knead the knots in your neck muscles. The touch is magical, as if by merely being there the hands can dissipate tightness from built-up tension. Before moving on, the hands shake the tension away from your body so that it is no longer a threat. Next the hands move to your lower back and massage the tightness out of your spine. The pressure is firm, and with each small circular stroke you notice your breathing gets more relaxed; it slows down and you are totally soothed by the comfort and compassion emanating from the hands. You can feel the muscles in your neck, shoulders, and back filling with blood, getting warm and supple under the gifted touch of the hands as they massage away fear and tightness. You feel release and a sense of freedom. You feel warm and protected. As you relax, say to yourself: "This is relaxation. This is how it feels to be loose. This is what I want."

Advantages of On-the-Spot Relaxation Exercises

Each of these brief but powerful relaxation strategies takes about a minute to experience. In that short time you can shift from tightness and fear to relaxation and a feeling of competence. Using these calming strategies will give you inner self-confidence. As you become aware of knowing when your body is relaxed, you will become even more skilled at calming yourself in the face of tension. Relaxation is a skill, a coordination of mind and muscles, and it can be learned by anyone who wants to do so and is willing to spend the time and effort (Percival, Percival, and Taylor, 1977).

STRETCHING YOUR BODY TO RELAXATION IN PREPARATION FOR A STRESSFUL INTERPERSONAL ENCOUNTER

When you have more warning about a stressful interpersonal encounter, you can add soothing stretches to augment the benefits of meditation and on-the-spot exercises. Before encountering a stressor, or at any time during your hectic day, break away from the busy pace of the unit and find a quiet place in which to relax your muscles for a minute or so. Find some privacy in the bathroom or an empty office. Here are some stretches you can do that take little space and can be done from the standing position, without any equipment.

These exercises involve tensing and relaxing the muscles until you feel the difference between the two sensations and learn to consciously relax any tense muscle. As your muscles learn the difference, they will develop a relaxation response (Percival, Percival, and Taylor, 1977).

High Stretch and Relax

Stand erect and stack your hands on top of your head. While taking a deep breath, reach high overhead, lifting your chest and moving your head back slightly. Stretch slowly until you have your hands as high as they will go. Hold for 3 seconds. Now exhale, letting the air out with a long, easy sigh, while dropping your arms slowly to your sides. Let your shoulders sag, your head fall forward, and your knees go loose and slightly bent. Remain in this relaxed position for 3 to 5 seconds. Allow all the tension to seep out of your neck, arms, shoulders, and your chest muscles. Repeat a few times before returning to work (Percival, Percival, and Taylor, 1977).

Shoulder Rotation

This stretch improves shoulder flexibility and relaxation of your shoulder girdle. Stand with your feet comfortably apart. Raise your elbows to shoulder height, allowing your forearms and hands to dangle loosely. Rotate elbows forward in large circles at a medium pace, keeping your hands and arms loose throughout. Move the shoulders in as large an arc as possible for about 20 rotations (Percival, Percival, and Taylor, 1977).

Shoulder Shrug and Relax

This relaxation exercise can even be done while you are talking on the phone. Stand with your feet comfortably apart. As you take a deep breath, shrug your shoulders up to your ears and moderately tighten the muscles throughout your body. Hold for 3 to 5 seconds. Now exhale with a long deep sigh, letting your shoulders drop down and your muscles go loose so that your knees bend slightly and your head drops forward to your chest. Repeat several times (Percival, Percival, and Taylor, 1977).

Arms Out, Up, and Relax

Stand erect with your feet comfortably apart. Lift your arms out to your sides and up over your head, simultaneously pulling your stomach in and lifting your chest. When you've reached as high as you can, let your arms drop loosely down. Allow your head to sag so your chin touches your chest and your knees go "soft." Try to get as loose and limp as you can. Feel the tension drain out. Repeat several times before returning to work (Percival, Percival, and Taylor, 1977).

With practice you will be able to call on your relaxation response at any moment. Being able to relax gives you the power to release tension in your muscles, reclaiming that energy for dealing with interpersonal stressors in your life. In the next few chapters, you will learn ways to prepare your mindset to handle difficult situations in your relationships with clients and colleagues.

 Moments of Connection...
Take Time

When asked how nurses can revitalize their practice, one nurse responded: "Take time to listen, to care, to share. Take time for yourself, especially. Life is too short to put it all into work. You have a lot to gain for yourself and can give more to others when you have energy and a meaningful life of your own."

Wit and Wisdom

It's not easy taking my problems one at a time when they refuse to get in line.

Ashley Brilliant, in *Potshots*

Think About It...
What, So What, and Now What?

Consider what you read about the importance of relaxation. What do you already do for relaxation? Which techniques in this chapter sound interesting to you? Answer the following questions.

What? . . . Write one thing you learned from this chapter.

So what? . . . How will this impact your nursing practice?

Now what? . . . How will you implement this new knowledge or skill?

THINK ABOUT IT

Practicing Relaxing

Exercise 1

During the next week, practice meditating for 10 minutes twice a day, perhaps once in the morning and again in the afternoon. After each of your meditations, keep notes of what the experience was like for you. Here are some questions to think about (but do not be limited by them): How does the experience of meditating make a difference to you? How does your mantra (sound) work for you? What thoughts or images occur? Are you able to let distracting thoughts float by and return to focusing on your breathing and on your mantra?

   Make an opportunity to talk about the practice of meditating with your classmates. Although meditation is a private event, you may feel comfortable exchanging ideas about how to make the process of meditation work more effectively so that it contributes to expanding your feelings of relaxation.

Exercise 2

Give the on-the-spot relaxation visions a try over the next few days. Focus on trying to stay with the relaxation that your vision creates in your body. Note when you get distracted and design a way of refocusing on your soothing internal technique. Note when you are able to distinguish the change from tension in your muscles to letting go in a relaxation response. As you practice you will get more and more astute at recognizing the difference, and soon it will be within your power to quickly and simply allow the tension to escape from your body.

Exercise 3

The next time you are on one of your clinical units take a moment away from the hectic pace to try out one of the relaxing stretch-release exercises. Time yourself to see how long it took to find a spot and complete a few relaxing stretch-releases. You will likely be surprised at how little time it takes. Just breaking away from the unit with the anticipation and intention of doing something good for yourself is beneficial, and the stretching and releasing reminds your body to relax. Note how refreshed you feel when you return to the unit.

   Make time in your class to talk about creative ways to incorporate a stretch-release exercise into your work day.

Wit and Wisdom

The growth of the human mind . . . is the highest adventure on earth.

Norman Cousins

Burke RJ: Stress and burnout in organizations: implications for personnel and human resource management, unpublished manuscript, 1985.

Calhoun GL: Hospitals are high-stress employers, *Hospitals* 54(12):171, June 1980.

Cormier WH, Cormier LS: *Interviewing strategies for helpers: fundamental skills and cognitive behavioral interventions,* ed 3, Pacific Grove, Calif, 1991, Brooks/Cole.

Freudenberger HJ: Burnout: contemporary issues, trends, and concerns. In Farber BA, editor: *Stress and burnout in the human service professions,* New York, 1983, Pergamon Press.

Johansen R, Swigart R: *Upsizing the individual in the downsized organization: managing in the wake of reengineering, globalization, and overwhelming technological change,* Reading, Mass, 1994, Addison-Wesley.

Pelletier KR: *Mind as healer, mind as slayer: a holistic approach to preventing stress disorders,* New York, 1977, Dell.

Percival J, Percival L, Taylor J: The complete guide to total fitness, Scarborough, Ontario, Canada, 1977, Prentice-Hall of Canada, Ltd.

Ramaswami S, Sheikh AA: Meditation east and west. In Sheikh AA, Sheikh KS, editors: *Eastern & western approaches to healing: ancient wisdom and modern knowledge,* New York, 1989, John Wiley & Sons.

Rasid ZM, Parish TS: The effects of two types of relaxation training on students' level of anxiety, *Adolescence* 33(129):99, 1998.

Roth B: Mindfulness-based stress reduction in the inner city, *Advances J Mind-Body Health* 13(4):50, 1997.

Rozman D: *Meditation for children,* Boulder Creek, Calif, 1976, University of the Trees Press.

Sweeney SS: Relaxation. In Carlson C, Blackwell B, editors: *Behavioral concepts and nursing interventions,* Philadelphia, 1978, Lippincott.

Titlebaum H: Relaxation. In Zahourek RP, editor: *Relaxation & imagery: tools for therapeutic communication and intervention,* Philadelphia, 1988, WB Saunders.

Vogler RW: Stress management, *Adult Health* 1(5):27, Sept 1998.

Weiss S: Using relaxation imagery with children, presentation at the 22nd annual seminar of The Florida Association of Pediatric Tumor Programs, Clearwater Beach, Fla, November 19, 1998.

 # Suggestions for Further Reading

American Nurses Association: *Survival skills in the workplace: what every nurse should know,* Kansas City, Mo, 1990, The Association.

This booklet, written by Lyndia Flanagan, provides nurses with a complete overview of the current issues creating stress in the workplace and lends practical strategies for coping with them. Strategies include enhanced self-awareness, finely tuned communication skills, and organizational know-how.

Breakwell GM: Are you stressed out? *Am J Nurs* 90(8):31, 1990.

In this brief article, Breakwell outlines the negative effects of stress and includes a test for checking your stress level. Salient advice is offered for controlling workplace stress.

Cohen S: De-stress for success, *Training Devel* 51(11):77, 1997.

Guzzetta CE: *Essential readings in holistic nursing,* Gaithersburg, Md, 1998, Aspen.

Harp D: *The new three minute meditator,* Oakland, Calif, 1990, New Harbinger Publications.

Jason LA, Wagner LI: Chronic fatigue syndrome among nurses, *Am J Nurs* 98(5):16B, 1998.

Klatz R: 25 strategies for coping with stress, *Total Health* 19(3):33, Jul/Aug 1997.

Mandle CL, Jacobs SC, Arcari PM, et al: The efficacy of relaxation response interventions with adult patients: a review of the literature, *J Cardiovasc Nurs* 10(3):4, 1996.

Stevens A: 12 sure tension tamers, *Heart Soul* 1(1):69, June/July 1997.

Turkington CA: *Stress management for busy people,* New York, 1998, McGraw-Hill.

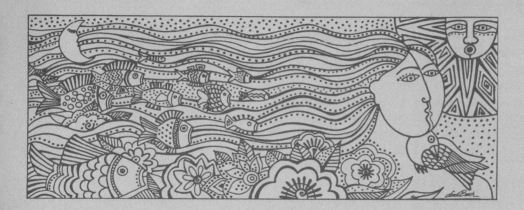

26

Imagery

Seek the ways of the eagle, not the wren.

Omaha Indian proverb

WHAT IS IMAGERY?

An image is defined in the *New Webster's Dictionary and Thesaurus* as a mental picture (1993). The term *visualize* or *visualization* is interchangeable with the term *imagery*. *Visualize* is defined as follows: to form a mental picture of something invisible, absent, or abstract (Barnhart, 1975).

Imagery or visualization is a process of mentally picturing an event we wish to occur in the present or future. It is a process of actually experiencing a picture that we hold in our mind's eye. In

405

visualizing our picture we may incorporate our senses to taste it, smell it, feel it, and imagine the sounds and emotions associated with it. For example, when we visualize a freshly baked apple pie we can actually smell it, taste the apples, and visualize eating the pie.

Try this experiment: The Tart Lemon

Close your eyes and imagine you are in your home. Picture yourself walking into your kitchen and looking at the refrigerator. In your mind's eye see the refrigerator. Open it and pull open the fruit and vegetable drawer. You see a large, bright, yellow lemon. Pick it up and notice the yellow, shiny, bumpy surface. Feel the weight of the lemon in your hand. Now take the lemon to a cutting board. Squeeze the lemon before you cut it. Already you can smell the citrus scent. Cut the lemon and inhale its fragrance. Open your mouth. Now squeeze a few drops of the cold, tart lemon juice onto your tongue. Open your eyes. Did your mouth pucker? Could you see the lemon, smell it, taste it?

NOTE: Not everyone images the same way. Some people report being actively involved in the scene. Some see it as actors on a stage. Others get sensory impressions, but not a clear image. Don't be concerned if you can't "see" things. Practice helps. This experiment helps you understand the behavioral applications of imagery.

Wit and Wisdom

Everyone who is successful must have dreamed of something.

Maricopa Indian proverb

When we visualize ourselves communicating, such as by listening actively, we can hear ourselves articulating empathic words, feel ourselves being warm, genuine, and natural, and enjoy observing a positive interaction between ourselves and our clients or colleagues.

Imagery is a process similar to daydreaming; however, imagery is combined with a conscious purpose. It is much more than mere fantasy. The key to successful visualization is to be clear about what you want and then commit to that course of action in your imagery. This is a crucial step for producing successful results. In your mind's eye there need be no limitations or constraints.

This chapter will focus on how you can use imagery to positively influence your interpersonal communication. You will learn the steps required to formulate a clear image of how you want to communicate with your clients or colleagues. You can then use that visualization to help you actualize your vision in reality.

Imagery has been used in physical healing for a long time. You may be interested in the history of visualization in medicine.

History of Imagery

Imagery may be the oldest healing technique used by humans. Early records of these techniques have been found on cuneiform tablets from Babylonia and Sumeria. Greek, Egyptian, Oriental,

Wit and Wisdom

Just Imagine

Take me away
To a beautiful place.
Let's get away
From this awful rat race.

They say a vacation
I can take in my mind.
Close your eyes, relax,
Leave your tension behind.

Pay attention to each sense.
See, smell, hear, taste and feel.
Let your mind go, just travel.
Your own stress, you'll heal.

It's OK to daydream.
They always said, "NO!"
Now it's OK to daydream.
Just let your mind flow.

Copyright 1995 Julia W. Balzer Riley.

and ancient Indian civilizations used visualization. Even today Navaho Indians and Canadian Eskimos practice imagery for healing purposes (Samuels, 1975).

In all these cultures disease was seen as a demonic force that had incorporated itself into the ill person's being. The shaman or physician-priest would heal through rituals or ceremonies by confronting the disease-causing demon with a positive force and exorcising the demon from the patient. The shaman derived his power from visualizing a higher authority, god, or spirit. At that time medicine was controlled by religion, mysticism, and magic (Samuels, 1975).

Paracelsus, a Renaissance physician, is known as the father of scientific medicine and modern drug therapy. A man opposed to the notion of separating the healing process from the spirit, he said: "The spirit is the master, imagination the tool, and the body the plastic material. The power of the imagination is a great factor in medicine. It may produce diseases in man and in animals, and it may cure them . . . Ills of the body may be cured by the physical remedies or by the power of the spirit acting through the soul" (Hartmann, 1973). The views of Paracelsus differed from the early shaman's views because Paracelsus believed that people's own thoughts, as well as gods and spirits, could be healing (Samuels, 1975).

It was during the Renaissance that the mind-body dichotomy was first conceived. The French philosopher Descartes helped establish the split with his attempts to free scientific questions from arguments concerning God. Scientists could then be concerned about the body without theological debate, and the philosophers and theologians were left to study the spirit and mind (Flynn, 1980).

Since the Renaissance, techniques of healing were divided into two systems: scientific and religious. Our Western society has adopted scientific healing—surgery and drug therapy. With increasing scientific investigation and medical specialization, the body-mind-spirit split continued into the twentieth century. By 1900, however, a number of medical scientists began investigating how the mind affects the body and healing (Samuels, 1975).

Jacobson (1942), searching for effective methods of relaxation, has demonstrated that the imagery we use in thought processes produces a muscular reactivity that resembles what occurs during the actual performing of the act. That is, if we imagine ourselves in our mind's eye as running, the muscles we normally use when we run will contract slightly.

Many scientists, as well as members of the medical profession, have continued to accept that the autonomic nervous system is unconscious, automatic, and not within conscious control. In the late 1960s physiologists DiCara and Miller demonstrated that parts of the autonomic nervous system can be conditioned and controlled. Using animals, they determined that rats could learn how to alter their stomach acidity, brain wave patterns, blood pressure, and blood flow (Miller, 1969). Furthermore, in their work with humans, scientists have verified the ability that yogis have to control specific processes of the body such as metabolic rate and heart rate (Lauria, 1968).

Groundwork laid by these scientists has been revolutionary in the current shift away from the body-mind-spirit split to body-mind integration. The implications of these findings for nursing and medicine are extraordinary and exciting!

Application of Imagery in Health Care

Imagery is used to clinically for such purposes as to promote relaxation, to alter physiologic responses, to alleviate pain, and to promote comfort during and after procedures. Some imagery techniques are end-state, the image of a healed state; process, step-by-step to a goal, such as successful, comfortable completion of a procedure; receptive, in which images for healing arise from the person's own mind; active, having a conscious choice of a healing image such as a healing white light directed to the affected area; and an anatomical image, such as the opening of constricted vessels (Dossey, 1995). Here is a specific example: a client with excessive gastric secretions was asked to gaze at the dryness and texture of blotting paper while imagining absorbent dryness. Tests indicated that after 10 days of doing these visualizations, the client's excessive secretions normalized (Luthe, 1969). The use of imagery empowers the client to promote wellness when disease produces a sense of loss of control.

One hypothesis is that the feelings of hope and anticipation are recorded by the limbic system in place of the hopelessness and despair. Psychoneuroimmunology (PNI) is the field of study of the "mulitidirectional interactions among behavioral, neuroendocrine, and immunological process of adaptation. Thoughts, emotions, and information are reciprocal stimuli to sensory and motor neurons, glandular tissues, and immune cells via chemical transmitters (Giedt, 1997). Clients who are enthusiastic about feeling better using imagery and who implicitly follow instructions show dramatic relief of their symptoms and marked improvement in their condition.

There is evidence that visualization can influence a person's heart rate, blood flow, immune response, and total physiology. Visualization is a noninvasive, cost-effective intervention. Knowing this, what then are the implications of imagery?

Implications of Imagery

How does the knowledge that it is possible for us to voluntarily affect our autonomic nervous system using visualization influence us in our nursing care? First, we as nurses can adopt a holistic philosophy of body, mind, and spirit integration. A holistic perspective emphasizes the interrelationship of the parts that make up the whole person. It acknowledges that the mind affects the body and vice versa. Accepting this notion of interdependence means understanding the power that exists within our whole body-mind-spirit beings to heal ourselves. This internal power can be used to maintain and increase our level of wellness, either alone or in conjunction with an external source of healing (Samuels, 1974). The American Holistic Nurses' Association offers a forum for the discussion of research and practice of holistic nursing, while nurses in other states conduct workshops on such interventions as therapeutic touch.

A simple application of imagery in nursing is the use of alternative language when performing procedures, language that while still truthful, suggests a different sensation than anticipated. When giving an injection, say, "You may feel a stick." This language decreases anxiety and shifts the pattern of response to "pain" to response to "a stick" (Kron, 1983). Imagery is also gaining increasing acceptance in the areas of corporate finance and sports. Researchers have discovered, for example, a frequent characteristic of executives of major U.S. corporations: "These people knew what they wanted out of life. They could see it, taste it, smell it, and imagine the sounds and emotions associated with it. They prelived it before they had it. And that sharp, sensory vision became a powerful driving force in their lives" (Mayer, 1984).

In an experiment at the University of Western Australia, one basketball team practiced 20 minutes longer a day while a second team used their 20 minutes to imagine themselves playing the game and mentally correcting themselves each time they missed a basket. After a period of weeks, the group that physically practiced the game improved 24%, and the group visualizing themselves as practicing improved 23% (Mayer, 1984).

Professional golfer Jack Nicklaus uses visualization to improve the muscle memory and motor skills involved in golf. Nicklaus has said that good golf requires one-half mental rehearsal and one-half physical coordination. He never hits a shot without first seeing a sharp, clear picture of that shot in his mind's eye (Mayer, 1984).

Imagery has been used in medicine, athletics, and business. It is a process that can be used by people in various walks of life to achieve success in whatever they value. We will now look at how imagery can be used by nurses to improve their interpersonal communication skills.

The Relationship Between Imagery and Interpersonal Communication

If we are clear about what is important to us, and if we are committed to creating what we value, imagery is an invaluable tool for self-direction (Mayer, 1984). This idea is the key to how imagery can be used by nurses to improve their interpersonal communication skills. If you are clear that it is important to be an effective communicator, and you are committed to creating that outcome, then imagery can help you achieve that goal.

As a professional nurse you will want to implement the interpersonal communication skills you will be learning in this book in a way that is beneficial to your clients, your colleagues, and yourself. Imagery will grant you a visualization of yourself implementing these skills in a helpful and effective way. It will provide you with a picture of yourself as a nurse who can handle a variety of interpersonal situations confidently and competently. These images will act like a beacon, beckoning you to achieve the goal of being a competent communicator.

As you read about each of the interpersonal communication behaviors, you will learn the correct way to implement each one with your clients and colleagues. You will develop a vision of yourself executing the communication behavior you are studying. When using imagery, some people experience themselves participating, while others observe themselves as actors on a stage. Some people get impressions without clear images. Some clients report better success with the use of the word *pretend* rather than *imagine*. Your perception may be fuzzy and vague at first. It is essential that you work at making this image of yourself as clear as possible. You need to create an image that envisions you communicating in a positive, effective, and competent manner. The more detailed and specific you can make your visualization, the more effective it will be to guide your actual communication.

Imagining yourself being successful is much like a rehearsal. This mental dry run helps cement an image of yourself carrying out the skill correctly. When the "dress" rehearsal goes well, it gives you confidence that your live performance will also be positive. You may find that the actual visualization process may take you 1 minute or less. The more you use this process, the more proficient you will become.

Seeing yourself perform the way you want to is just one more step toward successfully carrying out your performance in public. Having a visualization of yourself communicating well makes the future reality a viable possibility. Imagery helps you become familiar with your desired outcome so that you start accepting the notion that achieving your ideal is possible and forthcoming. Imagery makes you believe that you can achieve your goals.

Imagery can be influential in helping us communicate in a way that is in keeping with our goals as a nurse. If golf scores and management strategies can be improved through visualization, so can nurses' interpersonal communication skills.

Consider, too, the use of imagery to explore how mental models, which are deeply ingrained, can negatively influence the nurse's performance. Krejci (1997) helps students examine their images to such words as *nurse, doctor, power,* and *caring*. Sometimes these mental models are outdated and can affect nurses' abilities to grow professionally. Krejci cites the example of students in imagery about the word power, depicting the female nurse as a bystander watching a male figure wielding power. Reflecting on the importance of caring and advocacy roles of the nurse, nurses can reframe their views of power and claim the power of their role.

How to Use Imagery to Improve Your Ability to Communicate

Here are some of the essential points of effective imagery. First of all, imagery requires discipline; that is, the willingness to briefly stop what you are doing and proceed with the visualization process. Imagery is most effective when you are relaxed, so begin your imagery with three deep

Moments of Connection...
Just Imagine . . . Helping the Family Find Peace in Death

Nurses related stories of how they offer comfort to a dying person, using touch or song or prayer or their silent presence. The family members, too, need comfort, and this requires energy and creativity and the openness to differences in needs and ways of communication at this time. One nurse reflects on preparing to help a troubled family by imagining previous successes at such times and suggests nurses think back to how other families have grieved and coped and learned from the letting-go of a loved one. Remember vividly past successes to build confidence that the nurse has an active role in helping the family deal with suffering and emotional pain. For the nurse with less experience, imagine the family able to communicate with each other, to reach out to use support systems, and moving successfully through the experience. Use these images to prepare for intimate contact with the family.

breaths to facilitate relaxation. (Refer to Chapter 25 for other relaxation exercises.) Relaxation will help you let go of the thoughts swimming around in your head. This enables you to focus on becoming clear about what you want to create with your imagery. Once you are clear about your goal or purpose, commit to creating it with no reservations and with complete faith that your goal or purpose will be attained. Using all your senses, allow yourself to feel the experience of your goal being attained as though it were happening at the very moment of your visualization.

Although this may sound complex at the outset, with practice you will be able to go through these steps quickly and effectively.

You might think that the practice of visualization is quite abstract since it occurs unseen inside your head. On the contrary, there are concrete and specific steps you can take to ensure that your visualization influences your future performance in the way you intend. Here are some systematic steps you can take to make sure that your visualization has the desired results:

Be Clear About Your Desired Outcome

Before you envision how you will communicate, you must be clear about what it is you are trying to achieve. Is it your aim to be warm and comforting? Do you want to obtain specific information from your client or colleague? Is it your intention to get a point across? Whatever your purpose is in communicating, you must be clear about what you want to happen. The more tailored your mental rehearsal is to reality, the more positive influence it will have on your subsequent performance.

It might be helpful for you to compare a poorly articulated goal to a clearer, more detailed one.

Barb and Jane are both nurses working on a burn unit. Both nurses are concerned about Mrs. Charter, who has become withdrawn and weepy in the last 48 hours. Each nurse decides on her own desired outcome for this unhappy client situation.

Barb makes it her goal to help Mrs. Charter overcome her blue mood. This goal is not as clear as it might be because it does not provide Barb with many clues about how to proceed. Not only is it not specific, but it is unlikely that it is a logical place to begin without more data.

Jane's aim is to find out if Mrs. Charter is aware of what might be causing her mood change and to discuss with her whether there is anything that can be done to lift her mood. Her aim is to put Mrs. Charter at ease so that she can talk more freely about her feelings. This clearer desired outcome provides Jane with some guidelines on how to proceed.

Mentally Outline From Beginning to End the Whole Interaction

You will feel more prepared for your interaction if you complete this step in your mental imagery. For instance, if you are going to be teaching a client to care for a colostomy, do not limit your visualization to the time when you will be talking. Bring into your vision your preparation time, post-session time, and the direct teaching time. When you visualize your preparation you will anticipate all the equipment you will need and consequently have it ready. You might become aware that you fear embarrassment discussing the hygiene and sexual aspects of colostomy care with a male client. This awareness will prompt you to talk over your concerns with a more experienced colleague before the session so that you will feel less uncomfortable.

When imagining the actual teaching session, consider the beginning, middle, and end. Find out how much time you have and imagine yourself using the time effectively and productively for both you and your client. Envision the conclusion of the lesson: will you want time to debrief and discuss the session with a colleague afterward? Is it likely that you will have follow-up assignments after the session for which you must allow time—making referrals, for example, writing records, or securing information for the client? By mentally going through the whole encounter, you will be much better prepared.

Concentrate on Visualizing Details

Envision the most ideal environment for your encounter and take in all its details. In reality try to approximate this location in terms of privacy, lighting, warmth, accessibility to equipment, or whatever other criteria are important.

Visualize how you would like to be dressed for your interaction. If it is a play session with the children on the pediatric medical unit, you will likely envision yourself in a brightly colored pantsuit uniform. If you are mentally preparing yourself for your job performance interview with your manager, envision yourself wearing a uniform in which you feel your best. Pay attention to your posture and facial expressions. If you want to be businesslike with a serious middle-aged client, then picture how you will move to convey your intentions. If you wish to appear relaxed and confident as you present your case at your first nursing rounds, mentally see and feel yourself carrying off this composure.

As you direct yourself in your visions to create a positive impression, notice in your mind's eye that others are responding favorably. You may observe, for example, that you are being listened to and taken seriously and that your client or colleague seems interested in what you have to say.

In addition to your visual imagery, use your other senses. For instance, listen to what you are saying and how you are saying it. If what you are saying does not come across in the way you intended, then roll back the reel and replay it. On the rerun visualize yourself communicating more closely in line with how you would ideally like to. The beauty of mentally rehearsing is that you can repeat it as many times as you like until you get it right! Tune into your words and the way you are saying them, striving to hear the content and quality you desire.

Envision how you want to feel during your communication and be sure to concentrate on the positive. Engender feelings of calmness, confidence, competence, or compassion—or however you want to be feeling in reality. It is important to pause and actually experience these good feelings in your rehearsal, so you will be more likely to recognize them and allow them to surface in the real situation. Also visualize your client or colleague having feelings that are appropriate for the situation.

Using your wide-angle lens, see the whole interaction going as you planned. For example, your bereaved colleague feels relieved to have shed a few tears with you after the death of her long-term client; your skeptical supervisor seems positively impressed with your suggestion for a new staffing schedule; and your once worried client is able to drop off to sleep after your reassuring preoperative teaching session.

Envision the Best and Plan for the Unexpected

There are times when we are concerned about an interaction with a client or colleague for fear we will not be able to communicate in the way we want. Envisioning a positive rehearsal helps relieve some of that worry. To augment your confidence, it is a wise plan to envision some of the unexpected turns of events you might possibly encounter in reality and practice how to cope with them. For example, if it is your first time to teach prenatal classes and you are afraid that there might be questions about labor and delivery that you cannot answer, it would be wise to imagine a scene where you are asked one of these questions and then rehearse the best way to respond. You may gain comfort with saying, "I don't know . . . but I'll find out for you" if you visualize it in advance. Or an angry colleague might unnerve you with her hostility. If you visualize her attack in advance, you can prepare yourself with effective ways to cope with the anger.

Practicing in this way expands your repertoire and prepares you for many contingencies. If you have prepared yourself for several versions of what to expect and rehearsed for several options, you will feel more confident when you find yourself in the actual situation.

Rehearse Repeatedly When Necessary

Each of us has interpersonal situations in which we lack confidence. Some of us shudder at having to interact with angry hostile people, whereas others remain calm and empathic with volatile clients and colleagues. Some of us dread taking charge of teaching sessions, whereas others love that opportunity. Some of us feel we relate better on a one-to-one basis, and others prefer groups. For those interpersonal situations in which you feel uncomfortable, it is wise to repeat your positive visualization several times. Repeatedly go over the picture of yourself performing successfully in your difficult area. A one-shot visualization may not allow you to register all the things you must do to make your communication successful. Seeing yourself handling things well in many visualizations will more thoroughly prepare you for the event. Repeating the scene in your mind's eye will prevent you from being caught off guard in the actual event—you will be able to act instead of react.

When we are concerned about a situation, we can lapse into forecasting the worst or we can choose to concentrate on seeing a positive picture. A positive visualization attracts like a magnet, getting you closer to your goal. If you repeat your positive visualization enough times, you will perform well in reality.

Review Your Live Performance and Update Your Visualization

After you have completed your interaction, take time to evaluate how the session went. If there were parts of your interaction that you were less than pleased with, think positively about how you could improve your next exchange and visualize that happening. For example, envision how you could rephrase your words, arrange the room differently, or include gestures such as touch. This rehearsal will prepare you for the next time.

Do not put yourself down for your errors. Instead, give yourself credit for your improvements. Remember that you are learning and consider that each practice will get you closer to the way you want to communicate to clients and colleagues. Think back to your rehearsal and notice where you met or even surpassed your ideals. Visualize patting yourself on the back and congratulating yourself on your successes. Taking time to commend yourself will increase your self-confidence.

Think About It...
What, So What, and Now What?

Consider what you read about the importance of imagery as a tool to build communication skills. Do you already use imagery techniques? Which techniques in this chapter sound interesting to you? Answer the following questions.

What? . . . Write one thing you learned from this chapter

So what? . . . How will this impact your nursing practice?

Now what? . . . How will you implement this new knowledge or skill?

THINK ABOUT IT

Practicing Using Imagery

Exercise 1

McKim (1972) has adapted a psychological test to help assess the vividness of your images. Rate the following items using these criteria.

Rate as follows: **C** = Clear, **V** = Vague, **N** = No image at all

- The face of a friend
- A rose
- A playful puppy
- A full moon
- The sound of rain on a window
- The taste of pepper
- The smell of peppermint
- The sound of fingernails scraping on a chalkboard
- The smell of coffee brewing
- The feeling of stretching to reach for an item on a tall shelf

Exercise 2

McKim (1972) suggests that it is even more important to be able to control imagery than to evoke clear pictures.

Rate your ability to control an image using these criteria.

Rate as follows: **C** = Controlled the image well, **U** = Unsure, **N** = Not able to control the image

- A rose unfolding into full bloom
- A flat rock skipping across the surface of a lake
- A pinwheel spinning clockwise, then reversing
- A car racing forward, then running backward
- A sofa moving unaided up to the ceiling and back to the floor
- A balloon drifting up into the sky and then returning to the ground
- A wave crashing onto the shore and then reversing itself
- Yourself sitting down in a chair and then standing
- Words appearing on a computer screen and then disappearing as if deleted
- A cake rising as viewed through a glass oven door and then going back to uncooked cake batter

McKim cautions you not to be disappointed if you do poorly, but to repeat the exercises after you have practiced imaging. Look at this like a pretest that is administered before you learn the course content.

Exercise 3

In your everyday life take the opportunity to use imagery to help you communicate more effectively with others. For example, if you would like to invite a classmate to go shopping with you, visualize how you would like to extend the invitation and envision her enthusiastic response. Pre-

Continued

Practicing Using Imagery—cont'd

pare yourself for a refusal by hearing her extend her regrets, and watch yourself respond smoothly. Or you may have an upcoming test of your nursing care practice. Take time to see yourself successfully completing each part of the test, and imagine your instructor giving you top grades.

After a few days of using imagery, take stock of the ways in which it has helped you. What personal adaptations to the process of imagery have you made that might be useful for your colleagues to apply? In the class as a whole, compare reflections on the benefits of imagery.

Visualize yourself as successful! As you practice imagery you will discover it is a skill that requires discipline and concentration. It is self-constructive to develop the power of concentration in order to visualize yourself communicating in an effective way. If we want to be self-destructive, we can let our thoughts take control of us by allowing visions of making mistakes, embarrassing ourselves, or failing to communicate effectively to dominate our visions. If we permit negative and unproductive thoughts to worry and plague us, we might fall into the trap of acting out the failure. On the other hand, our chances for success are augmented by mentally rehearsing a positive outcome. If you have seen yourself succeeding in your mind's eye, it is but one more step to performing well in reality.

As you practice you will discover that imagery does not require much time and can be done anywhere. In the shower, on the bus, as you walk to your meeting, at the nurses' station—you can visualize anywhere because your imagination is always active. What imagery emphasizes is taking control of your thinking so that you create positive, self-enhancing pictures of yourself that facilitate more hopeful and confident feelings. Because imagery can be done conveniently, you can repeatedly bring into your awareness the image of the successful you.

As you learn each of the communication behaviors in this book, practice a positive visualization of yourself using them correctly. Rehearsing with the valuable assistance of imagery will help you feel confident and facilitate the integration of the skill into your communications repertoire.

Wit and Wisdom

The debt we owe to the play of imagination is incalculable.

Carl Gustav Jung

References

Barnhart CL, editor: *World Book dictionary,* Chicago, 1975, Doubleday.

Bolen J: Meditation and psychotherapy in the treatment of cancer, *Psychic* p. 20, July 1973.

Flynn P: *Holistic health: the art and science of care,* Bowie, Md, 1980, Robert J. Brady.

Dossey et al: *Holistic nursing: a handbook for practice,* Gaithersburg, Md, 1995, Aspen.

Giedt JF: A psychoneuroimmunological intervention in holistic nursing practice, *J Holistic Nurs Pract* 15(2):112, June 1997.

Hartmann F: *Paracelsus: life and prophecies,* Blauvelt, NY, 1973, Rudolf Steiner.

Jacobson E: *Progressive relaxation,* Chicago, 1942, University of Chicago Press.

Kron ER, Johnson K: *Visualization: the uses of imagery in the health professions,* Homewood, Ill, 1983, Dow Jones-Irwin.

Krejci JW: Stimulating critical thinking by exploring mental modes, *J Nurs Educ* 36(10):482, Dec 1997.

Lauria A: *The mind of a mnemonist,* New York, 1968, Basic Books.

Luthe W: *Autogenic therapy,* vol II, New York, 1969, Grune & Stratton.

Mayer AJ: Visualization, *En Route* 48(50):30, Jan 1984.

McKim RH: *Experiences in visual thinking,* Monterey, Calif, 1972, Brooks/Cole.

Miller N: Learning and visceral and glandular responses, *Science* 163:434, 1969.

New Webster's dictionary and thesaurus of the English language, Danbury, Conn, 1993, Lexicon.

Samuels M, Bennett HZ: *Be well,* Toronto, 1974, Random House.

Samuels M, Samuels N: *Seeing with the mind's eye,* New York, 1975, Random House.

Suggestions for Further Reading

American Holistic Nurses' Association: P.O. Box 2130, Flagstaff, Arizona 86003-2130. (520)526-2196. http://www.ahna.org.

> Membership includes a subscription to the *Journal of Holistic Nursing.*

Chapman EN: *Life is an attitude: staying positive during tough times, how to control your outlook on life,* Menlo Park, Calif, 1992, Crisp Publications.

Naparstek B: *Staying well with guided imagery,* New York, 1994, Warner Books.

Paul, AM: Reality goes under the knife, *Psychology Today* 31(2):14, 1998.

Rancour P: Interactive guided imagery with oncology patients, *J Holistic Nurs* 12(2):148, June 1994.

Rees BL: An exploratory study of the effectiveness of a relaxation with guided imagery protocol, *J Holistic Nurs* 11(3):271, Sept 1993.

> Relieve pain with imagery, *Prevention* 50(5):160, 1998.

Samuels M, Samuels N: *Seeing with the mind's eye: the history, techniques, and uses of visualization,* New York, 1975, Random House, Inc.

> Although an older publication, its coverage of imagery is comprehensive. In addition to unraveling the history of imagery in religion, healing and psychology, it provides visualization techniques and demonstrates application of imagery in all aspects of our lives, including healing.

Shames, KH: Harness the power of guided imagery, *RN* 59(8):49, 1996.

Sheikh AA, Sheikh KS: *Eastern & Western approaches to healing: ancient wisdom and modern knowledge,* New York, 1989, John Wiley & Sons.

> This book examines the achievements of Eastern and Western medicine and how Eastern practices are being integrated into Western medicine. Aness Sheikh offers workshops on guided imagery and is past president of the American Association for the Study of Mental Imagery.

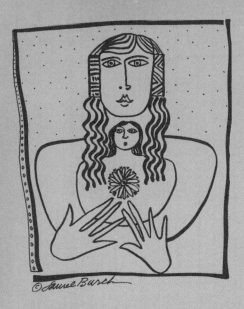

27

Positive Self-Talk

*Man is disturbed not by things but the views he takes
of them.*

Epictetus

1. Define self-talk and its influence on behavior.
2. Discuss the relationship between self-talk and interpersonal communications.
3. Practice positive self-talk to develop confidence in communication skills and nursing practice.

WHAT IS SELF-TALK?

Self-talk is not unlike the conversation that occurs between two people. Meichenbaum (1977) suggests that we have an ongoing internal dialogue—we speak to ourselves and we listen to ourselves. Self-talk is also known as self-verbalization, inner thought, inner speech, self-instruction, or that "little voice" in your head that forms a self-communication system. A familiar childhood story tells us that this skill is time-tested. Remember "the little train that thought he could," the tale of an old train that was being replaced by a shiny new model. The new train refused to climb a steep hill to deliver toys to the children. The old train met the challenge with positive self-talk. He repeated, "I think I can . . . I think I can . . . I think I can . . ." and sure enough, he was successful.

"Casual remarks made unintentionally by those around us can become self-prophecies" (Helmsetter, 1998). In response to the book, *What Do You Say When You Talk to Yourself,* which sold more than a million copies, thousands of letters were sent to the author to relate that they had believed something totally false about themselves throughout their lives based on something someone else had said (Helmsetter, 1998). Turkington calls negative self-talk the "evil within" and points out that we would seldom talk that way to others (Turkington, 1998).

Cognitive behaviorists have learned that internal dialogue has a powerful influence on our behavior. Our thoughts are our interpretations of the world, our judgments about our own behavior, and our assumptions about others' reactions to us. Our feelings are directly influenced by our thoughts, and how we construe our world provides the blueprint for our actions. It is not what is happening to us that is so significant, but how we interpret what is happening to us and what we do under the influence of these thoughts.

For any situation or interpersonal encounter we have, our self-talk determines the following:

- Our attitude toward the situation
- What we see, hear, and attend to
- How we interpret what we take in
- What we think the outcome will be
- How we act (including what we feel, say, and do)
- How we appraise the consequences of our actions

It is important that our internal dialogue be in our own best interests because it is a continuous and powerful influence on our well-being and performance. Cognitive behaviorists believe our internal dialogue causes problems when it is irrational, unrealistic, or ineffective (Meichenbaum, 1977).

Our internal dialogue can be constructive or destructive. A simple example is a person whose mother has always told her that she is clumsy. Believing it to be so, the woman's self-talk is not positive. She says, "I'm so clumsy. I am always bruising myself." She finds that she truly seems to be clumsy. By changing her self-talk, however, to "I am graceful and move easily and carefully," her awkwardness decreases.

Following are several clinical examples of positive and negative self-talk. As you read the examples, think about their possible effects on the nurses in the situation.

Tanya and Deirdre are nursing students in their senior year. As they anticipate their forthcoming clinical placements in a public health department, these thoughts go through their minds:

Tanya: "I've heard that the new director of the agency is a tyrant. I hate people like that. They have miserable dispositions that grate on my nerves. I just know I'm not going to like working with her. Team conferences will be a pain. She's sure to pick on me, and knowing me I'll probably make some blunder that'll be a red flag for her to show me up. I'll be glad when this rotation is over."

Tanya has set herself up for an unhappy and unfruitful clinical placement. Her negative thoughts about the director have entrenched the notion that she will be miserable in the public health rotation. This negative self-talk is destructive. Thinking the way she does, Tanya will likely act defensively and be so on edge that she will make a mistake. Her attitude will probably isolate her from friendly sources of support from staff.

Deirdre: "I've heard that the new director is a real stickler for good nursing care and demands a lot from her staff. It's great that I get to go to a health department where the home care is so good. I'm sure I'll learn a lot. I'm looking forward to making home visits and seeing how nursing care is given there. I'm also nervous because this is new and I don't know what we'll face, but I know I'll have the best teachers and get a lot out of the experience. Too bad it's only a brief rotation."

Deirdre has mentally prepared herself for a happy and rewarding clinical experience. Her interpretation of the excellence of the nursing care makes her keen to observe the nurses and reap the benefits of their experience. Her positive self-talk sets her up to risk interacting with the staff, and she will most likely get a lot out of the experience.

Our self-talk goes on continuously in our heads and is so automatic that we have to carefully listen to hear whether it is exerting a negative or positive influence on our feelings and behavior. If we want to have control of this habitual process, we need to listen to our thoughts, decide how we want to change, and systematically convert our thinking so that it influences our behavior in the intended direction.

Here is an example of a typical situation many student nurses encounter in the clinical area. As you read the scenario, put yourself in the position of the student nurse and write down your reactions.

You are a nursing student just entering your senior year after your summer vacation. To date, your clinical experience has been on the specialty units of your hospital: ophthalmology, gynecology, and the day-stay surgical unit. You are assigned to the intensive care unit and will be working with more complicated equipment. You are sure the patients will think you are clumsy and are afraid you'll make a terrible mistake. You hear the staff is discouraged because they have to cut back hours temporarily due to budget problems. You know the unit has a full census of clients, and you fear the staff will not have the time or energy to help you. Your clinical instructor told you the staff is looking forward to students, because last year's seniors were so eager to learn.

After you have written your reactions, put the list aside for the moment and review the following example of Suzanne's negative self-talk as she encounters the same situation.

Suzanne: "I'll never cope! Who can ever have enough experience to prepare for intensive care? I hear the patients are all so sick that most of them die. I can barely think of all the scary equipment. What about the families? They won't want a student when their family member is so sick. I'm nervous already thinking about it. I feel nauseated. Why did I ever come into nursing? I don't like the idea of being compared to last year's seniors. I know they had some real brains. I can see it now. I'll be feeling panicky the whole time. I'll go home depressed because of the deaths. I'll feel so inadequate."

Suzanne's self-talk is destructive. It is escalating her anxiety and focusing on all the things that could possibly go wrong. Suzanne is drowning in a flood of catastrophic thinking. With a mindset like hers, she will be tuned into anything negative and may force a self-fulfilling prophecy. Her self-talk dismisses any self-confidence and makes her anxious before, and likely during, the experience.

Take a moment to write down a constructive internal dialogue that Suzanne could use in the same situation.

Here is an example of positive self-talk for Suzanne. Compare your suggestions with this example.

Suzanne: "This is going to be difficult. There's a lot of new equipment to learn, but I know the prediction is most inpatient beds will be in critical care and I plan to work in a hospital. I need to learn this. This experience might help me get a good recommendation. Everyone has to learn something new sometime. I'm bright, and I'll just make it a point to let the staff know I'm eager to learn. This is the best time to learn to deal with dying patients. These nurses have so much experience. I'm sure they can give me some help if I ask them how they cope. I know I can do this . . . . The staff nurses know that I'm a student and will not expect miracles from me. They will be glad for the contribution I can make to the unit. I must find out more about the unit from Betty so that I can prepare myself as much as possible for the experience."

This self-talk is constructive. Suzanne's internal dialogue in this example is realistic and hopeful. By acknowledging her assets, Suzanne will go onto the unit feeling confident. She is likely to approach the staff in a friendly way, eager for new opportunities. Thinking about her situation as a challenge provides Suzanne with a positive goal for her career as a nurse. By deciding to seek out information beforehand, she is increasing her chances of success.

Now go back to your own internal dialogue that you generated earlier in this exercise. Determine whether it is positive or negative. Would your self-talk facilitate your best interests, or is it potentially destructive?

Positive Self-Talk Is Assertive and Responsible

The previous examples demonstrate how self-talk can be harmful or helpful to us. Positive self-talk is helpful because it emphasizes our strengths and our ability to handle the situations confronting us. This mental preparation makes us feel hopeful and confident. We have the right to feel good about how we handle situations we encounter, and positive self-talk is one technique we can use to ensure that our rights are realized. It is assertive to keep our internal dialogue positive.

Positive self-talk is not unrealistic or wishful thinking. It involves an accurate assessment of our abilities and the situation we are facing. Not having the knowledge or skills to effectively handle an interpersonal situation is no reason to think less of ourselves or to put ourselves down. Admitting our lack of experience and acknowledging our willingness and ability to learn realistically prepares us to tackle the situation. This positive kind of mental assessment is responsible because it takes into account the facts of the situation. Mentally putting ourselves down or discrediting our abilities is not responsible thinking.

Butler (1981) warns us that when our self-talk is negative, we are carrying around a toxic environment for ourselves everywhere we go. Negative self-talk is harsh and judgmental, demanding superheroic achievements, chastising us for failing, and generally making us feel tense and dissatisfied with ourselves. Butler encourages us to develop a positive, supportive way of talking to ourselves to cushion us from negative events. Chapman (1992) comments that "positive people are far more likely than others to face up to problems, make tough decisions, and refuse to look back." He says those with a positive outlook are often mistaken for people who just let things happen as if by fate. "Not so! Positive people often have more problems, because they take more risks and live life more fully" (Chapman, 1992).

Becoming aware of our self-talk is the first step to discovering if it is in our best interests. Learning how to change our self-talk starts with such an assessment. Butler (1981) suggests we ask ourselves the following questions:

- What am I telling myself?
- What negative thoughts am I generating that are destructive to me?
- What positive thoughts am I generating that are constructive for me?
- Is my self-talk helping me?

Moments of Connection...
Moving From "Not One More Patient" to "Make Time for Joy"

"Let's get this over with," the nurse thought to herself. After 15 hours of a 24 hour on-call day in the Post Anesthesia Care Unit (PACU) with only a brief break, the nurse was dreading the "one-more" case, a dislocated hip. Expecting a long recovery time and an admission to Short Stay, the nurse was surprised to learn the client was young, the procedure would be short, and he would be dismissed as an ambulatory client. The nurse was tired and crabby and wanted to "get this over with." After talking with the family, the nurse learned they were all headed to a special event: Mom and Dad's 50th anniversary. They were to have had photos taken. Instead they missed the photo appointment and had to eat in the hospital cafeteria. The nurse was instantly humbled and got to work to create a celebration. The family was invited into the PACU, the staff made punch and retrieved an instant camera from the OR to take pictures. What a mental shift. This was an opportunity to remember that joy can come when you least expect it!

The answers to these questions will point out how our thinking can work in our best interests and when it does not. This assessment alerts us as to whether we need to change our self-talk. Whenever you feel overwhelmed by negative self-talk and the accompanying anxiety, consider the thought-stopping technique of silently yelling to yourself "Stop!" to interrupt the barrage and derail your negative thinking (Redford and Redford, 1998).

Our next step is to specify how we need to change our internal dialogue so that it is more positive. At first this planning will require considerable effort, but then it will become part of our awareness, enabling us to tune in to our internal dialogue and adjust it quickly. Later in this chapter you will get experience in reformulating self-talk.

The Relationship Between Self-Talk and Interpersonal Communication

In Part One you learned about behaviors that are essential for caring communication. Parts of your self-talk will be about your ability to implement these behaviors with your clients and colleagues. How you construct your internal dialogue can enhance or diminish your skill level.

Here are examples in relation to the communication behaviors of empathy and confrontation.

Example 1: Self-Talk About Empathy

Here is what one nurse said to herself about empathy:

"I can't be empathic and sound natural. I'll trip over my words. If I try using empathy I'll sound artificial. My colleagues will laugh at me if I change my style and try to be empathic. I don't think I can think up an empathic response fast enough in a 'real' conversation to make it sound sincere. I'll look and feel awkward trying to be empathic."

Examine this nurse's self-talk.

1. What is she telling herself? She is telling herself that she will feel uncomfortable, silly, and unnatural if she attempts to be empathic. She is convincing herself that her friends will not admire her attempts and that she will lose their respect.
2. What negative thoughts is she generating that are destructive? She is convincing herself that she will not be effective in her use of empathy. She expects that she should be perfect the first time she is empathic. She is not permitting any failure, nor is she hopeful that her colleagues will support her.
3. What positive thoughts is she generating? This nurse is not generating one positive thought that might give her the hope and encouragement to try being more empathic.
4. Is her self-talk helping her? This self-talk will likely stop her from including empathy in her communication strategies. These thoughts will make her feel bad on two counts: she will miss providing the benefits of empathy to others and she will feel disappointed in her lack of willingness to try. She is left feeling convinced that neither she nor her colleagues have confidence in her ability. Her thoughts are nonassertive and irresponsible and not in any way helpful to her.
5. How can she change her self-talk so that it is more positive?

Here are examples of how her self-talk could be more positive.

"I'm going to try to use empathy even if I am a little stilted and awkward at first. I am convinced of the importance of empathy and know that my colleagues and clients will appreciate my efforts to show them that I understand, even if I am not perfect in my attempts. Some of my colleagues may teasingly comment on the change when I try to be more empathic; I will not let them deter me from including empathy in my communication. It may take me a while to find the right words, but that's okay. It will likely seem longer to me than to the other person. I really want to improve my communication, and I know that something new takes time to learn. I can be patient with myself until empathy comes more naturally in my interactions with others."

This positive self-talk is assertive and responsible. It underlies the importance this nurse places on being empathic and gives her encouragement to try being more understanding. It is not a glib dialogue, but rather a realistic assessment of her ability to weather the struggle of trying something new until it becomes a natural part of her communication. This positive self-talk is helpful because it boosts confidence and facilitates the incorporation of a new skill into her repertoire.

Example 2: Self-Talk About Confrontation

Here is one nurse's self-talk about confrontation:

"I think it's better to keep peace by not saying anything to the boss about his abrasive manner to me these past few days. If I confront him he'll think I'm being too sensitive and he'll be wary of me after this. He'll pull rank on me and get angry if I confront him. The more I think about it, the crazier it seems for me to be upset about his manner; he's probably got something on his mind and doesn't realize he's taking it out on me. What if I get all upset and mix up my words? I'd really look like a fool then."

Examine this nurse's self-talk.

1. What is she telling herself? She is convincing herself that she would be better off not to confront her boss about an issue important to her. She is arguing that her feelings are not as important as those of her boss.
2. What negative thoughts is she generating that are destructive? This nurse is denying her own feelings by deceiving herself that it might be better to let this episode pass. This self-

deception undermines her judgment. She is creating bad feelings about herself by suggesting that being sensitive or expecting to be treated politely is undesirable. She attempts to frighten herself with the assumption that her boss will get angry and, furthermore, that she would not be able to handle his anger. She imagines the worst scenario and tries to convince herself that she is likely to fail.

3. What positive thoughts is she generating? This nurse's self-talk is entirely negative and contains nothing positive for her.

4. Is her self-talk helping her? This negative self-talk would only deter her from standing up for something that is important to her: her desire to be treated with respect. This approach makes her doubt her ability to confront and to handle one possible consequence of a confrontation: her boss' possible anger. Her negative self-talk is nonassertive and irresponsible in that she is allowing herself to be mistreated and refuses to accept her responsibility for letting the behavior continue.

5. How can she change her self-talk to make it more positive? Here are examples of how her self-talk could be more positive.

"I don't like to confront my boss, but I don't like to be treated disrespectfully, so I will confront him. I know I can make my points clear to him without seeming like a whiner. My boss may become angry or hostile when I confront him, but I can handle this reaction without backing off or becoming defensive. I have practiced confrontation and feel confident that I can carry it off. If my confrontation isn't perfect, it doesn't matter; that I make my point as clearly as possible is what counts. Just because he's my boss is no reason to treat me so badly. I have the right to be treated with respect. He is more likely to respect me in the future if I set limits now."

This positive self-talk is assertive and responsible. It encourages the nurse to stand up for herself and it takes into account her ability to handle several possible outcomes. It is encouraging and supportive and would set this nurse up with the comfort and confidence to carry out her confrontation.

In Part Two of this book you learned how to communicate assertively and responsibly in the following situations where nurses are known to have difficulty:

- When clients or colleagues are distressed
- When clients or colleagues are aggressive
- When there is team conflict
- When evaluation anxiety is experienced
- When encountering unpopular clients

In all these situations, positive self-talk is important. Here are examples of self-talk in two of the above situations.

Example 3: Self-Talk When Colleagues Are Distressed

Here is one nurse's self-talk when encountering a colleague who is distressed and crying:

"I hate it when colleagues cry; I mean, with clients it's okay, I expect them to be upset. I don't know what to do when staff at work cry. Whenever anyone at work cries I get tearful, too, and I'm useless to them. If anyone cries, I don't know what I'll do. I just can't cope when grown people cry. I don't know what to do to make her feel better. What if she won't stop crying? If I can't help her to calm down then I'm not much good."

Examine this nurse's self-talk.

1. What is she telling herself? This nurse is telling herself that staff members do not have the same feelings and reactions as clients. She is telling herself that a lot is expected of her and that if she does not perform adequately by calming her upset colleague then she is not an effective person. She is convinced that if she cries too it will be detrimental to her colleague.
2. What negative thoughts is she generating that are destructive? She is putting considerable pressure on herself to perform in the only way that she thinks is acceptable. She is assuming that she will not be helpful to her colleague and gives no credit to herself. Her denial of a normal range of feelings in her colleagues prevents her compassion from surfacing in a way that would be helpful. Her impending sense of failure if she does not perform perfectly is likely making her tense.
3. What positive thoughts is she generating? This nurse is not saying anything comforting or encouraging to herself.
4. Is her self-talk helpful? Her self-talk is nonassertive because it downplays her potential to be helpful. It is not responsible because it distorts reality. Her self-talk would hinder her ability to reach out to her colleague and communicate in a helpful way. The restrictions imposed by this negative thinking would leave her feeling inadequate.
5. How can she change her self-talk so that it is more positive?

Here are examples of how her self-talk could be more positive.

"Everybody gets upset and staff are no exception. I may not be able to stop her from crying but I think I can comfort her. I always cry when any other staff member cries; but that's okay. It just shows how compassionate I am. My crying doesn't interfere with my ability to be helpful. She may not respond to my efforts to calm her down, but that doesn't mean I'm a bad nurse. Each of us has someone special we can relate to when we are upset. I don't have to do a lot to be helpful. Just listening and being there is often enough."

These inner thoughts are reassuring and confidence-building. They are responsible because they do not distort the reality of the situation. They are assertive because they acknowledge the nurse's desire and ability to help. This positive self-talk is helpful.

Example 4: Self-Talk When There Is Team Conflict

Here is an example of one nurse's thinking about the conflict situation on her nursing unit.

"All I want is a peaceful place to work. Wherever I go there are power struggles and I hate it. I just know this conflict is going to drag on; I wish I worked in Dr. Session's office. They never have any conflicts there. Maybe I should apply for a position in another office; I can't do anything about the conflicts between the support and clinical staff. I thought we had dealt with this conflict once and for all; I just hate these drawn-out disagreements. Whenever we discuss upsetting issues, my stomach gets in a knot and I feel like exploding; I don't know how much more I can take. I'm useless when there's conflict. I just let it tear me apart, and that's no good. I'm afraid I'm going to give the office manager a piece of my mind. She should get this conflict under control."

Examine this nurse's self-talk.

1. What is she telling herself? This nurse has the erroneous notion that conflict is brief, easily resolved, and nonrecurring. The false expectation that there are some places where conflict

does not occur is self-defeating. She is trying to convince herself that there is little she can do about the conflict. She feels that the office manager or the doctor should magically control the conflict.

2. What negative thoughts is she generating that are destructive? Her unrealistic ideas about the nature of conflict are causing her grief. Her image of herself as someone with little control in conflict situations makes her feel hopeless and ineffective. Her anticipation of unpleasant physical signs and symptoms in conflict situations initiates her anxiety at the slightest indication of conflict.

3. What positive thoughts is she generating? There is nothing reassuring and hopeful about her thinking.

4. Is her self-talk helpful? Her self-talk is nonassertive because it does not grant her any power to contribute to the resolution of the conflict. Her distorted perception about her lack of influence to affect change is irresponsible. These thoughts are not helpful because they immobilize her and increase her tension about the conflict.

5. How can she change her self-talk so that it is more positive?

Here are examples of how her self-talk could be more positive.

"Every office staff has conflict; it is an unavoidable part of working with others. Sometimes creative and effective ways of handling situations can come out of conflict. Maybe there are some positive benefits to this conflict. I can keep my cool to express my feelings about the conflict on our unit. My ideas will have more impact if I remain calm. Each thing I do to diminish the conflict goes a long way to resolving our problems. No one person can eliminate the conflict alone, but each contribution is significant. I get anxious when there's conflict on the unit, but it is not overwhelming. I can keep it under control."

This positive self-talk is assertive and responsible. Admitting that conflict is a normal part of working with others removes the sting of disagreement and makes her more apt to tackle the problem. Believing that whatever steps she takes to manage the conflict are significant promotes positive action on her part. Putting her anxiety in perspective allows her to function without being ashamed or overwhelmed. She is responsible in her assessment of the situation and her ability. This positive internal dialogue is assertive in its acknowledgment of her desire to handle situations effectively.

In his book, *Pulling Your Own Strings,* Dyer (1978) challenges us by suggesting that several ideas we take for granted do not exist in reality. Some examples are "disasters," "a good boy," "a stupid person," and "a perfect person." Each of these concepts represents a judgment about reality. Negative self-talk about our ability to communicate or handle interpersonal situations is our destructive and self-defeating judgment. Dyer advises us not to be victimized and encourages us to subscribe to thoughts that are reality-based and self-enhancing. If we can apply this advice to our intrapersonal communication, it will stand us in good stead for our interpersonal encounters with clients and colleagues. Talking to ourselves in encouraging, realistic ways increases our ability to communicate with others in assertive and responsible ways.

Bach and Torbet (1983) purport that we have two voices in our inner life: our "inner enemy" and our "inner ally." Our inner enemy keeps a running inventory of our weaknesses, maintains a certain misery level, and keeps all joyless, negative information on file and can display it at a moment's notice. Our inner ally is interested in action, growth, and change and prevents us from getting bogged down in doubts and fears. Our ally reassures us of the benefits and rewards of success and the pleasures of trying, encouraging us to take risks that will help get us where we want to go. When we make mistakes, it is our inner ally that comforts us and helps us view our mistakes in perspective.

As you practice enhancing and augmenting your interpersonal communication skills, focus on what your inner ally tells you. Allow comforting and realistic thoughts to support and encourage you while learning.

Using Positive Self-Talk to Enhance Your Interpersonal Communication

Positive self-talk can help you at three phases of interpersonal communication: before, during, and after.

Before your interaction with a client or colleague, you can take control of your thoughts and focus on realistic and encouraging inner dialogue that will make you feel more confident about your forthcoming encounter. This preparation makes you focus on your strengths rather than worrying about potential catastrophes. When you feel prepared, you will likely act more competently.

For some encounters you have hours or days to prepare your positive self-talk. At other times you get little preparation time. However, even for surprise encounters you can quickly tune into your internal dialogue (it is continuously active) and talk to yourself in encouraging ways.

For example, when you take a call from an angry family member, you can be saying these words to yourself:

Positive you: The unit secretary tells you there is a call from an angry family member. Tell yourself: "He's impatient and angry, and it could get me upset. But I will stay calm and collected." Slow down, relax your breathing, and loosen up your shoulders. You will find out what is troubling him and be able to handle it. Haste makes waste, so just remain steady and pay attention to each thing he says.

This preparation will prime you to handle this aggressive client situation calmly and effectively.

During your conversation you can tune into your inner voice and concentrate on supportive dialogue. For example, if the caller's voice is getting louder, and his language is getting more hostile, you can say to yourself:

Positive you: "He's getting angry. That's okay. I can handle his outburst. I will remain calm and find out what is so upsetting for him. My breathing is regular, my posture is relaxed, and I will keep my voice steady. There's no point in getting upset. I can take this professionally not personally!"

This positive self-talk will remind you to stay in control and handle the situation effectively. The comfort provided by your own supportive thoughts helps you to act the way you want.

After an encounter you can use positive self-talk to constructively review your performance. Noting your successes and the areas where improvement is needed are both important. This example of a constructive review would be helpful:

Positive you: "I thought I controlled my fear of his hostility really well. I actually remained calm and kept my voice tone on an even pitch. I think what I said to him helped to calm him down, but next time I'd like to achieve a relaxed body posture. My fists were clenched and my shoulders were pretty tight and I could feel that my knees were locked. When I can relax my body that will be one more positive message going out that I am in control and confident."

Positive self-talk is a tool you carry with you and is available at a moment's notice. When you have yourself on your side, you are never alone and you always have an encouraging supporter on whom to call.

Think About It...
What, So What, and Now What?

Consider what you read about the role of self-talk in communication. Do you already pay attention to your self-talk? What messages do you find you give yourself? Answer the following questions.

What?... Write one thing you learned from this chapter.

So what?... How will this impact your nursing practice?

Now what?... How will you implement this new concept or skill?

— THINK ABOUT IT —

Wit and Wisdom

The basis of optimism is sheer terror.

Oscar Wilde

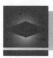 **Practicing Positive Self-Talk**

Exercise 1

Any time you encounter a difficult interpersonal situation, whether in practice or in real life, try talking positively with yourself to augment your ability to communicate assertively and responsibly.

Exercise 2

As a class compare your experiences with employing positive self-talk after you have practiced using it as suggested in the above exercises. What difficulties did you encounter in employing positive self-talk? What successes did you have by keeping your internal dialogue positive?

Exercise 3

For this exercise work in groups of three. One of you will be the nurse interviewer, another the client, and the third the feedback giver. The client and nurse will determine the purpose of their interview in advance. It is important to be clear about your roles and to keep the role-play situation simple. After 5 minutes of interaction, the feedback giver will comment on the nurse's communication skills.

Before each person begins the role-play, stop and tune into your self-talk. Ask yourself if your self-talk is helping you. Change any negative thoughts into constructive ones. During the role-play, try to focus on the voice inside your head and generate encouraging thoughts about your role performance (of nurse, client, or feedback giver).

After the interaction, pause and listen to the voice in your head. If you hear negative or destructive thoughts about your role performance, then make your internal dialogue more supportive.

After you have completed this exercise, pool together your reflections about employing positive self-talk. What have you learned about your own self-talk? How does your self-talk influence your performance?

Wit and Wisdom

Positive Self-Talk for Just One Day

Try an experiment
In your head.
Count all the negative
Things you've said.

Things you say
Just to you
If others said
You would sue!

Talk to yourself
In a positive way,
Holding negative
Thoughts at bay.

It makes a difference
Try it and see
Ask any therapist,
But that isn't free!!

Copyright 1995 Julia W. Balzer Riley.

References

Bach G, Torbet L: The everyday slow torture of self-hate, *New Woman* 1983.

Butler PE: *Talking to yourself,* New York, 1981, Stein & Day.

Chapman EN: *Life is an attitude: staying positive during tough times, how to control your outlook on life,* Menlo Park, Calif, 1992, Crisp Publications.

Dyer WW: *Pulling your own strings,* New York, 1978, A Funk & Wagnalls Book, published by Thomas Y. Cromwell Co.

Helmsetter S: What is self-talk? http://www.selftalk.com, 1998.

Helmsetter S: *What to say when you talk to yourself,* New York, 1997, Fine Communications.

Meichenbaum D: *Cognitive-behavior modification: an integrative approach,* New York, 1977, Plenum Press.

Turkington, CA: *Stress management for busy people,* New York, 1998, McGraw-Hill.

Williams V, Williams R: LifeSkills, *Mind/Body Health* VII(2):3, 1998.

Suggestions for Further Reading

Cormier WH, Cormier LS: *Interviewing strategies for helpers: fundamental skills and cognitive behavioral interventions,* ed 3, Pacific Grove, Calif, 1991, Brooks/Cole.

Chapter 16, Cognitive Restructuring, Reframing, and Stress Inoculation, is written to explain the theoretical underpinnings of these therapies and provides guidelines for practitioners to use these approaches in practice.

Ellis A, Lange A: *How to keep people from pushing your buttons,* New York, 1994, Birch Lane Press.

Jeffers, SJ: Feel the fear and do it anyway, Westminster, MD, 1996, Fawcett Books.

Williams V, Williams R: *LifeSkills,* New York, 1998, Time Books.

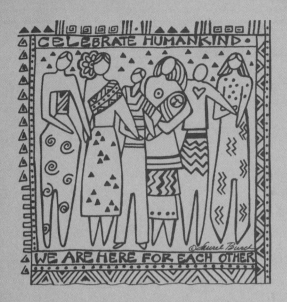

CELEBRATE HUMANKIND •

WE ARE HERE FOR EACH OTHER

28

Continuing
the Commitment

Life is full of wonder . . . are you looking for it?

Julia Balzer Riley

OBJECTIVES

1. Identify three competencies for life balance.
2. Identify strategies for renewal.
3. Discuss the importance of commitment to nursing to continue to build communication skills.

PUTTING IT ALL TOGETHER

As you become more comfortable with your ability to communicate, you soon become increasingly aware of how complex a venture it is. Beyond the technique comes the art, the intuitive application of what you know. This concluding chapter asks you to consider the commitments necessary to move on in your chosen profession: to remain open and sensitive to the human condition; to renew your energy; and to embrace change. To do these, you must find balance in life.

GENERATIVE BALANCE

Guterman proposes a model he calls *generative balancing,* which focuses on three competencies: "creating success, finding meaning, and renewal" (1994). "All three competencies are necessary for balancing, and the real thrill, the excitement of the ride—just as in life—comes from the movement, not from finding a steady-point" but from balance.

In a classic column, Ann Landers relates an essay that compares life to a journey on a train. The essay advises that the focus of life should not be the station, or the destination, but rather the journey itself.

Creating Success

To create success is to set goals, to see the station or the destination. Guzzetta (1998) compares her own journey toward holistic nursing practice to the weaving of a tapestry. ". . . master weavers of a tapestry have described the weaving of a tapestry as a calling, as transformation, as healing, or as a sacred work." What would your tapestry of success as a nurse contain? How would you embellish and color it to reflect your unique contribution?

Success achieved, however, is often not enough in itself. Balance comes from a life view that provides joy along the way. Says Rabbi Harold Kushner, author of *When Bad Things Happen to Good People,* "No man on his death bed ever says, 'I wish I'd spent more time at work.'" Nursing provides many opportunities for success: clinical practice, administration, teaching, research, advanced practice, and many emerging roles for the nurse entrepreneur. Balance comes from attention to all three components of the model.

Finding Meaning

Meaning for the Nurse

To find meaning is essential for the nurse. Arnold sees this process as crucial to prevent burnout, which she proposes is an existential crisis, and for the patient who needs the nurse in the role of "meaning maker" (1989). Arnold's work confirms what many career nurses have come to view as the essence of nursing.

Arnold (1989) suggests that many nursing students grow up with a set of values and beliefs that translate rules and regulations. Faith may be seen as a gift that is tied to good behavior. Do the right things, and all will be well. When nurses are faced with seemingly meaningless tragedies, "or an accumulation of stressors, the nurse's spiritual perspective is thrown off balance. Beliefs previously used no longer provide an accurate internal guide on which to base decisions." It may become hard to pray or attend religious services. Traditional passive beliefs in a higher power may "not necessarily lend any understandable meaning to life experience. If one thinks of spirituality in such narrow terms, the essence of spirituality as a relationship with a higher power is lost." Through the resolution of this existential crisis comes "a total acceptance and commitment to stewardship, anchored by a reasoned loyalty and trust in a higher purpose. What is needed is a broader perspective, a transcendent level of meaning that reorders the incomprehensible circumstances of pain and suffering that a nurse experiences on a daily basis."

Kushner faced just such an existential crisis when his own child died of progeria, a disease of premature aging. He questioned his own beliefs . . . how could he, a rabbi, a good person, have such a senseless tragedy occur in his life? In his book, *When Bad Things Happen to Good Peo-*

ple (1986), he concludes that you cannot control the events in your life, only the attitude that you hold to face life. Kushner discusses three ways that he found to give meaning to life: belong to people; accept pain as a part of life; and know that you have made a difference. These are all a part of your life as a nurse if you remain open and sensitive to the human condition.

To belong to people is to have a few people in your life who are a permanent part of your life, people with whom you share yourself. Nurses sometimes lament their poor relationships with family members. Until you can work these relationships through, claim close friends as new relatives.

To accept pain as a part of life is also to be able to experience the contrasting joy. To be fully present with a client or family member is to be open to sharing suffering, but also to be open to rejoicing in the triumph of coping and changing in the face of crisis.

To know you have made a difference can be a comfort when you feel unable to control the course of life's events. Savor the thank you's you get. Save the notes and cards you receive and place them in a book. Later, these notes will resurface and bring you renewed joy and pride.

The Nurse as Meaning Maker

The ability to develop a belief system, an inner process, as a way of understanding or explaining events that seem beyond human understanding, is reflected in interpersonal communication with clients and family. A nurse who isn't exactly sure what she believes reports that when a client's family was distressed, she spontaneously said, "There are some things that are beyond our understanding, but I believe that life has a purpose." Listen to colleagues as they comfort family and clients and you will hear a demonstration of their belief system.

Arnold advocates involvement as a part of life but recognizes that detachment and renewal of energy are necessary to maintain personal wellness and the continued ability to nurture one's own interpersonal relationships. Loss of meaning can cause spiritual distress, but setting impossible standards of perfection in professional and personal life can be overwhelming and exhausting. The level of intimacy in communication in nursing can take its toll on energy reserves; thus attention to renewal is essential.

Moments of Connection...
Nursing . . . Days of Wonder

I worked in the ICU and took care of an elderly man who was dying. He was a brilliant philosopher and teacher. We spent many evenings talking, and he touched me in ways I did not think were possible. He died one evening when I was not working. I was sad for days. One morning I saw his surgeon, who asked me if I would like to see the autopsy results. When I went with him, I was shocked to see we were in the actual autopsy. When I saw the body I realized for the first time what death was all about. This body was just a shell and his eyes were vacant. I knew all his experiences and stories and brilliant knowledge were with me and everyone else with whom he came into contact. The experience allowed me to accept my father's death a few years later and to help me in my work with the dying.

RENEWING ENERGY

Having discussed the inevitable stressors that nurses face today, it is time to actively consider how you will add energy, fun, and laughter to your life. Consider a body, mind, and spirit approach.

The Body

Find a physical activity you like and do it on a regular basis, but not obsessively. Dance, play tennis, walk, run; the list is endless. Start with 10 minutes twice a day—just move. Look in the mirror. Do you like what you see? Are you a role model for health and wellness? Do you see your body as sacred?

The Mind

Like a computer, the functioning of the mind is only as good as the data taken in. Choose music or movies or reading material that renew your energy. Add play and laughter and humor to your life. (Review Chapter 14, Humor, and note the boxes on comic vision and building a humor kit.) Embellish your world with beauty. See Stoddard's work for specific suggestions.

The Spirit

Nourish your spirit by taking time to read inspirational material or stories. Take time to be silent and to just be and not do. Practice a regular time to contemplate life. Review the chapters on imagery and relaxation. Write your own mission statement for your personal and professional life (Kenney, 1998). Mine is to "Respirit, reinspire, and revitalize nurses to provide sensitive care and find humor and joy along the journey." See Jones' *The Path* for specific directions to help you write your mission statement.

CONTINUING CONNECTIONS

A few final stories to demonstrate continuing the commitment and the risks and joy it entails.

Moments of Connection...
Daring to Be Yourself

A former patient came up to me in a restaurant and thanked me for helping her to remember what she had considered important in her life and what had worked for her in the past. After leaving the hospital where I had cared for her, she had started back to church. She remembered me years later.

Moments of Connection...
Pass It On!

I was able to speak to a group of high school students about careers in health care and talk about my job responsibilities and education. I shared the path I had taken and how good nursing had been to me and the rewards it has brought. Later that week, I received a note from one of the students thanking me for helping her to solidify her decision to become a nurse.

One nurse concludes that although nurses may wear many hats, they maintain the "commitment to the art of nursing" (Schettle, 1998). Nurses are taking on many expanded clinical and administrative roles to make an impact on health care delivery in complex integrated delivery systems, and yet they maintain the commitment to quality care to clients and families, to the promotion of wellness for individuals and communities, and through electronic communication move onto global concerns for health care. Nurses are asked to develop education for house-wide hospital education. Nurses are moving into industry to design corporate wellness programs. These new roles demand new skills and a commitment to the goal of being a lifelong learner.

The examples in this text deal with one issue at a time. Clinical situations present the complex lives of real people struggling with many of life's challenges at once. To face this complexity and what may seem like impossible situations, nurses must grow with their clients and families. Honest, clear communication takes a commitment to continue to grow, to deal with change, to stay connected with people. The rewards are substantial. Work can bring joy, but the cost is too great if you lose the joy that comes from having a rich personal life, interests to pursue, and people to whom you are connected. Consider these final exercises to help you along the journey.

Good-bye and good luck!

Wit and Wisdom

Happiness is not a goal. It is a by-product of something you do.

Author unknown

Practicing Continuing the Commitment

Exercise 1

List all the roles you play in your life, such as nurse or student, daughter or son, spouse, parent, community volunteer, etc. Then draw two circles four inches in diameter. Divide the first circle into portions like a pie, as many pieces as you have roles, each portion sized in proportion to the amount of time you spend in each role. When you are finished, consider if your use of time reflects your values. After this reflection, divide the second circle into portions according to how you would prefer to spend your time. If there are discrepancies between the two distributions of your time, consider alterations you might choose to make.

Exercise 2

Begin a journal to record the ups and downs in your daily nursing practice. Make daily recordings for two weeks. Review your journal to regain perspective. Continue your journal if this is helpful or try it again when times are tough. To start, answer just one question: "What brought me a sense of wonder, a sense of awe today?"

Exercise 3

Begin a "joy" book in which you write the joyful things that happen in your life. Review your joy book when you do not feel joyful. If you do not see how you make a difference, choose a worthwhile cause or activity and volunteer your services.

Exercise 4

Begin a "joy box," an "antidepression" kit, to collect mementos, motivational clippings, thank-you notes, small toys, things that lift your spirits. Encourage a child in your life to do the same thing. Call it a treasure box.

References

Arnold E: Burnout as a spiritual issue: rediscovering meaning in nursing practice. In Carson VB, editor: *Spiritual dimensions of nursing practice,* Philadelphia, 1989, WB Saunders.

Guterman MS: *Common sense for uncommon times: the power of balance in work, family, and personal life,* Palo Alto, Calif, 1994, CPP Books.

Guzzetta CE: Weaving a tapestry of holism, *J Cardiovasc Nurs* 12(2):18, Jan 1998.

Jones LB: *The path: creating your mission statement for work and for life,* New York, 1996, Hyperion.

Kenney EG: Creating fulfillment in today's workplace: a guide for nurses, *Am J Nurs* 98(5):44, 1998.

Kushner H: *When all you've ever wanted isn't enough: a search for a life that matters,* New York, 1986, Summit Books.

Kushner H: *When bad things happen to good people,* New York, 1983, Avon Books.

Schettle S: A nurse's reflection: Nursing in the 90's—old hat, new ways, *Am J Nurs* 98(5):16j, 1998.

Suggestions for Further Reading

Balzer Riley J: From the heart to the hands: keys to successful healthcaring connections, Ellicott City, Md, 1998, Integrated Management and Publishing Systems.
   To order call Constant Source Seminars, (800) 368-7675.

Byham WC: *Zapp! Empowerment in health care: how to improve patient care, increase employee job satisfaction, and lower health care costs,* New York, 1993, Fawcett Columbine.

Cohen M: Caring for ourselves can be funny business, *Holistic Nurs Pract* 4(4):1, 1990.

Covey SR: *The 7 habits of highly effective people: powerful lessons in personal change,* New York, 1989, Simon & Schuster.

DeAngelis B: *Real moments,* New York, 1994, Dell.

Fox W: *The reinvention of work: a new vision of livelihood for our time,* San Francisco, 1994, Harper.

Hannaford MJ, Popkin M: *Windows: healing and helping through loss,* Atlanta, Ga, 1992, Active Parenting.

Johansen R, Swigart R: *Upsizing the individual in the downsized organization,* Reading, Mass, 1994, Addison-Wesley.

Koerner JG: The power of place: career transformation through stability, *Nurs Admin Q* 19(4):44, 1995.

Kushner H: *When all you've ever wanted isn't enough: a search for a life that matters,* New York, 1986, Summit Books.

Kushner H: *When bad things happen to good people,* New York, 1983, Avon Books.

Perlman D, Takacs GJ: The 10 stages of change, *Nurs Manage* (21)4:33, 1990.

Stoddard A: *The art of the possible: the path from perfectionism to balance and freedom,* New York, 1995, William Morrow.

Stoddard A: *Daring to be yourself: create beauty, harmony, and individuality in your life by developing your unique personal style at home, work, and play,* New York, 1990, Avon Books.

Stoddard A: *Living a beautiful life: 500 ways to add elegance, order, beauty and joy to every day of your life,* New York, 1986, Random House.

Whyte D: *The heart aroused: poetry and the preservation of the soul in corporate America,* New York, 1994, Currency Doubleday.

Appendix

Self-Assessment Tool

How would you rate me on a scale of wonderful to marvelous?

Ashleigh Brilliant

In the changing health care climate we are beginning to understand that our clients have a choice of providers of care. Other industries are ahead of us in the focus on customer service. Your ability to communicate clearly and with compassion, to meet and even exceed your clients' expectations, is the essence of customer service. Many complaints are not about clinical issues but about perceived rudeness or lack of caring. Remember that you also have internal customers: your colleagues and staff from other departments and disciplines. Let's combine a look at communication skills and attention to customer service. Complete this self-assessment not only as a quick check of your skills, but also as a tool to teach the tenets of customer service.

COMMUNICATION: THE KEY TO CUSTOMER SERVICE

Instructions: Rate yourself from 4 (very skilled) to 1 (not skilled).

1. I feel good about my communication skills.	4	3	2	1
2. I smile at clients, families, and staff.	4	3	2	1
3. I make eye contact.	4	3	2	1
4. I introduce myself and wear my name badge.	4	3	2	1
5. I learn names and use the correct pronunciations.	4	3	2	1
6. If I don't understand, I seek clarification.	4	3	2	1
7. I take a moment to calm myself before interacting with clients.	4	3	2	1
8. I take responsibility for finding answers to questions.	4	3	2	1
9. I answer the telephone promptly and with a smile (that helps!)	4	3	2	1
10. I explain procedures clearly.	4	3	2	1
11. I encourage clients and their families to ask questions.	4	3	2	1
12. I encourage feedback about my work.	4	3	2	1
13. I receive positive feedback about my work.	4	3	2	1
14. I thank a colleague who helps me.	4	3	2	1
15. I offer to help my colleagues.	4	3	2	1
16. I listen, knowing it is OK to be quiet and not have all the answers.	4	3	2	1
17. I respect the clients' confidentiality.	4	3	2	1
18. I apologize for delays.	4	3	2	1
19. When I touch a patient, I do it gently.	4	3	2	1
20. I dress professionally and pay attention to my grooming.	4	3	2	1
21. I try to do something extra for clients, families, and colleagues.	4	3	2	1
22. I am learning to deal with multiple demands on my time.	4	3	2	1
23. I give compliments to clients, family, and colleagues (yes, doctors, too!)	4	3	2	1
24. I understand that I am still learning and that it is impossible to be perfect.	4	3	2	1
25. I try to be myself, bringing my own special gifts to my nursing practice.	4	3	2	1

Scoring: Add the numbers you have selected. Remember that this is a self-assessment, and feedback from your instructor, peers, and clients adds more data.

77-100	High awareness of necessary skills.
52-76	Average awareness of skills. Review your lower scores and select areas for growth.
25-52	Low awareness of necessary skills. Pay more attention to skill development.

Wit and Wisdom

Consider how you inhabit your job.
When you move into an apartment or a dorm,
you hang pictures, you decorate it to suit you.
It is a reflection of who you are and of your interests.
Do you bring yourself to your job?
Do you fill the role in your own special way?
Your uniqueness is part of you
and helps make your relationships more genuine.

References

Leebov W: *Customer service in healthcare,* Chicago, 1990, American Hospital Association.

Matza BR: *Becoming a customer service star,* King of Prussia, Penn, 1993, BRM Enterprises. Order from *The HRD Quarterly.*

Index